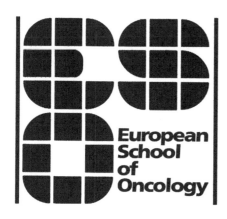

Monographs
Series Editor: U. Veronesi

The European School of Oncology gratefully acknowledges the educational grant for the production of this monograph received from SNAM, Italy

L. Tomatis (Ed.)

Indoor and Outdoor Air Pollution and Human Cancer

With 4 Figures and 23 Tables

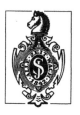

Springer-Verlag
Berlin Heidelberg New York
London Paris Tokyo
Hong Kong Barcelona
Budapest

LORENZO TOMATIS
International Agency for Research on Cancer
150, cours Albert-Thomas
69372 Lyon Cedex 08, France

ISBN-13: 978-3-642-78199-5   e-ISBN-13: 978-3-642-78197-1
DOI: 10.1007/978-3-642-78197-1

Library of Congress Cataloging-in-Publication Data
Indoor and outdoor air pollution and human cancer/ L. Tomatis (ed.).
  (Monographs / European School of Oncology)
Includes bibliographical references.

1. Cancer–Environmental aspects. 2. Air–Pollution–Health aspects. 3. Indoor air pollution–Health aspects. 4. Carcinogenesis. I. Tomatis, L. II. Series: Monographs (European School of Oncology) [DNLM: 1. Air Pollution–adverse effects. 2. Air Pollutants–adverse effects. 3. Neoplasms–chemically induced. QZ 202 I41 1993] RC268.25.I53 1993 616.99'4071–dc20 DNLM/DLC for Library of Congress

This work is subject to copyright. All rights are reserved, whether the whole or part of the material is concerned, specifically the rights of translation, reprinting, reuse of illustrations, recitation, broadcasting, reproduction on microfilms or in any other way, and storage in data banks. Duplication of this publication or parts thereof is permitted only under the provisions of the German Copyright Law of September 9, 1965, in its current version, and permission for use must always be obtained from Springer-Verlag. Violations are liable for prosecution under the German Copyright Law.

© Springer-Verlag Berlin Heidelberg 1993
Softcover reprint of the hardcover 1st edition 1993

The use of general descriptive names, registered names, trademarks, etc. in this publication does not imply, even in the absence of a specific statement, that such names are exempt from the relevant protective laws and regulations and therefore free for general use.

Product liability: The publishers cannot guarantee the accuracy of any information about dosage and application contained in this book. In every individual case the user must check such information by consulting the relevant literature.

Typesetting: Camera ready by editor

23/3145 - 5 4 3 2 1 0 - Printed on acid-free paper

Foreword

The European School of Oncology came into existence to respond to a need for information, education and training in the field of the diagnosis and treatment of cancer. There are two main reasons why such an initiative was considered necessary. Firstly, the teaching of oncology requires a rigorously multidisciplinary approach which is difficult for the Universities to put into practice since their system is mainly disciplinary orientated. Secondly, the rate of technological development that impinges on the diagnosis and treatment of cancer has been so rapid that it is not an easy task for medical faculties to adapt their curricula flexibly.

With its residential courses for organ pathologies and the seminars on new techniques (laser, monoclonal antibodies, imaging techniques etc.) or on the principal therapeutic controversies (conservative or mutilating surgery, primary or adjuvant chemotherapy, radiotherapy alone or integrated), it is the ambition of the European School of Oncology to fill a cultural and scientific gap and, thereby, create a bridge between the University and Industry and between these two and daily medical practice.

One of the more recent initiatives of ESO has been the institution of permanent study groups, also called task forces, where a limited number of leading experts are invited to meet once a year with the aim of defining the state of the art and possibly reaching a consensus on future developments in specific fields of oncology.

The ESO Monograph series was designed with the specific purpose of disseminating the results of these study group meetings, and providing concise and updated reviews of the topic discussed.

It was decided to keep the layout relatively simple, in order to restrict the costs and make the monographs available in the shortest possible time, thus overcoming a common problem in medical literature: that of the material being outdated even before publication.

UMBERTO VERONESI
Chairman Scientific Committee
European School of Oncology

Contents

Introduction
L. Tomatis 1

Outdoor and Indoor Air Pollution and Cancer: An Old and New Problem
L. Tomatis and L. Fishbein 3

Sources, Nature and Levels of Air Pollutants
L. Fishbein 17

Sources, Nature and Levels of Indoor Air Pollutants
L. Fishbein and K. Hemminki 67

Environmental Carcinogens: Assessment of Exposure and Effect
K. Hemminki, H. Autrup and A. Haugen 89

Experimental Evidence for the Carconogenicity
of Indoor and Outdoor Air Pollutants
J. Lewtas 103

Epidemiological Evidence on Indoor Air Pollution and Cancer
L. Simonato and G. Pershagen 119

Epidemiological Evidence on Outdoor Air Pollution and Cancer
G. Pershagen and L. Simonato 135

The Economics of Controlling Outdoor and Indoor Air Pollution
J. D. Graham 149

Introduction

Lorenzo Tomatis

International Agency for Research on Cancer, 150 cours Albert Thomas, 69372 Lyon Cedex 08, France

The present volume is a revised and expanded version of the European School of Oncology Monograph on Air Pollution and Human Cancer which was published in 1991. The 1991 version dealt only with outdoor air pollution, and the authors proposed for the subsequent volume to consider also indoor pollution because it may be as relevant or even more relevant as outdoor pollution in certain circumstances. This is related to particular characteristics of indoor pollution as well as to the fact that most people today spend more time indoors than outdoors.

In the present version the information on outdoor pollution has been updated and additional information is provided on indoor air pollution. The individual chapters were circulated among the authors and subsequently discussed in a meeting in London in April 1992. The spirit that dominated our meeting and our collaboration was fully collegial and collaborative and each of us freely and gratefully accepted criticisms and suggestions. Each author, however, remains responsible for his/her own chapter which expresses his/her own views. As the editor of this volume, I would like to express my gratitude to all collaborators who have kindly borne with me, even when my views diverged considerably from theirs. It has been a real privilege to interact with such a distinguished group of scientists.

I would like to express my gratitude, also on behalf of my colleagues, to Vlatka Majstorovic for her kind and very efficient assistance and to Marije de Jager for her competent and always helpful editing.

Outdoor and Indoor Air Pollution and Cancer: An Old and New Problem

Lorenzo Tomatis [1] and Lawrence Fishbein [2]

1 International Agency for Research on Cancer, 150 cours Albert Thomas, 69372 Lyon Cedex 08, France
2 Office of Toxicology Sciences, Center for Food Safety and Nutrition, Food and Drug Administration, Washington, D.C. 20204, U.S.A.

The history of mankind can be divided into 3 periods: the period of hunters-gatherers, the period that followed the agricultural revolution and the period that followed industrialisation. In his latest book, McKeown [1] observed that "in the first period there was no effective control either on the environment or on reproduction; in the second period there was some control on the environment but not on reproduction and in the third period there was further control on the environment and, for the first time, on reproduction but there was insufficient control on the conditions of life created by industrialisation."

McKeown's definition of the third period should perhaps be slightly altered, to read "further control but also further abuse of the environment", since, in fact, having imposed ourselves on the environment, we are at present concerned with the difficulty or the incapacity to control or reverse the modifications we have induced.

Air pollution is certainly not a new phenomenon [2]. Indoor pollution was probably experienced by the inhabitants of caves and of primitive houses, which had no or insufficient evacuation of fumes, and natural phenomena like volcanic eruptions and the accidental or voluntary burning of woods and forests have certainly contributed to the immission of pollutants into the air since time immemorial.

There is little doubt, however, that air pollution has increased particularly in the last century; the pollution of air near certain industrial plants and in big cities is one of the alterations to human existence brought about by industrialisation. René Dubos [3] observed that, although air pollution is an old phenomenon, the introduction of more of the same and of new pollutants on a large scale has transformed it during the last century and this century into an important health problem. Trends in estimated emissions of some of the most important air pollutants have been calculated for the world [4] and for individual countries [5]. These show that air pollution has become a planetary problem, and there is now no area of the earth that has been spared the presence and consequences of air pollution, as pollutants can cause damage far away from their point of emission into the atmosphere [6]. While in some industrialised countries there have been some successful initiatives to reduce the emissions of SO_2, polycyclic aromatic hydrocarbons (PAHs) and suspended particles, in many developing countries as well as in large areas of Central and Eastern Europe the situation would seem to be getting worse.

In contrast to the general reduction in OECD countries of sulphur dioxide, carbon monoxide, lead and particulate emissions, nitrogen oxides and VOC emissions have continued to increase or at best remain stable in the OECD regions (with the exception of Japan), principally due to the growth in vehicular traffic and total mileage driven since 1970 as well as other energy uses and industrial processes. It is further projected to remain a problem for the foreseeable future [7], since OECD countries remain responsible for 45% of the world CO_2 emission, 40% of sulphur oxides and 50% of nitrogen oxides [8].

In 1990, the population in industrialised countries was 1.21 billion, contrasted to 4.08 billion in the developing nations and the global population was 5.29 billion [9]. The global population in 1992 was 5.5 billion people. It is projectd by UN demographers that the global population in the year 2050 would be approximately 9.7 billion with more than 90% of this figure attributed to the developing nations [10]. Energy demand growth for the period 1973-1987 in the developing countries averaged 5.3% per year compared to 0.7% per year in the OECD countries and 3.2% in the former USSR and Eastern Europe together [11]. Hence these projected increases in energy demand alone are anticipated to lead to future increases in atmospheric pollutant emissions unless stringent emission constraints are in place.

This monograph will address the possible association between air pollution and human cancer and touches only briefly and marginally on adverse effects other than cancer. In a previous edition of this monograph [12], we concentrated on outdoor air pollution. However, exposure to air pollutants occurs both outdoors and indoors. Depending on the occupation, age, season, climate, personal habits, the proportion of time spent indoors and outdoors may vary very considerably but in many instances about 80% of the time is spent indoors [13]. Among the most important ambient air pollutants are suspended particles, SO_2, CO, NO, ozone and aerosols and a number of carcinogenic agents such as various polycyclic hydrocarbons, benzene, asbestos and certain metals. Ambient air pollutants almost inevitably end up indoors and add to those generated by indoor sources, even if pollution of indoor air by ambient air can be reduced considerably by minimising air exchange, by sealing buildings and using filters [14]. Reports concerning adverse health effects in non-industrial workplaces, such as office environments, have recently greatly increased [15]. Multiple chemical sensitivity (MCS) is also widely discussed but the extent to which it can be solely related to indoor air chemicals is at present uncertain [15,16]. Important sources of indoor air pollution have been in the past, and continue to be in many developing countries today, heating fuels and fumes from cooking without adequate ventilation, which may generate very high concentrations of suspended particles, of polycyclic hydrocarbons and of CO. In addition, radon, tobacco smoke, the importance of which cannot be underestimated [17-19], materials resulting from abrasion from surfaces, including asbestos, biologic organisms and volatile organic compounds as well as pesticides [20] may contribute to various degrees to indoor air pollution [21]. In spite of the campaign against the use of tobacco, in 1988 5.2 trillion cigarettes were produced worldwide, 40% of which were produced by 6 transnational tobacco companies. The 4 largest U.S. cigarette companies showed a sale of 32.5 billion U.S. dollars for cigarettes in 1988, with a profit of 7.2 billion. Half of the sales were international [22].

The exposures to air pollutants occur almost inevitably under the form of complex mixtures of gazeous and particulate matters so that an accurate assessment of health risks is particularly difficult [23]. Sources and routes of exposure to these agents other than air and through air, e.g., the presence of polycyclic aromatic hydrocarbons in certain foods or beverages [20], will not be considered in detail here.

Air pollution may have many indirect health effects which are not covered in this volume, including those associated with the increased mobilisation of metals, such as aluminium, cadmium and mercury, due to the increasing acidification of soil and water.

Evidence for Severe, Acute Effects

The worst effects of outdoor air pollution were seen in the U.K., probably due to the combination of early introduction of coal for heating and cooking purposes and early and rapid spread of industries, in a country where climatic conditions favour the formation of smog. R. Dubos [3] quoted an anecdote about William Harvey, who performed an autopsy on the centenarian "Old Parr" and concluded that he had probably died because he was exposed to the heavily polluted air of London after having lived all his life in the country. John Evelyn [24] described the filthy air of London in 1661 and associated the exposure to the thick London smog with a variety of health problems.

More recently, the severe adverse effects that can be caused by air pollution were demonstrated dramatically by a series of disasters, the best known of which are those that occurred in Liège, Belgium, in 1930, in Donora, Pennsylvania, in 1948 and in London in the winter of 1952 [2,25,26]. In Belgium, 63 people died following what was called a "smog incident". In Donora, due to an infrequent (but not exceptional) phenomenon of thermal inversion, the smog persisted and accumulated for several days, causing severe health effects in almost 600 inhabitants, of whom 17 died. In London, in a little over a week of the winter of 1952, more than 4000 people died due to the heavy smog. It was this last episode that finally triggered the introduction of severe measures to reduce air pollution. The Clean Air Act was approved and rigidly enforced in the U.K. in 1956, with subsequent considerable reduction in air pollution in London and in several other large cities. There is some evidence that further decreases in the present level of air pollution, in particular of suspended particulates, in cities like London could probably contribute to reducing mortality further [27]. In the spring of 1991 about 4.6 million barrels of oil were burning per day with a daily emission of soot of about 3,400 metric tons [28]. The emission in the ambient air of massive quantities of smoke, SO_2, hydrocarbons and NO_2 following the burning of oil wells in Kuwait is affecting air quality in a vast region, although apparently not on a global scale [29]. No reliable information is available at present on the short-term health effect on the population living in the region.

A 10-year follow-up of the residents of Donora indicates higher mortality and morbidity among people who were exposed during the smog episode as compared with non-exposed persons [30]. While this increase might be attributable to a considerable extent to a worsening of pre-existing heart and lung conditions, there is some evidence of increased morbidity among exposed individuals who had no pre-existing heart or lung conditions.

The Effects of Relatively Low Levels of Exposure

Adverse effects due to low levels of exposure may be much more difficult to ascertain, especially in the case of long-term chronic effects, such as cancer.

In many instances cancer is the result of a subjectively symptomless sequence and accumulation of pathological events which may begin early in life or even prenatally. This is one important reason why exposures involving entire populations, from the youngest to the oldest age groups, are of particular public health concern. On the one hand, even low levels of exposure may be acutely harmful to individuals who are particularly fragile with regard to health effects - like the very young and the very old; on the other hand, even low exposure levels may be harmful in the long term, and the more so the longer the duration of exposure.

As will be better explained in the two following chapters, much progress has been made in the development of analytical methods to detect chemicals in our environment. Specific chemicals can now be detected at levels lower by orders of magnitude than those that could be detected 20 years ago. Progress in toxicology and in the understanding of the mechanisms of carcinogenesis has not, however, kept the same pace. One of the main unresolved problem is the assessment of risks related to very low levels of exposure (as low as the levels of detectability of the available analytical methods) to a toxic agent. The problem is amplified by the fact that people are always exposed to several agents at the same time.

This paradoxical situation - that technological progress, instead of improving our decision-making capacity, has apparently widened our uncertainties - will hopefully be resolved with the development and continuous improvement of methods for the biological monitoring of individual exposures.

The recent worsening of the problem of air pollution has both quantitative and qualitative components: chemical pollutants that occurred at limited concentrations or in limited areas now occur in greater amounts and are more widespread, and newly synthesised chemical compounds are being emitted. The cumulation of these 2 components began during the last century and has not ceased. Furthermore, photochemical reactions in the atmosphere may engender new chemical species.

Two major types of outdoor (ambient) air pollution have been described: a "reducing" form, often called "London smog", resulting mainly from the incomplete combustion of coal and oil, the main components of which are soots, sulphur dioxide, nitrogen oxides and sulphuric acids; and an "oxidising" form, often called "Los Angeles smog", the main components of which are carbon monoxide, hydrocarbons and photochemical decomposition products. The urban atmosphere in which various particulates and pollutant gases accumulate, react and interreact under the influence of sunlight, has been described as "a giant chemical reactor" [31]. For a review of the acute effects on health of winter- and summer-type smog, see also [32].

Chemical agents that were present in the environment before the industrial revolution began - such as asbestos and certain metals - have been massively exploited only since the last century but increasingly during the present one. While these agents have been present for a long time, it is only since their massive industrial use that they have become a conspicuous source of hazardous exposure of both occupational groups and the general population.

Asbestos is found over almost the entire planet. For example, Japan, where there was no domestic production of asbestos, began to import it in growing quantities in the 1950s. A retrospective survey on the presence of asbestiform bodies in the lungs of the general population showed an impressive correlation between the increased importation and increase in the percentage of individuals with these bodies [33]. Japan is probably the only country in which a specific law allows compensation of pollution-related health damage. At the beginning of 1988, there were over 100,000 individuals in Japan receiving compensation for diseases related to air pollution [34]. Exposure to asbestos in the environment outside the working place may generate a very considerable risk of cancer, as is shown by the impressive mortality rates of pleural mesotheliomas observed in residents in and around a town where there was an asbestos-cement plant, and for whom an occupational exposure could be excluded [35]. The widespread presence of asbestos in urban areas is shown by the results of a survey carried out in New York City. There are asbestos-containing materials in about 68% of the buildings in this city. While these materials are mainly used for thermal insulation, about 28% of tall office buildings, 15% of hospitals and 12% of theatres had asbestos-containing materials used for surfacing [36].

About 60 million tonnes of bitumens are produced worldwide annually [37], most of which is used to pave roads and airstrips and for roofing. Although we know that bitumens contain several carcinogens/mutagens and there is evidence of an increased cancer risk in individuals occupationally exposed to them [38], we have no way of knowing whether the millions of tonnes used every year contribute in any way to our load of carcinogens. Similar considerations could be applied to rubber, as more than half of the 13 million tonnes (1980) produced annually is used in tyres [39], a large part of which is rubbed off onto our bitumen-paved roads.

A more detailed account of the spectrum of hazardous inorganic and organic, natural and anthropogenic pollutants discharged into the atmosphere, and of those that are formed as a consequence of the dynamics of atmospheric reactions and photochemical transformations, is given in the next chapter (see also [40]). While the first experimental evidence that urban air pollutants are carcinogenic was produced half a century ago [41,42], we are still far from identifying all of the genotoxic and non-genotoxic compounds present in ambient air, in spite of the spectacular progress made in identification procedures [43]. Major components of urban air pollution are aerosols containing strong acids such as sulphuric acid and ammonium bisulphates [44].

The role of the urban factor in increasing the prevalence of respiratory symptoms and diseases is confirmed by recent investigations [45]. While there is evidence that higher levels of air pollution are related to more severe symptoms and diseases than lower levels and that the most severe adverse effects of urban air pollution are seen where industry contributes to air pollution [45], a steeper exposure-response association at lower air pollution concentrations has also been reported [46]. As individual difference in sensitivity to the effect of air pollutants undoubtedly exists, the inescapable conclusion is that a fraction of the population exposed composed of sensitive individuals or individuals with pre-existing illnesses, like the asthmatics, may respond and even overrespond at low levels of exposure that are much lower than those effective in the rest of the population [47].

In many states of the U.S., airborne toxic substances are controlled by the Ambient Air Level (AAL) guidelines, which are based on the Threshold Limit Values (TLVs) developed by the American Conference of Environmental Industrial Hygienists (ACGIH). However, the assumption that TLVs are health-based limits has been seen as potentially misleading. On the one side, TLVs were made under strong corporate influence and therefore possibly more inclined to compromise with certain industrial interests than to fully protect human health. Moreover, TLVs for the same substances may vary up to 100 times in different cities. If one were to adopt the EPA criteria for making a quantitative assessment of cancer risks, one could easily infer that AALs are far from reassuring [48] and significant adverse health effects have been reported to occur even at concentrations of ambient air particulates below the National Ambient Air Quality Standards [49]. Similarly, admissions to hospital with attacks of asthma in Helsinki, Finland, were significantly correlated with ambient air concentrations of SO_2, O_3 and TSP (total suspended particles), even when lower than those generally accepted in many countries [50] and daily mortality in Detroit was reported to be significantly correlated to concentrations of TSP well below ambient air quality standards [51].

A detailed study carried out in the South Coast Air Basin of California with the aim of evaluating the health benefits of cleaning the air [52], has yielded several interesting results: 1) by attaining national ambient air quality standards (NAAQS) for ozone (O_3) and particulate matter (PM-10), it has been estimated that the Basin-wide annual health benefits will be of about 9.8 billion dollars; 2) attaining the NAAQS will prevent approximately 1600 annual deaths attributable to PM-10 levels; 3) important benefits, such as preservation of lung function, but also improvements of visibility and protection of materials and vegetation, have not been included in the estimates; thus the benefit estimates currently made are likely to be underestimated. In a study carried out in 2 neighbouring counties in Utah, it was reported that 30 to 40% of all deaths from non-malignant respiratory diseases as well as from lung cancer were attributable to community air pollution in the county where a steel mill was implanted during World War II [53].

The possible adverse effects of air pollution in children are of particular concern [54]. Schwartz et al. [55] assessed the impact of short-term exposure to air pollution on respiratory illness in children in 5 German cities. Two of the communities studied were located in highly industrialised areas of the Northern Westphal, one from an industrialised city of the north, and 2 non-industrialised cities of South Germany. Environmental levels of TSP, NO_2 and SO_2 were significantly associated with cases documented by medical visits, with TSP apparently being of the greatest importance. Exposure to particulates for short periods has been related to an increased frequency of lower respiratory symptoms and cough in school children [56] as well as in preschool children [57]. Similar observations were reported in a study of 6-year-old children in a heavily polluted community in Brazil [58], while the results of a study on school children in Israel are more difficult to interpret [59].

An association between childhood cancer and residential traffic density has been reported [60], but in spite of the reported high level of benzene levels derived from gasoline in urban areas, no increased links between leukaemia and other childhood cancers and specific components of air pollution could be found. The reported increasing risk of childhood cancer with increasing traffic density is worrying, even if it still remains to be confirmed.

Indoor air pollution may be, in certain situations and in certain countries, of more relevance in terms of adverse health effects, than outdoor air pollution. For instance, the high prevalence of respiratory illness in relation to domestic fire pollution is well documented [61]. Indoor pollution from coal combustion and cooking fumes is reported to be in some instances the most important risk factor for lung cancer in certain counties in China [62] and in others an important risk factor in addition to smoking [63]. Adverse health effects of indoor air pollution in China include a high prevalence of respiratory diseases besides lung cancer, birth defects and fluorosis [64]. The multiple adverse effects of indoor air pollution in children are well documented [65]. Radon is an important indoor pollutant. About 100,000 homes in England have levels of radon above 200 Bq/m^3, which is the agreed U.K. government "action level". Some of these houses were found to have up to 10,000 Bq/m^3. It has been estimated that about 2000 lung cancer cases per year may be caused in England by radon in the home [66].

Measures to control ambient air pollution have been taken in certain countries where the emission of pollutants in the environment is controlled by special legislation. In comparison, very little control can be exerted over indoor air pollution in private homes, as an adequate legislation can only concern part of the pollutants (e.g. radon), while other pollutants, like environmental tobacco smoke (ETS), can only be regulated in public places.

Lung Cancer

Most studies on the carcinogenicity of air pollution have focused on the possible association with cancer of the lung, and only a few have addressed cancers at other sites. The emphasis on lung cancer derives naturally from the fact that exposure to air pollutants is primarily via the respiratory tract and that carcinogens, the exposure to which is related to air pollution, are logically expected to be most relevant to the occurrence of lung cancer, although not necessarily limited to it. Furthermore, the lung is one of the preferred target organs for those agents and complex exposures that have been established as carcinogenic to humans. While tobacco smoke is by far the most important lung carcinogen, a causal association with lung cancer has been demonstrated for 11 other carcinogenic agents, namely As and As compounds, Asbestos, BCME, Cr compounds, coal tars, coal-tar pitches, Mustard gas, Ni and Ni compounds, soots, strong inorganic acid mists containing sulphuric acid, talc containing asbestiform fibres, and 6 complex exposures, namely aluminium production, coal gasification, coke production, hematite mining (radon), iron and steel founding, and occupational exposure as painters [67,68].

The success rate of surgical and/or radio- and chemotherapy of lung cancer is still today rather discouraging. Similarly, screening procedures for early detection do not offer at present great hope for a relevant reduction in mortality. The detectable preliminary phase of lung cancer is relatively short [69], with only 50% of cases having a detectable preclinical duration longer than 6 months [70], implying that screening should be performed at an impractically frequent periodicity to detect lung cancer at an early stage. However, even with a semi-annual screening there does not seem to be any significant reduction in mortality [71]. Lung cancer, which is the most frequent tumour in men and the frequency of which is increasing in women, is one that typically will essentially benefit from primary prevention.

Carcinogens to which exposure is mainly by inhalation may, however, also induce tumours at sites other than the respiratory tract; for instance, bladder and pancreatic cancers, and possibly liver and kidney cancers, are causally related to the inhalation of tobacco smoke. Air pollutants may also be ingested or penetrate the skin [72-74].

While this monograph is clearly focused on cancer, it must be remembered that air pollutants also have subchronic and chronic adverse effects other than cancer. Since an increased frequency of respiratory tract diseases is observed most often in children [75], it is relevant that lower respiratory infections early in life are linked to an increased risk of chronic bronchitis during adult life [76]. Some experimental results point to other possible toxic effects: a variety of carcinogenic and non-carcinogenic polycyclic hydrocarbons that are air pollutants have been reported to promote the formation of arteriosclerotic plaques [77].

An accurate evaluation of the role of outdoor air pollution in increasing the risk for lung cancer is made particularly arduous because of confounding by other carcinogenic exposures, such as active and passive smoking, a number of occupational exposures, radon gas and other indoor pollutants.

Most of the studies on the association between air pollution and lung cancer have focused on the role of the urban environment. As a rule, mortality rates for lung cancer are higher in large cities and are directly correlated to the density of the population [78]. Although the highest urban:rural ratio for lung cancer was observed where emissions from the burning of coal for domestic purposes and industrial emissions coexisted for the longest time, urban air pollution is not limited to industrialised countries. The highest concentrations of suspended particulate matter, sulphur dioxide and smoke, have in fact been recorded in large cities in developing countries [79,80]. In China, for instance, although considerable efforts are being made to reduce emissions, levels of particulates in urban areas and in areas around industrial settings are still very high [81]. The use of smoky coals may result in particularly severe pollution of indoor air: the highest incidence of lung tumours in the world has been reported in women of a region in China who are exposed in their houses to smoke from coal used for cooking and heating [62]. Massive urbanisation in association with poverty, resulting in a huge increase in urban pollution and poor hygiene, is a growing problem in developing countries. In 1965, 17% of the total population of developing countries with low incomes lived in large cities; in 1987, this was the case for 30% of the population [82]. In 1990 73% of the total population in developed countries and 37% in developing countries were living in an urban environment. The largest number of megacities, that is, cities with more than 10 million inhabitants, as well as those growing at the fastest pace, are located in developing countries, namely 16 versus 5 in the industrialised countries [83]. The concentrations of particulate matter and of sulphur dioxide are high in certain large cities in developing countries [4]. Urban concentrations of suspended particulate matter are still increasing in cities of low income countries and it is estimated that about 1,345 million people are exposed to concentrations that according to WHO Guidelines are unacceptable [84].

Air pollution is particularly severe in central and eastern Europe. It has been reported that 16% of the population of the Confederation of Independent States live in cities where air pollution exceeds government-set limits and that estimated sums required to monitor and ensure pollution clean-up would be in the order of 4.4 trillion rubles [85]. Reports concerning the effect of air pollution on health, in particular on the health of children, in certain industrial cities of the ex-USSR are rather worrying [86]. Some of the worst pollution levels have been observed in Poland, where recent data suggest that the levels of exposure of the general population to air pollutants in certain regions are comparable with the highest ever observed in specific hazardous occupations [87,88].

Interactions Between Carcinogenic Agents

It is in situations of heavy air pollution that attempts to demonstrate, and possibly quantify, interactions between air pollution and carcinogenic exposures, such as smoking and certain occupational exposures, can be made with some probability of success. Interaction between carcinogens in increasing the risk for lung cancer is well documented in the case of asbestos and tobacco smoking, which appear to interact multiplicatively [89,90]. In addition, there is convincing evidence of an effect exceeding an additive (and perhaps multiplicative) effect between radon and tobacco smoke and arsenic and tobacco smoke [91]. In a case-control study, air pollution appeared to contribute to a significant increase in the risk for lung cancer among smokers who had had carcinogenic occupational exposures [92,93]. This finding contrasts with the results of case-control studies in which excesses of lung cancer could be explained entirely (or almost entirely) by smoking habits and occupation [94,95], although a more recent study points to an independent role of air pollution in increasing the risk for lung cancer [96]. A number of studies indicate an increased risk for lung cancer in passive smokers, that is, individuals who are exposed to tobacco smoke released into the ambient air by smokers [97,98]. The strongest argument to support the epidemiological findings is that persons exposed to environmental tobacco smoke are exposed to a chemical mixture containing known carcinogens, that is, substances known to cause cancer in smokers. Since there is a quantitative, non-threshold dose-response relationship in active smokers, one can reasonably conclude that exposure to environmental tobacco smoke must also increase the risk for cancer [91]. It is tempting to compare exposure to air pollution to that to environmental tobacco smoke and to see it as a particular type of air pollution. Urban air and the air in the proximity of certain factories contains substances that have been shown to be carcinogenic at exposure levels that can occur in occupational environments. Jedrychowski et al. [99] found that the joint action of air pollution, smoking and occupational exposures is well described by a multiplicative model. To what extent low levels of exposure to carcinogens may contribute to an increase in cancer risk is, however, far from clear. Nor is the question of the possible synergistic effect of exposure to multiple carcinogens at levels of concentration that would possibly have no effect *per se*.

The Problems of Ozone

Ozone can exert both deleterious and beneficial effects - acting as a significant pollutant locally, while providing a valuable photochemical screen against excess ultra-violet radiation at high altitudes. Ozone is a highly reactive, powerful oxidant which can react with virtually every class of biological substance, resulting in rapid reactions, particularly in the cells, fluids and tissues that line the respiratory tract. Its 2 major effects are alterations (usually impairment) in the mechanical functions of the lung, often accompanied by respiratory symptoms, and structural injury to or functional impairment of specific types of cells in the respiratory tract [40,100-103]. The primary source of excess tropospheric ozone is reactions between the hydrocarbons and oxides of nitrogen emitted from the burning of fossil fuels. It may also be produced biogenically from the reaction between nitric oxide made by soil microbes and terpenes and other hydrocarbons released from trees. The maximal ozone concentrations that are attained in polluted atmospheres are dependent on the absolute concentrations of volatile organic compounds and nitrogen oxides as well as their ratio [31,40,104-,105]. Photochemical ozone formation was first observed in Los Angeles in the 1940s and subsequently in other cities in the U.S. and Europe. Ozone levels in the free troposphere are believed to have doubled during this century [7,106,107]. Current levels of ozone in North America and Europe frequently exceed WHO ceilings for both short-term and long-term ozone concentrations by a wide margin on a large scale [7,106].

The last decade has witnessed an increasing number of studies that have confirmed earlier observations that human activities, particularly the extensive use of the important chlorofluorocarbons (CFCs), could modify the total column amount and vertical distribution of ozone in the lower stratosphere [7,108-113]. Precipitous ozone depletion has been most graphically illustrated in studies in the late 1980s that originally revealed "ozone holes" over the Antarctic which were largely attributed to the destruction of ozone by reactive chlorine species derived from the photochemical atmospheric reactions of the CFCs [108-113].

More recent studies have revealed additional substantial "ozone holes" over the Arctic as well as in the middle and high altitudes of the Northern Hemisphere covering Europe, almost all of populated North America, the former Soviet Union, northern China, Japan and the Koreas [112-116], suggesting that the process of ozone depletion could contribute to a global ozone reduction.

Even with an anticipated greatly restricted and ultimate cessation of the use of CFCs by the year 2000, the CFCs possess average atmospheric lifetimes of many decades and hence atmospheric chlorine will persist in the stratosphere for comparable periods. Although variations of the natural spatial and temporal atmospheric ozone concentrations make it difficult to predict with precision the extent of future global changes of ozone depletion, various computer models have suggested the present rate of change to be 1-2% per year [7,108-113].

Reduced stratospheric ozone results in an increased flux of biologically damaging mid-ultraviolet radiation (UVB, 290-320 nm) to the surface of the earth and to ecologically significant depths in the ocean affecting phytoplankton and algae productivity and more specifically Antarctic marine ecosystems [7,108,116-118]. Both epidemiological studies and the results of tests with animal models link squamous-cell and basal-cell skin cancers to exposure to ultra-violet radiation [119], and there is convincing evidence that it contributes to an increase in the risk for malignant melanomas. It is therefore possible that increased radiation may generate an increased risk for pigmented and non-pigmented skin tumours [109].

The Greenhouse Effect, Global Warming and Acid Rain

Atmospheric emissions in both developing and developed (industrialised) countries can have regional and global consequences, as evidenced by the depletion of the ozone layer, mentioned above, by the increasing problems related to acid rain and by the greenhouse effect, even though the mechanisms, rate and extent of possible damage remain to be fully elucidated or modelled.

Much of the current concern about the fate of the global environment is related to the increased concentrations of greenhouse gases (carbon dioxide, methane, nitrous oxide and the CFCs), largely as a result of human activities [7,108,118-128]. Greenhouse gases released anywhere in the world disperse rapidly in the global atmosphere.

Global warming is the predicted consequence of the greenhouse effect and arises because an increase in the concentration of greenhouse gases tends to warm the earth's surface by downward re-radiation of infrared rays. The greenhouse effect is, similarly to most if not all ecological problems, a consequence of a myriad of interconnected human endeavours involving population growth, energy use, life-style, agriculture, economics and politics [7,108,121-133]. Of the greenhouse gases, carbon dioxide is by far the most important. Since the industrial revolution, carbon dioxide concentrations have increased by 25% and are currently increasing at the rate of about 0.5% per year [7,121,126]. Approximately 80% of total emissions come from fossil fuel combustion, mostly from the industrialised nations [131]. The U.S. and the Commonwealth of Independent States (former USSR) are the largest contributors, together emitting nearly half of the world's carbon from fossil fuels [133]. Much of the remaining 20% are believed to come from deforestation, mostly in tropical nations with Brazil being the largest contributor [133].

Carbon dioxide accounts for about half of all global warming and the U.S., possessing approximately 5% of the global population, is responsible for approximately 25% of the world's annual atmospheric carbon emissions. In contrast, the entire developing world (80% of the global population) is currently responsible for approximately 35% of the world's carbon emissions. The global emissions for carbon increased from 4.8 billion tonnes in 1971 to about 6 billion tonnes in 1988 [7,125].

There have been numerous model projections of the emissions and resultant atmospheric concentrations of greenhouse gases during the next century and the consequences for global surface temperatures. Current interpretations of temperature records reveal that the global average temperature has increased between 0.3° and 0.6° C (0.5° F and 1.1° F) during the last decade [7,123-129]. Many climatologists believe that a doubling of carbon dioxide equivalents of all greenhouse gases above pre-industrialised concentrations would increase global mean temperatures by a best guess estimate of 2.5° C (about 4.5° F) with bounds of 1.5° C and 4.5° C [7,121]. Other assessments suggest that if greenhouse gas emissions continue to increase as they have in the recent past (without remediation), global temperatures will increase during the next century by 0.3° C per decade resulting in an increase of about 1° C above the present value by the year 2025 and 3° C before the end of the next century [7,123].

The consequences of climatic change and the rate of change have been suggested to include possible changes for agriculture, forestry, sea levels, the energy sector etc. However, it is broadly acknowledged that these changes are extremely difficult to predict with any reliability [7,123-129]. For example, one scenario would suggest that global warming induced by greenhouse gases will accelerate sea-level rise by about 20 cm by 2030 and 65 cm by the end of the next century (causing a cascade of events) and the rate of increase of sea level could be 3-10 times greater than the 0.01 meter decade long-term average recorded during the past century [7,123,129]. A recent report by UNEP [127] projects increases in global mean temperature by 1.1° C by 2030 and by 4° C by 2090. The resultant warmer and dryer conditions would result in losses in agricultural products as high as 10-30% in "bread-basket" regions such as the American mid-west, Ukraine, Argentine pampas and the Australian wheat belt.

In the last 2 decades it has been widely established that many atmospheric pollutants, particularly sulphur and nitrogen oxides, particulates, heavy metals, pesticides and some industrial halogenated chemicals, e.g., PCBs, can be transported over large distances from their original emission sites by global atmospheric circulation and exhibit a variety of negative impacts on the environment distant from their original source [7,108,117-145]. Acid deposition consists principally of acid substances and their precursors such as sulphur and nitrogen oxides, acids and salts and the products of their atmospheric transformation. Acid rain is believed to affect forest soils that could lead to long-term deficiencies in soil nutrients [138,141].

Acid rain has been recognised since the early 1970s as a major air pollution problem in Europe and North America, engendered to a large degree by transboundary transport of sulphur and nitrogen oxides [7,108,117]. For example, the domestic deposition of sulphur dioxide varies greatly across Europe: from 5% in Norway to 83% in the United Kingdom in 1988. The deposition depends on the prevailing winds, size of the country and density of the emission field. Countries in Europe not only receive acid rain from their neighbours but also "export" large amounts of sulphur dioxide [7,139]. Over 50% of the forests in Germany, Greece, the United Kingdom and Norway, 40% of those in Poland, Bulgaria, Switzerland, Belgium, the Netherlands and Denmark, and over 30% of the forests in Yugoslavia, Spain and Finland have been affected by acid rain [7]. Acid rain is believed to be also responsible for the thousands of lakes that have been found to be strongly acidified with severe ecological consequences in Canada, Finland, Norway, Sweden and the United States [7].

REFERENCES

1. McKeown Th: The Origins of Human Disease. Basil Blackwell, Oxford, 1988
2. Brimblecombe P: The Big Smoke. Routledge, London 1988
3. Dubos R: Man adapting. Yale University Press, 1965
4. UNEP Environmental Data Report 1989-1990. Basil Blackwell Inc Publishers, Cambridge, MA, USA, 1989
5. Bocola W and Cirillo MC: Air pollutant emissions by combustion processes in Italy. Atmospheric Environment 1989 (23/1):17-24
6. Derwent D: A better way to control pollution. Nature 1988 (331):575-578
7. OECD: The State of the Environment. Organization for Economic Co-Operation and Development. Paris 1991
8. Clayson A: The state of environment: A report card for OECD countries. Ambio 1991 (20):163-164
9. World Resources Institute: World Resources 1990-1991. Basic Books, New York 1990
10. Brown L: Ten years to save the world. New Sci 1992 (Feb 22)
11. Levine MD, Meyers SP, Wilbanks T: Energy efficiency and developing countries. Env Sci Technol 1991 (25): 584-589
12. Tomatis L (ed) Air Pollution and Human Cancer. European School of Oncology Monographs. Springer-Verlag, Heidelberg 1990
13. Leibowitz MD and Walkinshaw DS: Indoor air '90: Health effects associated with indoor air contaminants. Arch Environ Hlth 1992 (47):6-7
14. Spengler JD and Samet JM: A Perspective on indoor and outdoor air pollution. In: Samet JM and Spengler JD (eds) Indoor Air Pollution. Johns Hopkins University Press, Baltimore MD 1991 pp 1-29
15. Fishbein L, Henry CJ: Introduction: Workshop on the methodology for assessing health risks from complex mixtures in indoor air. Env Hlth Perspec 1991 (95):3-5
16. Hileman B: Multiple chemical sensitivity. C & EN 1991 (July 22):26-42
17. Saracci R and Riboli E: Passive smoking and lung cancer: Current evidence and ongoing studies at the IARC. Mutat Res 1989 (222):117-127
18. Trichopoulos D, Kalandidi A, Sparros L and MacMahon B: Lung cancer and passive smoking. Int J Cancer 1981 (27):1-4
19. Pershagen G and Simonato L: Epidemiological evidence on outdoor pollution and cancer. This Volume
20. Wallace LA: Comparison of risks from outdoor and indoor exposure to toxic chemicals. Env Hlth Perspect 1991 (95):7-13
21. Spengler JD: Sources and concentrations of indoor air pollution. In: Samet JM and Spengler JD (eds) Indoor Air Pollution. Johns Hopkins University Press, Baltimore MD 1991 pp 33-67
22. Counolly GN: Worldwide Expansion of Transnational Tobacco Industry. J Natl Cancer Inst Monogr 1992 (12):29-35
23. Samet JM and Lambert WE: Epidemiologic approaches for assessing health risks from complex mixtures in indoor air. Env Hlth Perspect 1991 (95):71-74
24. Evelyn J: The inconvenience of the air and smoke of London dissipated. London 1661 (cited by R. Dubos, 1965)
25. Lawther PJ, Martin A and Wilkins ET: Epidemiology of air pollution. WHO P.H. paper No 15, 1962
26. Wilkins ET: Air pollution and the London fog of December 1952. J Roy San Inst 1954 (74):1-21
27. Schwartz J and Marcus A: Mortality and air pollution in London: A time series analysis. Am J Epidem 1990 (131):185-194
28. Hobbs PV and Radke LF: Airborne studies of the smoke from the Kuwait oil fires. Science 1992 (256):987-991
29. Johnson DW, Kilsby CG, McKenna DS, Saunders RW, Jenkins GJ, Smith FB and Foot JS: Airborne observations of the physical and chemical characteristics of the Kuwait oil smoke plume. Nature 1991 (353):617-621
30. Ciocco A and Thompson D: A follow-up of Donora ten years after. Amer J Public Health 1961 (51):155-164
31. Seinfeld JH: Urban air pollution: State of the science. Science 1989 (243):745-752
32. World Health Organization: Acute Effects on Health of Smog Episodes. WHO European Series, No 43, 1992
33. Shishido S, Iwai K and Tukagoshi K: Incidence of ferruginous bodies in the lungs during a 45-year period and mineralogical analysis of the core fibres and uncoated fibres. In: Bignon J, Peto J and Saracci R (eds) Non-Occupational Exposure to Mineral Fibres. IARC Scientific Publications Series No 90. International Agency for Research on Cancer, Lyon 1989 pp 229-238
34. Quality of the Environment in Japan. Environment Agency. Government of Japan, 1988
35. Magnani C, Borgo G, Betta GP, Botta M, Ivaldi C, Mollo F, Scelzi M and Terracini B: Mesothelioma and non-occupational environmental exposure to asbestos. Lancet 1991 (338):50
36. Lundy P and Barer M: Asbestos-containing materials in New York City buildings. Environ Res 1992 (58):15-24
37. IARC Monograph on the Evaluation of Carcinogenic Risks to Humans, Vol. 35. Polynuclear Aromatic Compounds. Part 4: Bitumens, Coal-Tars and Derived Products, Shale-Oils and Soots. International Agency for Research on Cancer, Lyon 1985
38. Hansen ES: Cancer incidence in an occupational cohort exposed to bitumen fumes. Scan J Work Environ Hlth 1989 (15):101-105
39. IARC Monograph on the Evaluation of Carcinogenic Risks to Humans, Vol. 28. The Rubber Industry. International Agency for Research on Cancer, Lyon 1982
40. World Health Organization: Air Quality Guidelines for Europe. WHO Regional Publications. European Series No 23, Copenhagen 1987, pp 315-326
41. Leiter J, Shimkin MB and Shear MJ: Production of subcutaneous sarcomas in mice with tars

extracted from atmospheric dusts. JNCI 1942 (3):155-165
42. Leiter J and Shear MJ: Production of tumors in mice with tars from city air dusts. JNCI 1942 (3):167-174
43. Schuetzle D and Daisey JM: Identification of genotoxic agents in complex mixtures of air pollutants. In: Waters MD, Nesnow S, Lewtas J, Moore MM and Daniel FB (eds) Short-term Bioassays in the Analysis of Complex Environmental Mixtures, VI. Plenum Press, New York 1990
44. Chen LC, Miller PD, Amdur MO and Gordon T: Airway hyperresponsiveness in guinea pigs exposed to acid-coated ultrafine particles. J Toxicol Environ Hlth 1992 (35):165-174
45. Viegi G, Paoletti P, Carrozzi L, Vellutini M, Diviggiano E, Di Pede C, Pistelli G, Giutini G and Lebowitz MD: Prevalence rates of respiratory symptoms in Italian general population samples exposed to different levels of air pollution. Environ Hlth Perspect 1991 (94):95-99
46. Schwartz J and Dockery DW: Increased mortality in Philadelphia associated with daily air pollution concentrations. Am Rev Respir Dis 1992 (145):600-604
47. Leibowitz MD: Populations at risk: addressing health effects due to complex mixtures with a focus on respiratory effects. Environ Hlth Perspect 1991 (95):35-38
48. Robinson JC and Paxman DG: The Role of threshold limit values in U.S. air pollution policy. Am J Ind Med 1992 (21):383-396
49. Schwartz J and Deckery DW: Particulate air pollution and daily mortality in Steubenville, Ohio. Am J Epidemiol 1992 (135):12-19
50. Pönkä A: Asthma and low level air pollution in Helsinki. Arch Environ Hlth 1991 (46/5):262-270
51. Schwartz J: Particulate air pollution and daily mortality in Detroit. Environ Res 1991 (56):204-213
52. Hall JV, Winder AM, Kleinman MT, Lurman FW, Braier V and Colome SD: Valuing the health benefits of clean air. Science 1992 (225):812-817
53. Archer VE: Air pollution and fatal lung disease in three Utah counties. Arch Environ Hlth 1990 (45/6):325-334
54. Bobak M and Leon DA: Air pollution and infant mortality in the Czech Republic, 1986-1988. Lancet 1992 (340):1010-1014
55. Schwartz J, Spix C, Wichmann HE and Malin E: Air pollution and acute respiratory illness in five German communities. Environ Res 1991 (56):1-14
56. Schwartz J, Dockery DW, Ware JH et al: Acute effects of acid aerosols on respiratory symptom reporting in children. Air Pollut Control Assoc 1989 Preprint n° 89-92.1)
57. Braun-Fahrländer C, Ackermann-Liebrich U, Schwartz J, Gnehm HP, Rutishauser M and Wanner HU: Air pollution and respiratory problems in pre-school children. Am Rev Respir Dis 1992 (145):42-47
58. Spektor DM, Hofmeister VA, Artaxo P, Brague JAP, Echelar F, Nogueira DP, Hayes C, Thurston GD and Lippmann N: Effects of heavy industrial pollution on respiratory function in the children of Cubatao, Brazil: A preliminary report. Environ Health Perspect 1991 (94):51-54
59. Goren AI, Goldsmith JR, Hellmann S and Brenneer S: Follow-up of school children in the vicinity of a coal-fired power plant in Israel. Environ Health Perspect 1991 (94):101-105
60. Savitz DA and Feingold L: Association of childhood cancer with residential traffic density. Scand J Work Environ Health 1989 (15):360-363
61. Norboo T, Yahya M, Bruce NG, Heady JA and Ball KP: Domestic pollution and respiratory illness in a Himalayan village. Int J Epidem 1991 (20):749-757
62. Xingzhou He, Wei Chen, Ziyuan Liu and Chapman RS: An epidemiological study of lung cancer in Xuan Wei county, China: Current progress. Case-control study on lung cancer and cooking fuel. Environ Health Perspect 1991 (94):9-13
63. Qing Liu, Sasco A, Riboli E and Meng Xuan Hu: Indoor air pollution and lung cancer in Guangzhou, People's Republic of China. Amer J Epidem 1992 (in press)
64. Chen BH, Hong CJ and He ZX: Indoor air pollution and its health effects in China - A review. Environ Technol 1992 (13):301-312
65. Anon: Indoor air pollution and acute respiratory infections in children. Lancet 1992 (339):396-398
66. Anon: Home with radon. Lancet 1992 (339):1291
67. Tomatis L, Aitio A, Shuker L and Wilbourn J: Human carcinogens so far identified. Jpn J Cancer Res 1989 (80):795-807
68. IARC Monograph on the Evaluation of Carcinogenic Risks to Humans, Vol 54. Occupational Exposures to Mists and Vapours from Strong Inorganic Acids and Other Industrial Chemicals. International Agency for Research on Cancer, Lyon 1992
69. Geddes DM: The natural history of lung cancer: A review based on rates of tumour growth. Br J Dis Chest 1979 (73):1-17
70. Walter SD, Kubik A, Parkin DM, Reissigova J, Adamec M and Khlat M: The natural history of lung cancer estimated from the results of a randomized trial of screening. Cancer Causes and Control 1992 (3):115-123
71. Kubik A, Parkin DM, Khlat M, Erban J, Polak J and Adamec M: Lack of benefit from semi-annual screening for cancer of the lung: follow-up report of a randomized controlled trial on a population of high-risk males in Czechoslovakia. Int J Cancer 1990 (45):26-33
72. Sellers Storer J, DeLeon I, Millikan LE, Laseter JL and Griffing C: Human absorption of coal-tar products. Arch Dermatol 1984 (120):874-877
73. Jongeneelen FJ, Leijdekkers ChM and Henderson PTh: Urinary excretion of 3-hydroxy-benzo[a]-pyrene after percutaneous penetration and oral absorption of benzo[a]pyrene in rats. Cancer Lett 1984 (25):195-201
74. Yang JJ, Roy TA and Mackerer CR: Percutaneous absorption of anthracene in the rat: comparison of in vivo and in vitro results. Toxicol and Indus Health 1986 (2/1):79-84
75. Goren A, Brenner S and Hellmann S: Cross-sectional health study in polluted and nonpolluted agricultural settlements in Israel. Environ Hlth 1988 (46):107-119

76 Barker DJP, Osmond C and Law CM: The intrauterine and early postnatal origins of cardiovascular disease and chronic bronchitis. J Epidemiol and Community Health 1989 (43):237-240

77 Penn A and Snyder C: Arteriosclerotic plaque development is "promoted" by polynuclear aromatic hydrocarbons. Carcinogenesis 1989 (9):2185-2189

78 Muir CS, Waterhouse J, Mack T, Powell J and Whelan S (eds) Cancer Incidence in Five Continents, Vol V. IARC Scientific Publications No 88, Lyon 1987

79 Bennett BG, Kretzschmar JG, Akland GG and Dekoning HW: Urban air pollution worldwide. Environ Sci Technol 1985 (19):298-304

80 Böhm GM, Nascimento Saldiva PH, Gonçalves Pasqualucci CA, Massad E, De Arruda Martins M, Araujo Zin W, Veras Cardoso W, Martins Pereira Criado P, Komatsuzaki M, Sakae RS, Negri EM, Lemos M, Del Monte Capelozzi V, Crestana C and Da Silva R: Biological effects of air pollution in São Paulo and Cubatão. Environ Res 1989 (49):208-216

81 Assessment of Urban Air Quality. UNEP/WHO, 1988

82 World Development Report 1989. Oxford University Press, New York 1989

83 World Health Organization: Our Planet, Our Health. WHO, Geneva 1992

84 World Development Report. Oxford University Press, New York 1992

85 Brandt R: Soviet environment slips down the agenda. Science 1992 (255):22-23

86 Revich BA: Quality of air in industrial cities of the USSR and child health. The Science of the Total Environment 1992 (119):121-132

87 Hemminki K, Grzykowska E, Chorazy M et al: DNA adducts in humans environmentally exposed to aromatic compounds in an industrialized area of Poland. Carcinogenesis (1990) (II):1229-1231

88 Perera FP, Hemminki K, Gryzbowska E et al: Molecular and genetic damage in humans from environmental pollution in Poland. Nature 1992 (360):256-258

89 Hammond EC, Selikoff JJ, Seidman H: Asbestos exposure, cigarette smoking and death rates. Ann NY Acad Sciences 1979 (330):473-490

90 Saracci R: The interactions of tobacco smoking and other agents in cancer etiology. Epidemiol Rev 1987 (9):175-193

91 Cancer: Causes, Occurrence and Control. IARC, Lyon 1990

92 Vena JE: Air pollution as a risk factor in lung cancer. Am.J Epidemiol 1982 (116):42-56

93 Winkelstein W Jr and Levin LI: Air pollution and cancer. Rev Cancer Epidemiol 1983 ( ):211-239

94 Haenszel W, Loveland DB and Sirken MG: Lung cancer mortality as related to residence and smoking histories. JNCI 1962 (28):947-1001

95 Pike MC, Jing JS, Rosario IP, Henderson BE and Menck HR: Occupation: explanation of an apparent air pollution related localized excess of lung cancer in Los Angeles County. In: Breslow N and Whittemore A (eds) Energy and Health. SIAM, Philadelphia, PA 1979 pp 3-16

96 Buffler A, Cooper P, Stonnett S, Contant Ch, Shirts S, Hardy J, Agu U, Gehan B, Buraj K: Air pollution and lung cancer mortality in Hanis County, Texas, 1979-1981. Am J Epidemiol 1988 (128):683-699

97 Trichopoulos D, Kalindidi A, Sparos L, MacMahon B: Lung cancer and passive smoking. Int J Cancer 1981 (27):1-4

98 Saracci R and Riboli E: Passive smoking and lung cancer: Current evidence and ongoing studies at the International Agency for Research on Cancer. Mutation Res 1989 (222):117-127

99 Jedrychowski W, Becher H, Wahrendorf J and Basa-Cierpalek Z: A case-control study of lung cancer with special reference to the effect of air pollution in Poland. J Epi Comm Health 1989 (in press)

100 Tilton BE: Health effects of tropospheric ozone. Environ Sci Technol 1989 (23):254-263

101 US Environmental Protection Agency: Air Quality Criteria for Ozone and Other Photochemical Oxidants. 4 Volumes. Report No. EPA-700/8-94-0208. Washington, DC

102 Lippmann M: Health effects of tropospheric ozone. Environ Sci Technol 1991 (25):1954-1962

103 Zeliloff JT, Kraemer G, Vogel MC and Schlesinger RB: Immunomodulating effects of ozone on macrophage functions important for tumor surveillance and host defense. J Toxicol Environ Hlth 1991 (34):449-467

104 Ember LR, Layman PL, Lepkowski W and Zurer PS: Tending the global commons. Chem Eng News 1989 (Nov 4):14-64

105 McElroy MB and Salawitch RJ: Changing composition of the global stratosphere. Science 1989 (243):763-770

106 World Health Organization: Air Quality Guidelines for Europe. WHO Regional Publications. European Series No 23. Copenhagen 1986 pp 315-326

107 Penkett SA: Changing ozone: Evidence for a perturbed atmosphere. Environ Sci Technol 1991 (25):631-635

108 McElroy MB, Salawitch RJ: Changing composition of the global stratosphere. Science 1989 (243):763-770

109 Solomon S: Progress towards a quantitative understanding of antarctic ozone depletion. Nature 1990 (347):347-354

110 Anderson JG, Toohey DW, Brune WH: Free radicals within the antarctic vortex: The role of the CFCs in antarctic ozone loss. Science 1991 (251):39-46

111 Schoeberl MR, Hartman DL: The dynamics of the stratosphere polar vortex and its relation to springtime ozone depletions. Science 1991 (251):46-52

112 Roland EF: Stratospheric ozone in the 21st century: The chlorofluorocarbon problem. Environ Sci Technol 1992 (25):622-629

113 Folkins I, Brasseur G: The chemical mechanisms behind ozone depletion. Chem Ind 1992 (April 20):294-297

114 Kerr RA: Ozone destruction worsens. Science 1992 (252):204

115 Brune H, Andersonb JG, Toohey DW, Fahey DWL: The potential for ozone depletion in the Arctic polar stratosphere. Science 1991 (252):1260-1266
116 Smith RC, Prezelin B, Baker KS, Bidigare RR, Boucher NP, Coley T: Ozone depletion: Ultraviolet radiation and phytoplankton biology in Antarctic waters. Science 1992 (25):952-959
117 Seinfeld TH: Urban air pollution: State of the science. Science 1989 (243):745-752
118 Ember LR, Layman PKL, Lepkowski W, Zurer PS: Tending the global commons. Chem Eng News 1989 (Nov 4):14-64
119 IARC Monographs on the Evaluation of Carcinogenic Risks to Humans Volume 55: Solar and Ultraviolet Radiation. International Agency for Research on Cancer, Lyon 1992
120 National Academy of Science (NAS): Ozone Depletion, Greenhouse Gases and Climate Change. National Academy Press, Washington DC, 1990
121 National Academy of Sciences: Policy Implications of Greenhouse Warming. National Academy Press, Washington DC, 1991
122 Boyden S and Dovers S: Natural resource consumption and its environmental impacts in the Western world: Impacts of increasing per capita consumption. Ambio 1992 (21):63-69
123 Schneider S and Rosenberg N: The greenhouse effect: Its causes, possible impacts and associated uncertainties. In: Rosenberg N (ed) Greenhouse Warming: Abatement and Adaptation. Resources for the Future, Washington DC, 1989 pp 7-34
124 Philips VD: Living in a terrarium. Environ Sci Technol 1991 (25):574-578
125 Rosswall T: Greenhouse gases and global change: International collaboration. Environ Sci Technol 1991 (25):567-573
126 Hileman B: Web of interactions makes it difficult to untangle global warming data. Chem Eng News 1992 (April 27):7-19
127 UNEP/WHO: Climate Change and World Agriculture. Geneva 1991
128 UNEP: Intergovernmental Panel on Climate Change Working Group 1. Scientific Assessment of Climate Change. UN Environmental Program, Geneva 1990
129 Arrhenius E: Population, development and environmental disruption - An issue on efficient natural resource management. Ambio 1992 (21):9-13
130 Schneider SH: The greenhouse effect: Science and policy. Science 1989 (243):771-781
131 World Resources Institute: World Resources 1990-1991. Basic Books, New York 1990
132 Dickinson R and Cicerone R: Future global warming from atmospheric trace gases. Nature 1986 (319):109-115
133 Swisher J and Masters G: A mechanism to reconcile equity and efficiency in global climate protection: International carbon emission offsets. Ambio 1992 (21):154-159
134 Ballschmitter K: Global distribution of organic compounds. Environ Carcinogen Ecotox Revs 1991 (C9):1-46
135 Schroeder WH and Lane DA: Fate of toxic airborne pollutants. Environ Sci Technol 1988 (22):240-246
136 Travis CC and Hester ST: Global chemical pollution. Environ Sci Technol 1991 (25):814-1819
137 Oehme M: Further evidence for long-range air transport of polychlorinated aromates and pesticides: North America and Eurasia to the Arctic. Ambio 1992 (20):293-297
138 Schwartz SE: Acid deposition: Unravelling a regional phenomenon. Science 1989 (243):753-763
139 Hordijk L: Use of rains model. Environ Sci Technol 1991 (25):596-603
140 Saenger J (ed): The State of the Earth. Unwin Hyman, London 1990
141 Eriksson E, Karltun E and Lundmark JE: Acidification of forest soils in Sweden. Ambio 1992 (21):150-154
142 Roberts L: Learning from acid-rain program. Science 1991 (251):1302
143 Dunmore J: Acid rain in Europe. In: DocTer Institute for Environmental Studies - European Environmental Yearbook 1987. DocTer International, London 1987 pp 665-666
144 Kamari J (ed): Impact Models to Assess Regional Acidification. Kluwer, Dordrecht 1990
145 Streets DG: A Review of Acid Rain Models for Europe. Report-Task Force on Integrated Assessment Modeling. Economic Commission for Europe. United Nations, Geneva 1988

Sources, Nature and Levels of Air Pollutants

Lawrence Fishbein

Office of Toxicology Sciences, Center for Food Safety and Nutrition, Food and Drug Administration, Washington, D.C. 20204, U.S.A.

A broad spectrum of potentially toxic chemicals spanning many inorganic and organic structural categories, is released into local, regional and global atmospheres from both natural and anthropogenic sources and from both industrialised and developing countries [1-13]. In one data base compilation, more than 2,800 atmospheric compounds were identified of which more than 300 (about 11%) have been bioassayed [1]. More than 65,000 chemicals are used in commerce in the industrialised nations of the world. Many of these substances, e.g., industrial solvents, VOCs, polychlorinated biphenyls, pesticides, and aerosol products containing volatile propellants and active ingredients (as well as trace contaminants such as chlorinated dibenzodioxins and furans) are emitted directly or indirectly into the atmosphere because of human activities [3,11-13]. These atmospheric pollutants can be transported over great distances to further exhibit a variety of deleterious impacts on human health and the environment quite distant from their original emission sites [1-13].

Urban areas have long been considered the major locus of serious air pollution due to the relatively high density of pollution sources such as industries, residences and vehicular traffic, giving rise to 6 major priority pollutants of health and environmental concern: sulphur dioxide, nitrogen oxides, suspended particulate matter, ozone (photochemical smog), carbon monoxide and lead [1-3,11,12]. Because of the deleterious effects of these 6 pollutants, most industrialised and many developing nations have set legal air quality standards for some or all of them [2,3,11,12].

Motor vehicles cause more air pollution than any other single human activity, contributing nearly one-half of the human caused nitrogen oxides, two-thirds of the carbon monoxide, and about half of the hydrocarbons in industrialised countries as well as most of the airborne lead in developing countries [11,12].

Globally, fuel combustion (fossil, wood and biomass) is the principal cause of man-made air pollution as a consequence of increased energy demand, industrial activity and vehicular transportation. Energy production has expanded more than 20 times since the 1850s, following a tripling of world population and an average annual growth of 2-4% in economic output, resulting in the intensification of air pollution at all levels, local, regional, national and global [11,12].

A large number of both inorganic and organic agents, e.g., metals, VOCs, hydrocarbons and pesticides originating in outdoor air are also found in indoor environments, often at levels exceeding those found outdoors; these are believed to contribute substantially to indoor pollution, which is increasingly recognised as a potentially significant health problem [2,11,14-32].

Outdoor Environments - General Considerations

The introduction of toxicants into the atmosphere may be direct via the inadvertent or deliberate release from a particular mobile or stationary source, or indirect as a consequence of initial discharge or disposal of chemicals into other environmental media such as water or soil. Hazardous pollutants may be accidentally released into ambient air via escape of raw materials or finished products at their manufacturing site (e.g., release of methyl isocyanate in Bohpal, India), or by a chemical spill resulting from a transportation mishap such as a truck, cargo train derailment and/or barge or ship spillage or collision. Many toxicants are accidentally released from the thousands of chemical facilities and numerous small business establishments such as dry cleaning establishments and service stations.

Nitrogen oxides, carbon monoxide and VOCs (e.g., benzene, toluene and xylene) have been identified in many instances to be related to tailpipe emissions and, in the case of VOCs, to emissions from petrol stations as well [1-12].

Pollutants also occur in the atmosphere as a result of myriad atmospheric reactions and photochemical transformations. The resultant chemical species present vary with precursor pollutants, altitude, season and location [3-5,10-13].

Urban locations are increasingly plagued by complex mixtures of gases and particles with condensed organic matter primarily derived from the combustion of fossil fuels (e.g., coal, oil petrol, diesel fuel) from vehicle, industrial and power plant sources as well as from vegetative sources (wood and plant). Rural areas can also be afflicted with many of the above complex mixtures (perhaps to a lesser degree) but also be subjected in varying degrees to the products resulting from the combustion of biomass matter (especially in many underdeveloped areas) [2-4,11-14,18,33-37].

In recent years, there has been increasingly broadly expressed concern about the fate of the global environment as related to 3 principal areas: a) stratospheric ozone depletion [2-5,11,12,38-44]; b) induction of the greenhouse effect resulting from increased atmospheric concentration of greenhouse gases (carbon dioxide, methane, nitrous oxide and the chlorofluorocarbons) and their possible effects on global climate [4,5,11,12,44-58], and c) the global transport of air pollutants [4,5,10-13,49-53,56-61] with their subsequent effects (e.g., acid rain) [2-5,11-13,62-68] (see also chapter 1).

We have become additionally more aware that nature is often not benign, as witnessed by the recent volcanic eruptions such as Mt. Pinatubo in the Philippines in 1991 and its resultant huge emissions of sulphur oxides and particulates with both short and long-term implications [11,69-71].

Even more regrettably, we have become aware that catastrophic wartime events, however relatively "isolated", such as the recent Kuwait oil fires set during the Persian Gulf war and the subsequent emission of massive amounts of sulphur oxides, nitrogen oxides, particulate matter, PAHs and metals, may have the potential for deleterious local, regional and more distant acute and chronic human health and environmental effects [72-76].

Physical Properties, Stability, Fate, Transformation and Transport

Following emission into the atmosphere, individual pollutants possess characteristic residence times (lifetimes) which are a function of source parameters as well as the physical and chemical properties of the pollutant and/or its photochemical reactivity [3-5,7,10-13].

Although the earth's atmosphere is composed of principally inert molecules or chemically reducing gases such as nitrogen, hydrogen and methane, the atmosphere acts as an oxidizative system because of its overall composition and the relative chemical reactivity of natural atmospheric constituents and/or contaminants. The principal oxidants are ozone, the OH radical and hydrogen peroxide. Other chemically reactive species in the atmosphere include: atomic oxygen, the free radicals HO_2, CH_3O_2, peroxides such as CH_3O_2H, nitrogen oxides, sulphur oxides and a wide ariety of acidic and basic species. The total atmospheric burden of ozone, OH and hydrogen peroxide principally determines the "oxidizing capacity" of the atmosphere [77].

Hence, a broad spectrum of naturally occurring and anthropogenic pollutants, once emitted into ambient air, can be potentially converted at various rates into species characterised by higher chemical oxidation states than their precursor substances. The fate of toxic air pollutants is determined by a variety of physical, chemical and/or photochemical processes occurring in the atmosphere during their residence time in this environmental compartment. In addition to the concern of the direct action of atmospheric pollutants on human health, atmospheric input is believed to be the predominant source of a number of toxic pollutants in lakes and streams. For instance, 60-90% of the polychlorinated biphenyl (PCB) burden in the Great Lakes in the United States have been estimated to originate from the atmosphere [3-5,7,10].

The majority of emission sources release pollutants into the atmosphere close to (troposphere) or directly upon the earth's surface, and the height at which pollutants are released will determine the distance of their travel before their contact with the ground or another receptor surface [3-13]. It is important for an assessment of the impact of atmospheric emission sources on human health as well as natural ecosystems to quantify emissions to the extent possible, both spatially and temporally. Physical processes will act on pollutants immediately following their release from an emission source. This initial interaction is dependent on factors including the actual configuration of the emission source (area, height above the surrounding terrain) and initial buoyancy conditions [3-13]. Following emission, pollutants generally enter into a mixing layer in the lower region of the troposphere (which typically extends to 1-2 km during the day and a few hundred meters in the evening), where the pollutants circulate and disperse vertically and horizontally, promoting intimate contact between vapour-phase and aerosol-associated constituents [3,10]. This initial important contact ultimately results in chemical transformations of pollutants near their source while their concentrations are still relatively high and precedes dilution [10]. Diffusion and transport is dependent on air mass circulations effected by local, regional or global forces. Dispersion represents the combination of transport and diffusion processes. Compared to the major pollutants of an inorganic nature (e.g., SO_2, NO_2 and CO_2), considerably less is known of the movement and behaviour of many trace organic contaminants in the atmosphere [3-5,7,10-13].

During transport and diffusion through the atmosphere, many toxic pollutants, with the exception of the most inert chemicals, are likely to undergo complex chemical or photochemical reactions. These can potentially transform a pollutant from its primary physical and chemical state when entering the atmosphere to another state that may have similar or very different characteristics. Many volatile organic chemicals (VOCs) such as chlorofluorocarbons (CFCs), which have long residence times, are implicated in the depletion of the stratospheric ozone layer. Transformation products may differ from their precursors in chemical stability, toxic properties as well as other characteristics [3-5,10-13,38-45].

Atmospheric organic pollutants are found in both gaseous and particulate phases. The manner in which a given compound partitions will greatly influence the compound's atmospheric removal mechanisms and lifetime as well as its health effects due to inhalation. The vapour pressure of the compound in addition to the amount and type of particulate matter present and temperature will affect the extent of association with particulate matter. Airborne particulates of respirable size, whether of natural or man-made origin, form an important fraction of all atmospheric aerosols [3,13,78].

The atmospheric aerosol is a highly complex entity comprising mixtures of primary emissions such as soot and fly-ash as well as secondary species that constitute the "sink" of many atmospheric chemical processes. The prevalent compounds of urban aerosols include sulphates, nitrates, ammonium, carbonaceous material, trace metals and water [3]. Additionally, meat cooking operations have been recently found to be a major source of organic aerosol emissions to the urban atmosphere, comprising up to 21% of the primary organic carbon particle (diameter <2µm) emissions in the Los Angeles area. More than 75 organic compounds were quantified including a broad spectrum of n-alkanes, n-alkanoic acids, n-alkenoic acids, dicarboxylic acids, n-alkanols, n-alkanals, furans, lactones, amides, nitriles and PAHs [78]. Control of the fine particle component of the urban aerosols is a major problem in cities such as Los Angeles [3,78].

Although concentrations of toxic air pollutants near a source may be high, their air concentrations in urban, rural and remote locations may be several orders of magnitude lower than those of ubiquitous type of air pollutant.

Air concentrations of both vapour and particulate phases tend to decrease rapidly as a function of increasing distance from the emission sources. Atmospheric toxic air pollutants are generally present in the atmosphere at trace concentrations (parts-per-billion or parts-per-trillion) requiring specially stringent considerations and sophisticated equipment for their collection, separation and quantification [3-5,7,10]. It is also important to distinguish the chemistry of the urban atmosphere considered by Seinfeld [3] to be a "giant reactor in which pollutant gases such as hydrocarbons and oxides of nitrogen and sulphur react under the influence of sunlight to create a variety of products including ozone and submicrometer aerosols" from that of the natural troposphere. While ozone concentrations in unpolluted tropospheric air vary between 20 and 50 ppb, levels as high as 700 ppb have been found in polluted urban areas. The urban atmosphere contains relatively high concentrations of a large number of alkanes, alkenes, and anthropogenic aromatic hydrocarbons compared to the natural troposphere [1-3,35-37,78].

For practical purposes, organic pollutants can be divided into 3 phases accoring to the different sampling techniques: a) the particulate phase; b) semi-volatile compounds with boiling points higher than 100° C and c) the gas phase consisting of smaller and more volatile compounds [1,3,5,10].

Natural Sources of Airborne Pollutants

The major natural sources of toxic airborne pollutants and some representative examples of toxicants released [10-12,33,34,70,71] include:
a) crustal rock and soil - trace and heavy metals (As, Se, Cd, Hg, Pb, Mn);
b) volcanic emissions - heavy metals, trace gases and aerosols containing sulphur and nitrogen oxides, carbon dioxide, PAHs;
c) fires (forest, biomass) - methane, nitrogen oxides, particulates, CO, carbon dioxide, methyl chloride, PAHs;
d) vegetation and soil erosion - methane, Se, Zn, PAHs;
e) swamps - hydrogen sulphide, VOCs.

Anthropogenic Sources of Airborne Pollutants

The major anthropogenic sources of toxic airborne pollutants and some representative examples of toxicants released [2,3,10-13] include:
a) industrial processes (manufacturing and commercial operations) - VOCs, PCBs, trace metals, industrial solvents;
b) pesticide and fertiliser manufacture and use - chlorinated hydrocarbons, nitrogen and phosphorus organic compounds, trace metals;
c) transportation (land, sea, air) - VOCs, PAHs, sulphur and nitrogen compounds, trace metals;
d) waste treatment and disposal - organic and inorganic compounds, trace metals;
e) combustion processes (fossil fuel, biomass, municipal and industrial waste) - heavy metals, trace elements, PAHs, PCDDs, PCDFs, carbon dioxide, sulphur and nitrogen oxides, particulates, methane and methyl chloride.

Combusion emission products represent one of the major and most widespread sources of atmospheric pollution from both industrialised and developing countries. These emissions are very complex mixtures arising from the incomplete burning of materials derived from fossil fuels, vegetative sources or mixtures of these materials (e.g., garbage, waste and coal). The emission mixture can consist of gases such as CO, carbon dioxide, sulphur and nitrogen oxides, hydrocarbons and aldehydes, semi-volatile organic compounds (e.g., 2-3-ring aromatics), PAHs, polar substituted PAHs and other polar organic compounds as well as condensed inorganic matter absorbed onto small, usually sub-micron carbonaceous particles (soot) or non-carbonaceous particles such as silica [1-3,10-13,33-37].

A measure of the extent of air pollutants which can result from the combustion of fossil fuels can be gleaned from recent airborne studies of the smoke from the more than 600 oil wells which were ignited in Kuwait in February 1991 during the Persian Gulf war [72]. With about 4.6 million barrels of oil burning per day, the emissions (in metric tons/day) of the following pollutants were:

sulphur dioxide: 2.0×10^4 (equivalent to 57% of emissions from U.S. electric utilities); carbon monoxide: 1.03×10^4 (equivalent to 0.1% worldwide emissions from all sources); carbon dioxide: 1.8×10^6 (equivalent to 2% of global emissions from fossil fuel and biomass burning); soot (elemental carbon): 0.34×10^4 (equivalent to 13 times the soot emissions from all U.S. combustion sources); particles (including soot): 1.2×10^4 (equivalent to 10% of global emissions from biomass burning). The smoke from these fires absorbed about 75% to 80% of the sun's radiation in regions of the Persian Gulf.

A recent preliminary toxic release chemical inventory compiled by the U.S. Environmental Protection Agency (EPA) disclosed that some 2.4 billion pounds (approx. 1 billion kg) of toxic air pollutants are released annually into America's air supply [79,80]. This figure is based on reports of only 55% to 75% of the total number of companies responding to the questionnaire. Even the total emission figure may be a small percentage of the total since it does not include the thousands of small companies that emit these chemicals but were not included in the inventory. The largest single source of chemical air emissions by more than 4-fold is the chemical industry which reported release of some 886.5 million pounds (369 million kg). Other major sources of air emissions were: primary metals (approx. 90 million kg), paper products (94 million kg), transport equipment (87 million kg) and rubber and plastics production (60 million kg). Other major contributing sources of the toxic chemical emissions included: fabricated metals, electrical and electronics equipment, petroleum and coals, machinery, furniture and fixtures, instruments, textiles, stone, clay and glass, lumber and wood, food, leather and apparel [79,80].

The above toxic release inventory included more than 320 chemical toxicants (carcinogens, mutagens, neurotoxins and other substances associated with serious health effects) listed in the Superfund Law (hazardous waste site substances). Sixty of the substances in the inventory are listed as carcinogens by the National Toxicology Program (NTP) of the U.S. Public Health Service [80]. The releases of the listed carcinogens were estimated to be approximately 98 million kg nationally and included (million kg) dichloromethane (methylene chloride), 46.7; benzene, 10.3; chloroform, 9.8; formaldehyde, 6.3; butadiene, 4.1 and carbon tetrachloride, 1.8. Neurotoxins on the list include a number of the most prevalent chemicals in the inventory (million kg): toluene, 98.2; xylenes, 50; methyl ethyl ketone, 53 and trichloroethylene, 198.8 [80].

While comparable European estimations are not available, it is at least possible to compare production figures for certain compounds in different parts of the world. Dichloromethane yearly production in the U.S. was 226,000 tons in 1983 and 270,000 tons in Europe in 1980 [81]. As about 80% of all dichloromethane produced ends up in the atmosphere, Europe and the U.S. contribute approximately equally to its dispersion in the environment. Worldwide production of benzene is estimated to be about 19 million tons annually, of which about half was produced in Europe [81].

It is broadly recognised that there are severe air, water, and soil pollution problems in central and eastern Europe (particularly in Poland, the former East Germany (DDR), Czechoslovakia, Romania and Bulgaria) and the former USSR, largely resulting from the reliance of these regions on hard and brown coal, lignite and the heavy concentration of chemical, mining and metallurgical operations coupled with inefficient transport for periods ranging from at least 40 to over 70 years [11,12,82-89]. For example, the almost exclusive reliance on low-grade high sulphur coals for residential heating and power generation has resulted in massive atmospheric pollution problems, especially in the former East Germany, the northern Bohemia region of Czechoslovakia and the Silesian industrial region of Poland. Sulphur dioxide emissions have been estimated at about 5.2 metric tons in East Germany and 3.9 million metric tons in Poland in 1988. On a per capita basis, emissions in East Germany were estimated at 313.3 kg compared with 24.2 kg in West Germany (FRG) [11]. Coal burning also produces large quantities of particulates. East Germany emitted between 5 and 6 million metric tons of particulates and Poland emitted nearly 3 million metric tons in 1985. In contrast, Sweden had estimated annual emissions of 40,000 metric tons of particulates in 1982-1984 [11]. Central and eastern Europe and the former USSR also emit significant amounts of other atmospheric toxicants including nitrogen oxides, carbon dioxide, ammonia, chlorine, fluorine, phenol, arsenic, lead, hydrogen sulphide and many VOCs [11].

Most vehicles in these regions operate on leaded petrol averaging 0.3 to 0.56 grams of lead/litre. Several countries in these regions have substantial numbers of outmoded and inefficient two-stroke engines that emit relatively high levels of hydrocarbons, particles and aldehydes [11]. The full dimensions of the atmospheric emissions and the scope of pollution are yet to be fully defined [11,12,82-93].

Greenhouse Gases

Much of the concern about the fate of the global environment is related to the increased concentration of greenhouse gases (carbon dioxide, methane, nitrous oxide, the chlorofluorocarbons (CFCs) and tropospheric ozone), the resultant "greenhouse effect" and the potential for global warming and subsequent health and environmental sequelae. The greenhouse gases are released into the atmosphere largely as a result of human activities and once released anywhere in the world are dispersed rapidly in the global atmosphere [3-5,11-13,33,34,44-60] (see also chapter 1).

Carbon Dioxide

Of the greenhouse gases, carbon dioxide is by far the most abundant and important, accounting for about half of the increase in the greenhouse effect and projected global warming. It is emitted into the atmosphere by both natural and anthropogenic sources. Because of its long lifetime in air, carbon dioxide is relatively well mixed throughout the atmosphere. Since the industrial revolution (about 1850), carbon dioxide concentrations have increased by 25% largely due to the combustion of fossil fuels and, to a lesser degree, deforestation. Present average global concentrations of carbon dioxide are about 350 ppm compared to approx. 265 ppm in 1850 [11,12,33,34,45-51,58].

The total annual emissions of carbon dioxide have reached almost 22 billion metric tons and the emissions have increased by 260% since 1950 (on a per capita basis, a disproportionate share of carbon dioxide is emitted by industrialised and oil-producing nations). While the per capita emissions in the U.S., for example, were 19.7 metric tons in 1989, the per capita emissions in China and India were 2.2 and 0.8 metric tons, respectively. The European Community with 340 million inhabitants accounts for 13% of the global carbon dioxide while the U.S. with 240 million people accounts for approx. 23% [11,12,44,45]. The U.S. is the largest emitter of carbon dioxide, followed by the former Soviet Union, China, Japan, Germany, and India. The countries of the OECD account for 47% of the global total; the former Soviet Union plus central Europe accounted for 23% of the total carbon dioxide emissions in 1989 [11]. Energy consumption patterns for the last 30 years project that combustion of fossil fuels will increase globally by 0.4% (1.70 ppm) to 2% (8.50 ppm) per year for the next 50 years and with this rate of increase carbon dioxide concentrations in the lower atmosphere will double to about 600 ppm within the next 50 to 60 years [58,94].

Trend analysis shows that carbon dioxide emissions have generally increased in the OECD region compared to 1971 levels. However, this growth has been slower in Europe (and even negative in some countries) than in Japan and North America. OECD as a whole has experienced slower growth than the world, primarily reflecting structural changes in energy demands and fuel substitution as well as economic structural changes [11,12].

Deforestation is the second most important source of atmospheric carbon dioxide, accounting for approx. 25% of total anthropogenic emissions [11,12,33,34]. Although deforestation has declined in Brazil in recent years, it accounts for 15% of carbon dioxide emissions and is the largest single country source. The countries of south and southwest Asia, however, account for fully 40% of carbon dioxide emissions from deforestation [11]. It has been estimated that the annual emissions from deforestation and land use changes are in the range of 1.6 billion tons of carbon per year, which is considerably smaller than the annual emissions of carbon dioxide from fossil fuel combustion (about 6 billion tons of carbon in 1987) [12]. Emissions of carbon dioxide from fossil-fuel burning, cement production and gas-flaring now account for 22,000 million tons per year [71,95]. Additional sources of atmospheric carbon dioxide are volcanoes [70,71]. Active volcanoes on land typically pump out carbon dioxide at rates of approx. 0.1-2 million tons/year with a median rate of approx. 1.3 million tons/year [71]. Mount Etna emits carbon dioxide at an astonishing rate of 25 million tons per year, which equals the amount of four 1,000 MW coal-fired power stations [71]. While the global rate of carbon dioxide emissions from sub-aerial and submarine volcanoes is uncertain, a conservative estimate of 130-175 million tons a year has been made [71]. The major reservoirs for carbon are the atmosphere, the oceans, the terrestrial biosphere including soils and reserves of fossil fuels, although there is considerable uncertainty about reservoir sizes and transfers [4,5,11,12,44,45,96].

Methane

Methane plays an important role in atmospheric chemistry by influencing both the ozone concentration and the infrared radiative flux. Levels of methane, one of the fastest growing of the greenhouse gases, have risen dramatically in recent years and are currently increasing by about 1% each year [4,5,50,51,96,97]. The concentration of methane has doubled over the past 200 years, increasing from 750 ppbv to about 1700 ppbv [97]. While the annual rate of increase of methane has slowed down from 20 ppb in the late 1970s to the current rate of about 10 ppb, the absolute level of methane continues to rise [51].
The globally averaged concentration of methane increased from 1559 ppbv in September 1980 to 1685 ppbv in September 1988. This amounts to an additional 280 million metric tons of methane in the atmosphere during that period [98]. The total mass of methane in the atmosphere undergoes seasonal variations, with highest levels occurring during late fall and early winters of the Northern Hemisphere and lowest in the summers [98].
On a global scale, the annual flux of methane is estimated to be 400-600 Tg (1 Tg = 10^{12} g) [98]. Methane is emitted into the atmosphere from both natural and human activities. More than half of the methane released into the atmosphere originates from the action of anaerobic bacteria on plant material, in rice paddies and wetlands of all types in all latitudes and the stomachs of ruminants such as sheep and cattle. Methane is also released from the incomplete combustion of vegetation in forest, range or biomass fires or when land is cleared for agriculture. Additionally, methane is released from coal mines, leaks in natural pipelines, leaks of natural gas associated with oil production and decomposition of organic matter in landfills [4,5,11,50,51,96,97]. Altogether, these sources emit about 545 million metric tons/year [97].
Overall, China emits the most methane at 40 million metric tons, followed by the U.S. (37 million tons), India (36 million tons) and the former USSR (34 million tons) [11]. Animal husbandry is the largest source of anthropogenic emissions of methane with India, which has the largest number of cattle, emitting almost 14% of the global lifestock total. Wet rice agriculture is another major source of methane with India and China each emitting 26% of the methane attributable to this source. The former USSR is the largest emitter of methane from gas production and transmission (35%) and is second (19%) only to China (33%) in methane emissions from coal production. Methane is also emitted from solid waste disposal and large and populous countries are the major emitters, e.g., the U.S. leads with 37%, and the former USSR is the next largest emitter from this source [11].
Methane has an atmospheric lifetime of about 9 years and its primary sink is the reaction with hydroxyl radicals in the troposphere to produce primarily carbon dioxide and water through a series of steps, some involving the nitric oxide radical (NO°) and others carbon monoxide [50,51,97]. Approximately 50±20 million metric tons of methane escape to the stratosphere and 30±15 million metric tons are taken up by soil microbes, leaving 45±5 million metric tons as an annual addition to the troposphere [97]. Methane acts to increase ozone in the troposphere and lower

stratosphere. Its cumulative greenhouse effect is currently believed to be one-third that of carbon dioxide but on a molecule-by-molecule basis, its effect, ignoring any feedback or involvement in any atmospheric processes, is 20-30 times that of carbon dioxide [11].

Nitrous Oxide

Emissions of nitric oxide (N_2O) into the atmosphere are primarily due to microbial processes in soil and water and are part of the nitrogen cycle. Anthropogenic sources of nitrous oxide include combustion of fossil fuels (primarily from power plants) and biomass, as well as increased use of fertilisers [4,5,11,12, 46,97,101-105]. However, there is considerable uncertainty concerning the magnitude of nitrous oxide emissions from the combustion of fossil fuels such as oil, natural gas and coal, as well as wood and peat [11,100].

The concentration of nitrous oxide in the atmosphere is currently increasing at the rate of about 0.3% (0.060 ppb) per year, probably due to human activities [11,97,100,103]. The pre-industrial concentration of nitrous oxide in air was estimated to be 280 ppb contrasted to 306 ppb (which is about one-thousandth that of carbon dioxide) in 1989 [11]. This results from the emission of 5 million tons of nitrous oxide per year into the atmosphere. Based on an atmospheric residence time of over 100 years, the present imbalance of nitrous oxide sources and sinks is about 25% [100]. The only known atmospheric sink for nitrous oxide is its breakdown to nitric oxide in the stratosphere by ultraviolet light [4,5]. Nitrous oxide is an important depletor of stratospheric ozone. Present levels may contribute one-twelfth the amount contributed by carbon dioxide toward the greenhouse effect [11]. It has been suggested that doubling of the present nitrous oxide concentration would effect a 12% decrease in total ozone. It should be noted that the concentration of nitrous oxide is growing much faster in the Northern Hemisphere than in the Southern Hemisphere [97]. Anthropogenic sources now contribute about half as much nitrous oxide to the atmosphere each year as that contributed by natural sources [97,103,104]. Future emissions of nitrous oxide are expected to increase principally in industrialised countries as a result of increased use of catalytic convertors on automobiles and possibly of an increased use of fluidised beds in coal combustion [102,103]. Concentrations of nitrous oxide of 320-330 ppb were suggested to be likely by the year 2000 [46], regardless of which anthropogenic source is assumed to be growing.

Chlorofluorocarbons

Chlorofluorocarbons (CFCs) were first discovered in 1930 and the demand for these agents grew dramatically from 1946 through the mid 1970s due to their broad utility as aerosol propellants, blowing agents, solvents, refrigerants and for air conditioning [3-5,11,12,44,46,50,106]. Most of the world's CFCs are produced and consumed in the Northern Hemisphere. The U.S. is the world's largest producer and consumer of CFCs. The major chlorofluorocarbons, often referred to popularly by their trade names of "Freons", are: fluorotrichloromethane (CFC-11); dichlorodifluoromethane (CFC-12); 1,1,2-trichloro-1,2,2-trifluoroethane (CFC-13); 1,2-dichloro-1,1,2,2-tetrafluoroethane (CFC-14) and 2-chloro-1,1,1,2,2-pentafluoroethane (CFC-15) [4,5,11,12,46,50,106].

The worldwide CFC output in 1991 was 680,000 metric tons (60% of the 1986 level of 1.13 million metric tons) and the major use categories were: refrigeration and air conditioning, 33%; foam blowing, 27%; solvents, 19% and aerosols, 18% [107]. Outside of North America, a significant amount ($>1.5 \times 10^8$ kg) of CFCs have continued to be used as aerosol propellants although that application was essentially banned in the U.S. in 1978 [106].

The United States, European Community and Australia consume most CFCs, with an estimated per capita consumption in the U.S. alone of approx. 0.82 kg of CFC-11 and CFC-12 compared to Japanese consumption of approx. 0.5 kg per capita of CFC-11 and CFC-12. Because of their chemical stability, the CFCs do not decompose in the troposphere but rise to the stratosphere where ultraviolet radiation catalyses the release of chlorine atoms that destroy ozone [5,11,12, 38-51,108].

CFC-11 and CFC-12 were first measured in the atmosphere in 1971 and 1973, respectively [46]. In 1981, there were about 6.0×10^9 kg of CFC-12 in the atmosphere together with 5.0×10^9 kg of CFC-11. At 1981 release rates, these amounts represent the cumulative results of 15-20 years of global emissions. Atmospheric concentrations of these CFCs were observed to have increased by about 6% per year during the period 1978-1981. In the early 1970s, the annual emissions of the CFCs were a larger fraction of the amounts already in the atmosphere. Larger percentage annual increases were noted along with considerably more CFCs in the Northern Hemisphere than in the Southern Hemisphere. It should be noted that while most of the release of the CFCs continues to be in the Northern Hemisphere [4,5,11,12,46,50], the hemispheric difference has decreased to less than 10% [46].

Since the late 1970s, the non-propellant uses of CFCs have continued to increase by about 4% a year, while the propellant use decreased from 56% to 34% of total CFC production [12]. At the beginning of the 1980s, the atmospheric concentrations of CFC-11 and CFC-12 were increasing at about 6% per year [11,12,50]. Atmospheric concentrations of CFCs and halocarbons are rising faster than those of most greenhouse gases because their annual rate of release has been increasing in recent years [11,12,46,50]. In 1989, an estimated 580,000 metric tons of CFCs were emitted, with the U.S. (22%) and Japan (16%) as the principal users and emitters of these gases [11]. The atmospheric concentration of CFC-11 and CFC-12 in 1989 was 0.28 ppb and 0.47 ppb, respectively, with a present annual increase rate for CFC-11 of 0.010 ppb (3.4%) and for CFC-12 of 0.025 ppb (5.3%) [11]. The concentration of CFC-113, which is used extensively as a solvent for cleaning electronic microcircuits, is soaring at an annual rate of 11% [50].

An International Convention for the Protection of the Ozone Layer was drawn up in 1985 and a Montreal Protocol was signed by 36 nations in 1987 which stipulated a 50% reduction in CFC production by 1999. A subsequent London meeting in June 1990 led to a revision of the Montreal Protocol, pledging the elimination of CFC production by 2000 and also that of methyl chloroform by 2005 and carbon tetrachloride by 2000. Hydrogen-based CFCs (HCFCs) (Halons) would be restricted to applications where less ozone-destructive alternatives are not available and phased out by 2040 at the latest and developing countries were granted a 10-year grace period [11,12]. E.I. Du Pont de Nemours Co, the world's largest manufacturer of CFCs, said that it would phase out CFC sales to industrialised countries by 1996 and Halon sales by 1994.

Even if future release rates of the CFCs remained at present levels, their atmospheric concentrations would increase since the CFCs take roughly 10 years to reach the stratosphere and some CFCs have estimated atmospheric lifetimes in the tens to hundreds of years [5,46,50,51,109]. The major CFCs are believed to contribute approx. 15-24% to global warming [11,12,49,110].

Two additional greenhouse gases, CF_4 (CFC-14) and C_2F_6 (CFC-116), which arise from the primary smelting of aluminium, have recently been reported [111]. These gases have atmospheric residence in excess of 10,000 years. Of the chlorofluorocarbons, the radiative forcing of CF_4 and C_2F_6 during the 1980s was exceeded only by CFC-11,-12, 113 and HCFC-22. Global emission rates of 28,000 tonnes per year for CF_4 and 3,200 tonnes for C_2F_6 in 1987 have been reported [112], which suggests global average emission factors of about 1.6 kg CF_4 and 0.2 kg C_2F_6 per tonne of primary aluminium production [112]. Lashof and Ahuja [113] estimated that CF_4 was responsible for 1.7% of the total warming potential of all global anthropogenic greenhouse gas emissions in 1986.

Other Halocarbons

Other halocarbons such as methyl chloroform and the Halons are also considered as greenhouse gases although their contribution is considered minor compared to the CFCs; their atmospheric levels are, however, increasing rapidly [3,5,11,12,44,46,50,106,109]. These halocarbons include carbon tetrachloride, which is used in the production of CFC-11 and CFC-12 and had earlier extensive use as a solvent for cleaning sheet metal, as a solvent for paints and adhesives and as a cleaning agent in the electronics industry; and the fire retardants CF_3Br (Halon-1301) and CF_2BrCl (Halon-1211). The major CFCs are believed to contribute approx. 15-24% to global warming [11,12,49,110].

In the Northern Hemisphere, the "background" concentration of methyl chloroform was 158 ppt in 1985 and has been increasing at a rate of 8 ppt per year [114]. In southern California (Los Angeles urban area), some 13,000 tons of methyl chloroform are released every year. Methyl chloroform levels averaging 28 ppt have been recorded at 21 southern Californian locations during the period 1987-1990 [114].

Methyl chloroform has a much shorter lifetime (about 6.5 years) than the fully halogenated gases. Although halocarbons that have hydrogen atoms can be consumed in the troposphere by hydroxyl radicals, there are currently 130 ppt of methyl chloroform in the atmosphere and it is increasing at a rate of about 7% per year. Carbon tetrachloride, with a lifetime of about 50 years, has an atmospheric concentration of about 125 ppt that is growing at an annual rate of about 1% [4]. These halocarbons contribute to the destruction of the ozone layer and to greenhouse warming [4,5,11,12,46,50].

Even with the projected phase-out of the CFCs by the late 1990s, the stratospheric concentrations of chlorine will continue to grow. By the year 2010, chlorine concentrations are projected to be about 3 times as large as the current level of about 3 ppt, largely due to the projected increase in the use of carbon tetrachloride and methyl chloroform [113].

Since the signing of the Montreal Protocol, curtailing and eventually banning the production of chemicals that can destroy stratospheric ozone, many new compounds have been proposed as substitutes for the regulated compounds. Bromocarbons (Halons), for example CF_3Br and CF_2ClBr, which are used as fire-extinguishing agents, are major anthropogenic sources of stratospheric Br and will have to be eventually replaced. Among the proposed substitutes for the Halons is CHF_2Br, which has good fire-suppression characteristics and a calculated atmospheric lifetime of approx. 7 years, which is shorter by approx. factors of 10 and 2 than those for CF_3Br and CF_2ClBr, respectively [58,115,116].

Ozone - Natural and Anthropogenic Sources

Ozone is continuously being produced in the stratosphere by solar ultraviolet radiation. Radiation at wavelengths less than 242 nm dissociates molecular oxygen into atoms that attach themselves to O_2 to form ozone as shown:

$O_2 + h\nu \rightarrow 2O$ (a)

$O + O_2 + M \rightarrow O_3 + M$ (b)

where M represents another molecule of oxygen or nitrogen that is unchanged in the reaction [3-5,39,58]. At lower altitudes (lower than approx. 20 km), where only radiation with wavelengths greater than 280 nm is present, the only significant oxygen atom production is from photo-dissociation of nitrogen dioxide:

$NO_2 + h\nu \rightarrow NO + O$ (c).

The nitric oxide produced in this reaction reacts rapidly with ozone to regenerate NO_2:

$NO + O_3 \rightarrow NO_2 + O$ (d).

Reactions (b-d) occur rapidly, establing a steady state ozone concentration [3-5].

Ozone has been implicated, to varying degrees and under specified atmospheric conditions, to the chemical and physical processes in ambient air that produce such particulate and aerosol-related phenomena as acid precipitation and deposition, atmospheric visibility reduction and climate modification [2-5,11,12,39,58,117]. Ozone is a highly reactive gas and a strong oxidant that reacts rapidly and selectively with many organic compounds.

Ozone, the main component of photochemical smog, is principally formed in the troposphere through a series of complex photochemical reactions involving nitrogen oxides, carbon monoxide and reactive hydrocarbons produced by combustion of fossil fuels, vehicular emissions as well as a variety of anthropogenic and biogenic volatile organic compounds (VOCs) [2-5,11,12,58,117-119]. Tropospheric ozone is also a greenhouse gas as it absorbs infrared radiation near 9.6 μm [119].

The maximum ozone concentration that can be reached in polluted atmospheres appears to depend not only on the absolute concentrations of volatile organic compounds and nitrogen dioxides but also on their ratio. Conditions are favourable for the formation of appreciable levels of ozone at intermediate ratios of 4:1 to 10:1 [2,3,118]. There are no significant anthropogenic emissions of ozone *per se* into the atmosphere [2]. The concentration of ozone, a priority pollutant, is used to assess regional air quality [2,5,11,12] (see also chapter 1).

With respect to source emissions of ozone, there remains substantial uncertainty concerning the effect of naturally occurring (biogenic) organic precursor emissions on rural ozone concentration [120]. Biogenic organic species, mostly isoprene and several monoterpenes, are emitted by many types of forest trees and cultivated plants. There are seasonal and geographical differences between the biogenic organic emission rates. Isoprene can contribute as much as 50% of the overall reactivity of rural air even though its concentration is as low as 6% of the ambient hydrocarbon level [121]. These species (isoprene and monoterpenes) are rapidly oxidised into a number of intermediate species such as methyl vinyl ketone, methyl glyoxal and formaldehyde which are also highly reactive [120,121].

The concentrations of ozone range from a few parts-per-billion by volume to approx. 50 ppb in unpolluted air to more than 100 ppbv in areas polluted by industrial activity or burning biomass [2-5,11,12,33,34,58,117]. In polluted air, ozone concentrations have reached levels as high as 400 ppbv [58]. Photochemical ozone formation was first observed in Los Angeles in the 1940s and subsequently in other cities in the U.S. and Europe [2,11,12]. Current levels of ozone in North America and Europe frequently exceed WHO ceilings for both short-term and long-term ozone concentrations by a wide margin on a large scale [2,11,12]. During the summer, elevated ozone levels are common over most of Europe and North America for days at a time [12,122]. The problem is not restricted to urban areas, as there is increasing evidence that background levels of ozone are increasing over North America and Europe as a result of progressive increases in the levels of nitrogen dioxide and VOCs, the precursors of ozone.

The atmospheric concentration of ozone ranges from 0.02-10 ppm (volume), with an atmospheric lifetime of less than a few hours. However, the lifetime of O_X (ozone and oxygen atoms) depends strongly on location, varying from about an hour in the upper stratosphere to months in the lower stratosphere to hours to days in the troposphere [2-5,39,123,124]. Seasonal variations in ozone concentration occur which are caused principally by changes in meteorological processes, while diurnal patterns of ozone vary according to location, depending on the balance of factors affecting ozone formation, transport and decomposition [2,5]. Long-range transport of ozone and/or its precursors from upwind source areas or from a tropospheric origin is responsible when elevated ozone concentrations have been measured in rural areas having insignificant local sources of ozone precursors [2]. Long-range transport of ozone between urban areas has become increasingly evident [120].

There is good evidence to suggest that surface ozone has been increasing throughout much of the Northern Hemisphere (about 0.1 to 0.3% per year) over the past century in some locations [117,119]. More recently, dry-season ozone concentrations may be increasing in the tropics because of widespread biomass burning [33,34,117].

Increases in ozone concentration are believed to principally result from the increased global precursor methane since preindustrial time. Photochemical models suggest that increasing methane and carbon dioxide concentration could account for a doubling of tropospheric ozone since 1800. Continued growth in emissions of methane, NO, CO and hydrocarbons will tend to increase tropospheric ozone [117]. The sources of these precursors are varied and include power plants, vehicles, residential and small business emissions of solvents, paints, etc. Natural VOC sources such as trees can also contribute elevated ozone levels, particularly when vehicle exhausts keep NOx levels high [11,12].

Several model studies have been conducted to estimate the effects of ozone depletion on tropospheric ozone. The effect of increased penetration of u.v. radiation into the troposphere is to increase ozone formation in urban areas. However, on a global basis, lower tropospheric ozone concentrations are expected to result from stratospheric ozone depletion [117].

Stratospheric Ozone Depletion

Ozone exhibits a critical role in preserving global ecological balance due to its strong absorption of biologically damaging incoming ultraviolet light. Ozone exists in a dynamic equilibrium between its formation by solar ultraviolet photolysis (at wavelengths greater than 242 nm) of molecular oxygen ($O + O_2 \rightarrow O_3$) and destruction by a number of chemical processes including several chain sequences triggered by HOx, NOx and ClOx radicals and bromine oxide [4,5,11,12,38-51,106-108,119,125,126]. The ozone concentration peaks in the stratosphere at an altitude of 20-25 km. The transport of ozone is driven by the variable wind fields of the stratosphere, seasonal variations and intra-annual variability in ozone amounts.

It has been recognised from the early 1970s that chlorine could destroy stratospheric ozone [126] and that the broad and escalating use of the CFCs led to a pronounced increase in the stratospheric chlorine content [125,126]. Indeed, the observed rates of systematic increase of the CFCs, particularly $CFCl_3$ (CFC-11) and CF_2Cl_2 (CFC-12) in the atmosphere have been shown to be consistent with their known global anthropogenic production rates [46,125].

The natural concentration of the chlorine family is fairly low, around 0.7 ppb, largely due to the oceanic release of methyl chloride. By the early 1980s, the chlorine content of the stratosphere had risen to about 2.5 ppb [45,125] and in 1990 it was considered to be about 3 ppb. It is now well established that human activities represent the only source of the CFCs and their destruction occurs uniquely in the stratosphere. These extremely stable compounds may survive 50-100 years in the atmosphere. In only a few years, winds throughout the troposphere uniformly distribute CFC molecules released from a single point source and over the decades the molecules eventually reach the middle stratosphere (about 25 km or higher), where ultraviolet from the sun tears them apart. The fragments of the photodissociation of the CFC molecules augment the chlorine family concentrations [4,5,11,12,38-51,106-108,119,125,126].

As generally proposed by Molina and Rowland [108], the most important sink for atmospheric $CFCl_3$ (CFC-11) and CF_2Cl_2 (CFC-12) appeared to be the photolytic dissociation to $CFCl_2 + Cl$ and $CF_2Cl + Cl$, respectively, at altitudes of 20-40 km; each of the reactions creates 2 odd-electron species: one chlorine atom and one free radical. The extensive catalytic chain reaction leading to the net destruction of ozone and O occurs in the stratosphere according to this overall sequence [3-5,125,126]:

$CF_2Cl_2 + h\nu \rightarrow CF_2Cl + Cl$
$CFCl_3 + h\nu \rightarrow CFCl_2 + Cl.$

The odd nitrogen and hydrogen radicals and atomic chlorine participate in catalytic cycles that destroy the ozone such as the following:

$Cl + O_3 \rightarrow ClO + O_2$ (1)
$ClO + O \rightarrow Cl + O_2$

$O_3 + O \rightarrow 2O_2$ (net)
$NO + O_3 \rightarrow NO + O_2$ (2)
$NO_2 + O \rightarrow NO + O_2$

$O_3 + O \rightarrow 2O_2$ (net)
$OH + O_3 \rightarrow HO_2 + O_2$ (3)
$HO_2 + O \rightarrow OH + O_2$

$O_3 + O \rightarrow 2O_2$ (net).

Since the atomic oxygen that reacts in the second reaction in each of the above cycles otherwise would have formed ozone, the net effect of each cycle is the destruction of 2 ozone molecules [4,125,126].

An increasing number of studies during the last several years have confirmed earlier observations in 1985 [126], that human activities, particularly the extensive use of the

CFCs, could modify the total column amount of ozone in the lower stratosphere [5,11,38-43,125] (see also chapter 1). Precipitous ozone depletion has been shown most dramatically in studies commencing in 1985, that originally revealed changes in Antarctic ozone, now widely referred to as the "ozone hole". In the 4 subsequent years, ozone layers have continued to drop such that in 1989, 70% of the total column ozone content over the Antarctic (10% of the area of the Southern Hemisphere) was lost during the months of September and early October. This precipitous loss of 3% of the world's ozone in a period of just 6 weeks graphically illustrates how rapidly global-scale changes can occur [38].

The size of the "ozone hole" over the Antarctic and the amount of depletion vary from year to year, depending on the temperature and polar wind conditions. When the polar vortex (the strong atmospheric circulation centered over the polar area) is undisturbed and temperatures are especially cold, a larger decrease occurs. An important reason for concern about the Antarctic ozone hole is that processes that appear to be significant in the polar environment could be important at other latitudes and contribute to a global ozone reduction [12].

More recent studies have revealed additional substantial "ozone holes" over the Arctic as well as in the middle and high altitudes of the Northern Hemisphere covering Europe, almost all of the populated North America, the former Soviet Union, northern China, Japan and the Koreas [40,125,127,128], suggesting that the process of ozone depletion could contribute to a global ozone reduction. In the Northern Hemisphere there is evidence of a 5-8% decrease in total ozone, with the largest depletions in the highest latitudes and during winter and spring [129]. Estimates in 1991 suggest that about 3% of the stratospheric ozone has been depleted over the United States and other temperate countries which could result in an increase of 6% u.v. radiation striking the earth's surface [12]. Other recent projections suggested that northern mid-latitudes were losing ozone at the rate of about 4% to 5% per decade and globally ozone is decreasing at a rate of 2.3% a decade [127].

Recent findings reported by Stolarski and coworkers [39] based on both ground-based and satellite measurements established that there has been an apparent downward trend in the total column amount of ozone over mid-latitude areas of the Northern Hemisphere in all seasons. Decreases in ozone are occurring in the lower stratosphere in the region of the highest ozone concentration (below 25 km) and are suggested to amount to about 10% per decade [39].

It should be noted that record high amounts (exceeding 1.5 ppb) of chlorine monoxide radical were measured over Canada, northern New England in the U.S. and northern Europe in January, 1992 [128].

Numerous mechanistic studies have been reported illustrating the progress towards a quantitative understanding of Antarctic ozone depletion [38,39,41-43]. The causal link between surface release of CFCs and the massive loss of ozone in the Southern Hemisphere has been established by Anderson and coworkers [38], who utilised 3 lines of evidence. They observed containment in the vortex of ClO concentrations 2 orders of magnitude greater than normal and, utilising *in situ* observations obtained during high altitude flights, showed a decrease in ozone concentrations as ClO concentrations were increasing. Additionally, a comparison was made between observed ozone loss rates and those predicted with the use of absolute concentrations of ClO and BrO, the rate limiting radicals in an array of proposed catalytic cycles.

Recent studies have suggested that polar stratospheric clouds (PSCs) play a key role in the formation of the Antarctic ozone holes [38,39,41,42,130]. The frequency of PSCs is higher in the Antarctic stratosphere than anywhere else in the stratosphere. The presence of PSCs implied that chemical reactions taking place on the ice particles in the clouds freed chlorine from the CFC reservoirs [42,130]. The PSCs were also suggested to serve as a nitrogen sink and hence they would consist of a frozen form of nitric acid (nitric acid hydrate) [41]. Overall, PSCs are suggested to initiate chemical reactions that free molecular chlorine from the reservoirs. The ClO-ClO catalytic cycle begins once sunlight breaks Cl_2 apart. The chlorine atoms react with ozone forming ClO and oxygen; ClO forms its dimer (Cl_2O_2) which is quickly broken by sunlight to Cl and O_2; chlorine then attacks ozone again. PSCs also prevent reservoirs from forming by removing nitrogen from the atmosphere through the precipitation of nitric acid.

It has also been recently suggested that the recent Mt. Pinatubo eruption might intensify ozone depletion as a consequence of the initial large amounts of sulphur dioxide spewed into the stratosphere where it was subsequently transformed into a sulphate aerosol which is projected to remain in the stratosphere for 2-3 years. Sulphate aerosols furnish sites for chemical reactions that release chlorine atoms from CFCs and other halocarbons in the stratosphere. The eruption is projected to cause a possible 15 to 25% loss of ozone at high latitudes and a decrease in ozone in the tropics [11,69].

Reductions of Antarctic ozone due to synergistic actions of chlorine and bromine have also been proposed [41,129,131,132]. As noted earlier, the CFCs have been linked to the destruction of stratospheric ozone and are being phased out in accordance to the Montreal Protocol agreements. Many substitutes have been proposed, with the principal candidates being either hydrochlorofluorocarbons (HCFCs) or hydrofluorocarbons (HFCs) [58,106,132,133]. Recent studies have focused on computer model calculations of the relative effects of a number of the proposed HCFC and HFC replacements on their ozone depletion potential (ODP) [43,132-134,135] and their global warming potential [133]. Fisher et al. [132] reported that a significant fraction of the hydrohalocarbons are destroyed in the troposphere by reaction with the hydroxyl radical so that they deliver substantially less chlorine to the stratosphere per kilogram used and have shorter atmospheric lifetimes than the chemically inert CFCs and thus they have less ozone depletion potential (ODP) by an order of magnitude. However, these estimates were challenged by Solomon and Tuck [134], who suggested that the globally averaged ODP estimates provided by Fisher et al. [132] were probably lower limits.

Additional tropospheric lifetime studies and preliminary ozone depletion evaluations of 3 possible replacements of the CFCs and the Halons have been reported [136]. Halons 1201 (CF_2BrH) and 2401 ($CF_3CCFBrH$) are being considered as substitutes for CF_2Br and CF_2ClBr in fire extinguishers (which use is being phased out because of their ozone depletion potential) [116]. Halon 1201 has a calculated atmospheric lifetime of approx. 7 years which is shorter by approx. factors of 10 and 2 than those for CF_3Br and CF_2ClBr, respectively [116].

Greenhouse Effect and Global Warming

The greenhouse effect can be described as the reduction of the long-wave radiation to space as a result of the intervening atmosphere. Global warming is the consequence of the greenhouse effect since an increase in the concentration of greenhouse gases (carbon dioxide, methane, nitrous oxide and the chlorofluorocarbons) tends to warm the earth's surface by increasing the amount of heat that is trapped in the lowest part of the atmosphere [4,5,11,12,44-58,111,113,133, 139]. The greenhouse effect is a consequence of many interconnected and complex activities as well as naturally occurring events [11,12,45-59] (see also chapter 1). Despite all the recent controversy that surrounds the term, the greenhouse effect is one of the most well established theories in atmospheric science [47-51,58,145, 146]. What is controversial about the greenhouse effect is exactly how much the earth's surface temperature will rise given the increases in the greenhouse gases, particularly carbon dioxide, over a particular period of time; what are the projected consequences, i.e., changes in sea level, agriculture and forestry [11,12,45-59,113,137-142] and to what extent do the atmospheric, ocean and biosphere feedbacks impact on the greenhouse effects [49-51,137-148].

Human activities are affecting the composition of the global atmosphere in a major way and, as noted earlier, since the industrial revolution carbon dioxide concentrations have increased by 25% [11,12,45,49], largely due to the combustion of fossil fuels. The rapid rate of land use changes and deforestation that accompany human population growth especially in the tropics, is contributing to the further release of greenhouse gases.

The relative contributions of greenhouse gases to global warming in 1985 showed that carbon dioxide was by far the largest contributor (71.5%) and in decreasing order the other contributors were: CFCs, 9.5%, methane, 9.2%, carbon monoxide, 6.6% and nitrous oxide, 3.1% [113]. The contributions from each of the anthropogenic derived greenhouse gases to the changes in radiative forcing from 1980 to 1990 were as follows: carbon dioxide, 55%, CFC-11 and CFC-12, 17%, other CFCs, 7%, methane, 15%, and nitrous oxide, 6% [131,145].

Many investigators have noted that the combined effect on climate of increases in the concentrations of a number of trace gases, principally methane, nitrous oxide and the CFCs, could rival or even exceed that of the increasing concentration of carbon dioxide [113]. Although these trace gases are present at concentrations that are 2-6 orders of magnitude lower than carbon dioxide, they absorb infrared radiation much more strongly than carbon dioxide. An index of global warming potential for methane, carbon monoxide, nitrous oxide and the CFCs relative to that of carbon dioxide was recently proposed by Ahuja [113]. Methane has per mole a global warming potential 3.7 times that of carbon dioxide while CFC-11 and CFC-12 have 4,000 and 10,000 times, respectively, the global warming potential of carbon dioxide.

The global contribution to annual net emissions shows that the U.S. is the largest contributor at 18%, followed by OECD Europe, 12%, the former Soviet Union, 3% and the rest of the world, 34%. This index was based on annual emission of the 3 major greenhouse gases, carbon dioxide, CFCs and methane, and the heat trapping potential for each gas. The carbon dioxide emissions were net emissions since they take into account the effect of deforestation on the carbon dioxide flux into the atmosphere [11,12].

While our knowledge of greenhouse gases emitted by industrial, energy, agriculture and deforestation sources is fairly well documented, in contrast, our knowledge of the production rates of these gases produced through biological processes and the factors regulating emissions is still inadequate [11,12,49].

Rough estimates could be made for the percent of global warming between 1980 and 2030 arising from each of the greenhouse gases and both anthropogenic and natural source emission sectors [11,12]. The following conclusions could be drawn: a) if current trends were to continue, carbon dioxide would continue to contribute roughly half of the global warming over the next 40 years; b) in regard to the various sectors of human source emitters, energy use contributes about half of the greenhouse effect, deforestation and agriculture together contribute about 25% and industry the remaining 25%. This latter assumption depends on the belief that current trends of CFC emissions would continue. However, full implementation of the Montreal Protocol would reduce the CFC contributions to global warming by half of the projected value by 2030 [11,12].

Critical to an assessment of the greenhouse threat is the need to better resolve uncertainties in climate models that deal with atmospheric, ocean and biosphere feedbacks [5,51,138-151]. The greenhouse effect (a climate forcing by either human activities or natural sources) is in competition with other mechanisms for climate change. The natural forcings that appear to be the most significant based on systemic comparison of radiative effects, are changes of stratospheric aerosols arising from large volcanic eruptions (e.g., Mt. Pinatubo) and changes of solar irradiance [11,12,150]. For example, the massive eruption of Mt. Pinatubo in the Philippines in June, 1991, spewed an immense volume of ash and sulphur dioxide into the stratosphere that could have a significant short-term impact on the earth's atmosphere. The sulphur dioxide gas turns into an aerosol of sulphuric acid causing a haze which can reflect and scatter sunlight which could ultimately effect the lowering of the average global temperature by more than 0.3° C for 3 or 4 years, enough to temporarily mask global warming [11,69]. Additionally, emissions from the burning of up to 5 billion tons of plant material produces smoke and aerosols in the atmosphere which help block the sunlight from reaching the earth's surface. About half of the smoke is believed to result from the use of wood for fuel, burning agricultural wastes and slash-and-burn techniques of clearing forests [33,34,142], the rest comes from natural fires in grasslands and forests [142].

Additional feedbacks could result from stratospheric ozone depletion caused by the CFCs [152]. Studies by Ramaswamy et al. [152] suggest that a significant negative radiative forcing results from ozone losses in the middle to high latitudes in contrast to the positive forcing at all latitudes caused by the CFCs and other gases. Decreases in ozone which absorbs sunlight have led to lower temperatures in the stratosphere which leads to cooling in the troposphere. Averaged over the entire earth, the cooling from ozone loss almost completely offsets the calculated greenhouse warming from CFCs. At higher altitudes where ozone depletion is greatest, the cooling may even exceed the CFC warming effect [152].

The climate change that results from a change in the climate forcing depends on many feedback processes in the climate system, many of which, such as changes of clouds, water vapour, ice, and snow cover are complex and not well understood [50,51,137-142,150,151]. The single largest uncertainty in climate models appears to be the behaviour of clouds as the world warms [137,138].

There have been numerous model projections of the emissions and the resultant atmospheric concentrations of greenhouse gases during the remainder of this century and the next century and the resultant consequences for global surface temperature [11,12,47-53] (see also chapter 1). These predictions range from relatively modest to "catastrophic". For example, it is estimated that doubling the concentrations of carbon dioxide in the atmosphere could lead to an eventual global warming anywhere in the range of 1.5° C and 5.5° C [11,12,45,50,51,153,154].

The consequences of climatic change and the rate of change include a broad spectrum of effects on sea level, agriculture, forestry, the energy sector, etc. It is widely acknowledged that these changes are extremely difficult to predict with any reliability and are thus greatly dependent on the refinements of atmospheric mechanisms and models [11,12,48-53,56,59,137,150-152] (see also chapter 1). A new set of greenhouse gas emission scenarios has been recently produced by the Intergovernmental Panel on Climate Change (IPCC) [137], with as the main concern their effect on climate and sea level. The new scenarios differ from each other because they make different assumptions regarding population growth, economic growth, technological developments, resource limitations, fuel mixes, agricultural development, etc. The models also include the effects of carbon dioxide fertilisation feedback from stratospheric ozone depletion and the radiative effects of sulphate aerosols. Changes in temperature and sea level are predicted to be less severe than those estimated previously, but are still far beyond the limits of natural variability. Plausible estimates of the increase in surface temperatures between now and some points in the future (to the year 2100) lie within a range whose upper limit is 3 times greater than the lower, but with likely greenhouse emissions, both the lower and upper limits are positive [137].

Sulphur Oxides

Sulphur oxides (sulphur dioxide, acid aerosols resulting from oxidation in the atmosphere and sulphur dioxide plus particulate matter) are largely derived from human activities primarily involving stationary sources (the combustion of fossil fuels in energy production, and to a lesser degree ore smelting and industrial boilers) [2-5,7,11,12,155-159] and are major air pollutants in urban areas worldwide [2-5,7,11,12,155-158]. They contribute not only to local and urban air pollution but also to a much broader scale of pollution through long-distance atmospheric transport [2-5,11,12,156] (see also chapter 1).

Additionally, natural sources such as volcanoes can also contribute substantial levels of ash and sulphur oxide to the global atmosphere [2,4,5,11,12,69]. The Mt. Pinatubo eruption emitted 18 million metric tons of sulphur dioxide into the stratosphere, about twice the amount emitted by the eruption of El Chichon volcano in Mexico in 1982 (at that time the largest eruption in 50 years) and almost as much as the entire sulphur dioxide emissions in the U.S. in one year [11,12].

The combined population of the OECD countries, 849 million, which represents 16% of the world's population, released 40% of the global sulphur oxide emissions in 1989 [11,12]. Trend analysis shows that sulphur dioxide emissions have generally decreased in the OECD region compared to 1970 levels, reflecting structural changes in energy demands (energy savings and fuel substitution), pollution control policies and technical progress [11,12]. In Japan, annual average sulphur dioxide concentrations declined by 60% between 1975 and the late 1980s, where the maximum daily concentrations are exceeded in less than 0.5% of all cases [11]. Sulphur dioxide levels have declined by about 45% in Canada and the U.S. between the mid 1970s and the late 1980s. The number of areas not attaining the U.S. national ambient air quality standard declined by more than 40%. In the United Kingdom, ambient levels of sulphur oxide declined by 52% between the mid 1970s and the late 1980s. These reductions in sulphur dioxide concentrations are significantly larger than the emission reductions that took place over this period [11]. Sulphur dioxide emissions in OECD Europe have fallen more than 20% from 1980 to 1989. The largest decline occurred in Germany (formerly FRG), which reduced sulphur dioxide emissions by 53% during that period and plans to reduce these emissions further by 80% from 1983 levels by 1993 [11,12].

While the use of tall stacks has reduced urban sulphur dioxide levels in industrialised countries by increasing the dispersion of the exhaust gases at power generating facilities and industrialised sites, they have unfortunately resulted in the long-range transport of these emissions and their subsequent deposition in locations far from their initial source in Europe, North America and elsewhere [2,4,5,11,12] (see also chapter 1).

In the U.S. in 1985, nation-wide emissions of sulphur dioxide were 23 million tons, and 50% of these emissions were vented through smoke stacks taller than 145 meters, which enabled these pollutants to travel long distances [159].

The annual mean levels of sulphur dioxide in major cities of Europe are now largely below 100 $\mu g/m^3$ [2], having declined from an earlier range of 100-200 $\mu g/m^3$ [159]. The annual mean sulphur dioxide concentrations in most rural areas in Western Europe are between 5-25 $\mu g/m^3$. However, due to the use of high chimneys to disperse emissions, there are also large rural areas where average concentrations of sulphur dioxide exceed 25 $\mu g/m^3$.

While concentrations of sulphur dioxide have declined in most urban areas and in those cities where levels were highest in Europe in the early 1970s, many cities in southern Europe in particular have levels of sulphur dioxide that still exceed the European Community's air quality guideline of 130 $\mu g/m^3$ (daily mean during winter) [11].

As noted earlier, there are still severe air pollution problems in central and eastern Europe, particularly in Poland, the former East Germany (DDR), Czechoslovakia, Romania and the former Soviet Union, largely resulting from the regions' heavy reliance on hard and brown coal for periods ranging from at least 40 to over 70 years (in the case of the former Soviet Union) [11,12,82-93]. Sulphur dioxide emissions have been estimated at about 5.2 million metric tons in former East Germany and 3.9 million metric tons in Poland in 1988. On a per capita basis, emissions in East Germany were estimated at 313.3 kg compared with 24.2 kg in West Germany [11].

The United Nations-sponsored Global Environmental Monitoring System estimated in 1987 that some two-thirds of the world's urban population lived in cities where the ambient sulphur dioxide concentration was at or above the WHO limit and that 70% of the world's urban population lived in cities where the level of suspended particulates exceeded WHO guidelines [11,160].

In 1979, 35 nations of central and western Europe and North America signed the convention of Long-Range Transboundary Air Pollution. A protocol requiring 30% reduction in sulphur dioxide emissions from 1980 levels by 1993 was adopted in 1985 [11,161,162]. Although the United States did not sign the sulphur dioxide protocol, it has subsequently passed legislation (Clean Air Act) that will mandate the reduction of sulphur dioxide emissions by 35% to 8.9 million ton per year by 2000 (a 10 million ton reduction from 1980 levels) [11,163].

An agreement between the U.S. and Canada signed March 13, 1991, calls for action such as reducing sulphur dioxide levels in the U.S. as noted above to 10 million tons below 1980 levels by 2000 while sulphur dioxide levels in eastern Canada must be reduced by 2.3

million tons by 1994 and capped at that level through 1999. Canada would also impose a national sulphur emissions cap of 3.2 million tons per year by 2000 [164].

It should be noted, however, that global levels of sulphur dioxide (as well as nitrogen oxides) are expected to increase in the years ahead in developing countries as their energy demands continue to rise coupled with an expansion of vehicular traffic [11,12,161]. China is expected to double its coal use by 2000 [11,165]. Each year China mines more than a billion metric tons of coal, more than any other country in the world. By the end of this century, China plans to produce 1.4 billion tons of coal/year, almost all of which will be burned at home. By the year 2020, China could mine 2 billion tons/year, half of the world's production [166].

Sulphuric Acid (Acid Aerosol)

One of the major global atmospheric changes associated with increased combustion of fossil fuels is the release of acids and their precursors into the atmosphere. Principal concerns in this area involve acids arising from sulphur oxide and nitrogen oxide emissions, including sulphuric acid and bisulphate aerosols [2-5,11,12,155-163,167,168]. The major portion of sulphur emissions from combustion sources is emitted as sulphur dioxide, which is further oxidised to sulphur trioxide in the atmosphere at the rate of 0.5-1.0% per hour. The rates of sulphur dioxide oxidation depend on various factors, including: ambient temperature, humidity, concentration of oxidants and catalytic components of particles in the atmosphere and cloud droplets [2].

In the presence of moisture, sulphuric acid is formed which is present as an aerosol often associated with other pollutants in droplets or solid particles extending over a broad range of sizes [2]. Sulphuric acid and its partial atmospheric neutralisation product represent almost all of the strong acid content of ambient aerosol. Although most of the sulphuric acid in ambient air results from sulphur dioxide formed via the combustion of fossil fuels, other anthropogenic sources include other direct or primary point sources of sulphuric acid such as acid manufacturing plants and consuming industries such as fertiliser and pigment factories [2].

The principal natural sources of sulphuric acid are volcanoes, e.g., Mt. Pinatubo via the initial emission of sulphur dioxide [11,12,69]. The highest levels of acid aerosol are in the range of 20-30 µg sulphuric acid/m^3 (6-12 hour average) in various parts of North America and 28 µg sulphuric acid/m^3 (6-12 hour average) in Europe (West Berlin) [2,168]. The highest reported level in the U.K. was 680 µg/m^3 (1 hour average) in London in 1962. However, higher levels were believed to have been present in London in earlier years [2].

With decreased emissions of sulphur dioxide reported in North America, OECD Europe and Japan in the past decade, the sulphuric acid aerosols would also be anticipated to be lower [11,12]. However, as noted earlier, there has been severe air pollution over many decades in central and eastern Europe, principally Poland, the former East Germany (DDR), Czechoslovakia, Romania and the former Soviet Union as a restult of their overreliance on high sulphur-containing coals for power production, residential heating and industry. This has resulted in very high emissions of sulphur dioxide in these regions with undoubtedly commensurate high acid aerosols, particularly in urban areas as well as their transport to other regions distant from their initial emission source [11,12,82-93].

Nitrogen Oxides

Nitrogen oxides comprise a wide range of gases of which the most important atmospheric gases are nitrogen dioxide, nitric oxide and nitrous oxide. Of these species, nitrogen dioxide is the predominant form from the point of view of atmospheric significance on local, regional, national and global scales as well as its effect on human health [2-5,11,12]. The major source of emissions of NOx into the atmosphere is the combustion of fossil fuels in stationary sources (heating and power generation) and internal combustion engines in motor vehicles, and industrial processes such as the production of nitric acid and the use of explosives and welding processes [2]. Excluding the combustion of fossil fuels, the largest source of anthropogenic emissions of NOx is the burning of biomass [33,34] and natural fires.

About 50% of all man-made NOx emissions in OECD countries, mostly in the form of NO and, on average, up to 10% as nitrogen dioxide comes from road traffic, followed by power plants and industrial combustion [12]. In urban environments, vehicle emissions are the predominant source of NOx emissions [11,12]. Stationary sources such as coal-burning power plants, ore smelters and industrial boilers, are responsible for about 35% of the NOx emissions [11,12,160].

The nitrogen oxides which are emitted in the flue gas of power plants consist of about 95% of nitric oxide and 5% of nitrogen dioxide. After emission, nitric oxide is converted to nitrogen dioxide via oxidation with atmospheric ozone [2-5,169-171]. The oxidation rate depends on a number of important factors including: the molecular reaction rates and physical kinetics such as dispersion and mixing of the plume with ambient air, which are dependent upon meteorological conditions such as wind speed, solar radiation and concentration of the reactants [170].

Nitrogen-containing air pollutants such as nitric acid, aerosol nitrates and peroxyacyl nitrate (PAN), are formed as further reaction products of nitrogen dioxide in the atmosphere. In the lower atmosphere (troposphere), NOx reacting with VOCs in the presence of sunlight is instrumental in the production of photochemical smog (a mix of more than 100 different chemicals, dominated by ozone) [1-5,11,12]. Nitrogen oxides with sulphur oxides contribute to acidic wet and dry deposition [3-5,80,81].

Differences in NOx emissions in different countries can be attributed principally to differences in fossil fuel combustion. Global emissions of NOx in 1970 were estimated at approx. 53 million tonnes [2,85]. Annual mean nitrogen dioxide concentrations in urban areas throughout the world are generally in the range of 20-90 µg/m^3 (0.01-0.05 ppm) [2]. Urban outdoor levels of nitrogen dioxide vary according to seasonal, diurnal and meteorological factors with typically higher levels from peak traffic emissions of nitric oxide [2-5,11,12]. The maximal hourly mean value of nitrogen dioxide may be 3-10 times the annual mean [2].

Changes in combustion-generated emissions of NOx (and SOx) between 1966 and 1980 show that NOx and SOx are unevenly distributed globally, resulting in large local and regional variations from the global mean fluxes. The greatest rates of emission of NOx and SOx from fossil-fuel combustion between 1966 and 1980 occurred in the northern mid-latitudes while the greatest increases during this period have taken place in the tropics [169]. Emissions of NOx in the U.S. in 1985 were stated to be 20.6 million tons [159].

Average nitrogen dioxide levels in many OECD countries do not show a clear trend over the past 20 years. For example, in the U.S., average annual nitrogen dioxide values for 1988 were somewhat below those for 1977, while in countries such as western Germany and Japan, average nitrogen dioxide levels in 1988 were higher than or close to those in the early 1970s. Monitoring activities over the last 2 decades indicate an increase in NOx in urban areas throughout the world [11,12,160]. Concentrations of nitrogen dioxide in urban areas show large variations with time, with peak levels often several times higher than the average [2-5,11,12].

Emissions of NOx are not falling and they are even rising somewhat in most OECD countries. An increasing fraction of NOx emissions comes from the increased number of motor vehicles and the higher speeds driven [11].

Trend analysis shows that NOx emissions have increased in the OECD region compared to 1970 levels with the exception of Japan [12]. Contributions of various nations and regions to the global budget of anthropogenic emissions of nitrogen oxide in the late 1980s were as follows: North America, 31.9%; OECD Europe, 18.7%; Japan, 1.7% and the rest of the world, 47.7%. The tonnage of atmospheric emissions (tonnes) of NOx were: North America, 21,700,000; OECD Europe, 12,700,000; Japan, 1,176,000; world, 68,000,000 [12].

A protocol mandating a cap on NOx emissions at 1987 levels was adopted in 1988 by 35 nations from central and western Europe and North America as part of the Convention on Long-Range Transboundary Air Pollution. Additionally, 12 members of the European Community further promised 30% NOx reductions by 1988 [12,161,162]. Reducing NOx has proven to be more difficult than reducing sulphur dioxide emissions and emission increases of NOx have been the rule in all but a few nations.

There have been a number of technological advances that hold promise for a certain degree of further nitrogen oxide reductions. Advanced burners have reduced NOx emissions by 50% at some power generating facilities. Up to 70-90% of NOx and up to 95% of sulphur oxides can be removed by available scrubber technology [12].

Catalytic converters to treat exhaust gases can reduce emissions of NOx by about 60% over the life of a car and have been an important tool in controlling auto emissions in the U.S. and Japan for over a decade [12]. The U.S. EPA announced new standards in 1991 that will require large municipal incinerators to reduce overall air emissions 90% by 1994 using advanced pollution control technologies (APCT). New facilities will need to install scrubbers to further cut NOx emissions by about 40% [172].

Acid Deposition

Acid deposition is a collective term for "wet" (acid rain, snow) and "dry" (acidic particles and aerosols) deposition which originates from both natural and anthropogenic emissions of sulphur dioxide, oxides of nitrogen, and acids and salts of the products of their atmospheric transformation. The principal anthropogenic emission acid deposition precursor sources are the combustion of fossil fuels in energy production and vehicular traffic (generating 30-50% of total NOx emissions) [11].

Acid deposition can occur at a short distance from emission sources or thousands of kilometers distant. Smokestacks up to 300 meters tall can inject sulphur dioxide and NOx high into the atmosphere where most are converted to sulphate and nitrate particulates which may be transported to distant sites before being deposited [11].

Acid deposition can severely affect soils, forests, agriculture, aquatic habitat and the weathering of buildings [2,5,10-13,54,62-68,173-179] (see also chapter 1).

The phenomena of acid deposition became a major concern in the late 1970s and early 1980s in highly industrialised regions in Europe and North America where sulphur deposition in the most polluted areas is more than 10 times higher than the natural background rates [2-5,11,12,62,173,174]. China, the third largest emitter of sulphur dioxide after the U.S. and the former Soviet Union, has also begun to experience regional acid deposition in its eastern and southern provinces [11,12,173,174]. More limited incidents of acid deposition have also been reported in Japan [11].

Acid deposition is engendered to a large degree by transboundary transport of sulphur dioxide and nitrogen oxides [1,2,11,13,64, 173-177]. For example, the domestic deposition of sulphur dioxide varied greatly across Europe: from 5% in Norway to 83% in the United Kingdom in 1988. The deposition depends on a number of factors including: the prevailing winds, size of the country and density of the emission fields. Countries in Europe not only receive acid deposition from their neighbours but also atmospherically "export" large amounts of sulphur dioxide elsewhere [12,64] (see also chapter 1). For example, one three-stack nickel smelter in the Russian Arctic has been reported to emit more sulphur dioxide than all sources combined in Norway, which as acid deposition afflicts northern Norway [178]. Most acid deposition in Finland originates in Finland and to a considerable degree in Russia [179]. In North America, it is estimated that almost 40% of sulphur deposition (acid deposition) in the northeastern U.S. and Canada originates from midwestern U.S. (from primary power generating plants) [11,12].

Projections for increased emissions of sulphur dioxide and nitrogen oxides in the developing countries as a consequence of significant population growth, larger-scale industrialisation, increased use of fossil fuels and motor transport [11,12,165,166] would undoubtedly lead to enhanced acid deposition primarily in southeast Asia with the greatest impact on India and China [175].

Hydrocarbons

A large number of hydrocarbons (e.g., saturated and unsaturated aliphatic, aromatic, polycyclic and halogenated derivatives) have been found in the atmosphere [1,180]. For example, more than 130 alkanes have been identified; of those detected in ambient air, about two-thirds are found in the gas phase and about one-third in the aerosol phase. A large number of alkanes have been found in indoor environments and higher alkanes have also been found in rain and snow [180]. Nearly 150 alkanes and alkynes have been found in the gas phase more commonly than in the aerosol phase. By far the largest source of atmospheric alkanes, alkenes and alkynes is the combustion of fossil fuels. Nearly a hundred monocyclic hydrocarbons have been detected, about two-thirds in the gas phase with the great majority arising from the combustion of fossil fuel or biomass. More than 70 monocyclic arenes including benzene and its derivatives have been found in the atmosphere, most often in the gas phase and are produced by fossil fuel combustion as well as a broad variety of industrial processes [97,180].

Ethylene, Propylene and Butenes

Alkenes in urban air are of concern because of their potential for atmospheric transformations including photochemical conversion to genotoxic products in the presence of nitrogen dioxide [181,182]. Ethylene is extensively used in a broad spectrum of chemical and polymer production and dissipative losses to the atmosphere could be expected to occur. Ethylene is also produced by all plant tissues, by soil micro-organisms including fungi and bacteria and it has also been detected in marsh gases and gases desorbed from coals samples [183].

In the U.S., ethylene concentrations in air varied from 29-88 $\mu g/m^3$ (25-77 ppb) in downtown Los Angeles; from 21-24 $\mu g/m^3$ (18-21 ppb) in Azuza, California; from 805 $\mu g/m^3$ (700 ppb) in the centre of Washington, D.C., to 45 $\mu g/m^3$ (39 ppb) in an outlying suburb and from 7 $\mu g/m^3$ (6.1 ppb) to 8.2 mg/m^3 (7100 ppb) in the Houston, Texas area [183]. Ethylene concentrations in the air of rural areas in the U.K. varied over a 2-year period from 0.53-11.5 $\mu g/m^3$ (0.46-10 ppb) with a mean of 2.64 $\mu g/m^3$ (2.3 ppb). Ethylene concentrations in the air near Delft, the Netherlands, have been reported to average 18 $\mu g/m^3$ (15.5 ppb) [183].

Propylene is extensively employed in chemical synthesis, e.g., the production of propylene oxide, acrylonitrile, isopropyl alcohol and in polymer production, principally polypropylene. It has been detected in urban air at levels of 1-10 $\mu g/m^3$ and in rural air at levels of 0.10-8.2 $\mu g/m^3$ [183]. Propylene has been detected in vehicle exhausts [181]. Petrol vapours and exhaust are sources of a similar magnitude for the 2-butenes in urban air. Petrol vapours have been found to be sources of a similar magnitude for trans-2-butene, cis-2-butene, methylpropene and 1-butene. Among the 4 isomeric butenes, methylpropene is the most abundant in petrol vapours and exhaust [181].

Butadiene

1,3-Butadiene is a major industrial commodity in the U.S., western Europe and Japan, with broad utility in polymer production. According to a 1984 U.S. EPA survey, emissions of butadiene to the atmosphere from the production of 1,3-butadiene were approx. 3.8 million pounds (1.72 x 10^6 kg/year or 0.14% of the amount produced; about 99% of the emissions were due to equipment leaks) [184]. The EPA has estimated that the total emissions of butadiene to the atmosphere from the production of styrene-butadiene co-polymers is approx. 15 million pounds (2.27 x 10^6 kg/year or 0.3% of the amount produced) [185].

Low levels of butadiene (0.001-0.005 and 0.019-0.030 ppm) have been measured in urban air near industrial sites in the U.S. [186]. Butadiene has also been found in vehicle exhausts [181,186]. In one study of urban air in Goteborg, Sweden, butadiene was found in the range of 0.5 $\mu g/m^3$ [181].

Benzene

Benzene is a major industrial chemical produced in enormous quantities by many industrialised countries and is extensively utilised in the production of a large number of substituted aromatic hydrocarbons. The total global annual cycle, including benzene in fossil fuels, is estimated to be 32 million tonnes of which 4 million tonnes are believed to be lost to the environment [187]. Benzene emissions from 36 coke by-product recovery plants in the iron and steel industry in the U.S. were estimated at 18,700 tons per year in 1989. In 1989 the U.S. EPA ordered a 90% reduction in the industrial emissions of benzene over the next 5 years [188]. According to a recent EPA source survey inventory, 85% of benzene emissions in the U.S. are from mobile sources, of which 70% are from exhaust, 14% from evaporative emissions and 1% from vehicle refuelling [189,190].

Benzene emissions from vehicles are related to the benzene levels of the fuels, the total aromatic level of the fuel [190,191], as well as the catalytic converter catalysts to control hydrocarbons, carbon monoxide and nitrogen oxides [189]. (Catalytic converters were first introduced in the U.S. in 1981 [189].) U.S. petrols contain an average of 0.8% benzene while European petrols contain on average 5% benzene with occasional levels reaching 16% [2,186]. In one study [190], it was found that as fuel efficiency control improved, hydrocarbons, benzene and toluene emissions all decreased, and in 1987 cars emitted less than 6% of all benzene emitted by pre-catalyst cars. In other studies [189,190], benzene was found to comprise about 2.15% of total hydrocarbon emissions from a gasoline engine or about 4% of automotive exhausts.

Benzene emitted to the atmosphere has a half-life of less than 1 day [2,192]. Benzene concentrations in ambient air are generally between 3 and 160 $\mu g/m^3$ (0.001-0.05 ppm) and higher ambient benzene levels are found in metropolitan areas [2,186,191]. In the vicinity of petrol stations and storage tanks and benzene producing/handling industries, concentrations of benzene at levels of up to several hundred $\mu g/m^3$ have been reported [2,186,191].

Since 85% of human exposure to benzene in the U.S. is believed to originate from petrol [190], there has been recent increasing interest in the reformulation of fuels and to a much lesser degree the use of alternative fuels such as methanol or ethanol alone or in various blends with petrol [193]. In reformulated petrols, the average aromatics in unleaded fuels is about 20-30% to maintain a high octane rating. A variety of extenders and additives have been employed including methyl butyl tertiary ether (MBTE), ethyl butyl tertiary ether (EBTE), methanol and ethanol to reduce benzene and NOx emissions. The use of methanol is advocated as a straight replacement for petrol (M-100=100% methanol) or as a blend of 85% methanol and 15% petrol (M-85) to effect the lowering of benzene and butadiene emissions [194,195].

Methyl Chloride

Methyl chloride, widely employed in the production of alkyl lead anti-knock agents and methyl silicone polymers and resins, is the most abundant of the nearly 70 alkanic halogenated derivatives found in the troposphere. Its emission occurs from both natural and anthropogenic sources [180,196]. An average global atmospheric concentration is estimated to be in the order of 1 ppb (2.1 $\mu g/m^3$), with the lower concentrations (0.6-0.9 ppb) (1.2-1.7 $\mu g/m^3$) in rural areas and near localised sources [196].

The principal sources of methyl chloride are formed in the oceans by seaweeds and marine micro-organisms and by the various combustion processes of organic matter such as forest fires, biomass burnings, slash and burn agriculture, fossil fuels, incineration of municipal and industrial waste, accidental fires and cigarette smoke [196,197]. The principal source of atmospheric methyl chloride are the oceans which release 1000-8000 million kg/year. Urban sources and the combustion of vegetation are estimated to release 150-600 million kg/year while emission from the manufacture, processing and distribution of methyl chloride contributed about 20 million kg in 1980 [196,197]. It was estimated that 0.1 million tons of methyl chloride were emitted into the atmosphere from the Amazon biomass burnings in 1987 [34].

The primary mechanism for the removal of atmospheric methyl chloride is believed to be the reaction with hydroxyl radicals. The residence time of methyl chloride in an urban atmosphere is estimated to be 231 days with a daily rate loss (12 sunlit hours) of 0.4% [196]. Average levels of methyl chloride in air at 10 urban sites in the U.S. ranged from 0.7-3.0 ppb (1.4-6.2 µg/m^3) and the calculated average human exposures to methyl chloride at these sites ranged up to 140 µg/person/day [191,196]. Measurements of methyl chloride in the air of southern England between December 1974 and April 1975 showed a mean concentration of 1.1 ppb (2.3 µg/m^3) while the average concentration in the stratosphere over France in 1978 was calculated to be approx. 0.7 ppb (1.5 µg/m^3) [196].

Tetrachloroethylene

Tetrachloroethylene (perchloroethylene) is a broadly used solvent in dry-cleaning and metal cleaning, in processing and finishing operations in the textile industry, in grain fumigation and in the manufacture of fluorocarbons [2,198,199]. An estimated 85% of manmade tetrachloroethylene is released into the ambient air as a result of evaporation.
The annual production of tetrachloroethylene is estimated to be 100,000-250,000 tonnes in western Europe, about 265,000 tonnes in the U.S. and about 55,000 tonnes in Japan [2,198]. An estimated 85% of tetrachloroethylene are released into the ambient air as a result of evaporation. Global emissions are now estimated to be as high as 800,000 tonnes annually [2].
In southern California (Los Angeles urban area), 12,000 metric tons of tetrachloroethylene are released every year [114]. The highest concentration of tetrachloroethylene measured in 1987-1990 at 21 locations in southern California was 20 ppb with 24-hour averages of 12 ppb [114]. Average instantaneous concentrations of tetrachloroethylene in the ambient air of 62 out of 92 cities in Western Germany ranged between 1 and 10 µg/m^3 in the autumn of 1980 [2]. Levels of tetrachloroethylene in air fluctuate considerably on a seasonal, diurnal and spatial basis [2,114,199]. Global background levels of tetrachloroethylene are around 0.2 µg/m^3 [2,199].

In the troposphere, tetrachloroethylene is photochemically degraded, with reaction with hydroxyl radicals [2,11] the principal mechanism by which it is removed. The estimated lifetime of tetrachloroethylene in the troposphere is less than one year.

Carbon Monoxide

Carbon monoxide is one of the most common and widely distributed air pollutants whose total emissions are believed to exceed those of all other urban air pollutants combined [2,11,12]. Estimates of CO emissions vary from 350 to 600 million tonnes/year, with the principal sources of emissions resulting from incomplete combustion processes (e.g., in vehicles, industrial processes, heating facilities and incinerators) [2-5,11,12,198]. Carbon monoxide is emitted in OECD countries from the incomplete combustion of fossil fuels, up to 90% by road traffic and industry. However, in many urban areas, vehicle exhaust accounts for nearly all the CO emitted [11,160].
On a global scale, natural sources, chiefly decomposition of organic matter, biomass burning and forest fires constitute about 65% of total CO emissions [11,33,34]. The estimated global CO from biomass burning is close to 1,000 teragrams/year (1 teragram = 10^{12} grams) [33]. It has been estimated that 94 million tons of CO were emitted into the atmosphere from the Amazonia biomass burnings in 1987 [34].
Additionally, CO is produced by natural sources as well as chemical reactions in the troposphere (e.g., in the oxidation of methane) and biospheric processes [2-5,11,12]. Carbon monoxide is the principal component in the complex tropospheric photochemical reactions leading to the formation of ozone, the main component of photochemical smog [2-5].
The principal biosphere CO production processes are based on the oxidation from plant material, photo-oxidation of organic matter, in ocean water, and chemical oxidation of organic carbon in soil. Additionally, there is evidence that CO is produced by biological reduction of carbon dioxide due to the activity of anaerobic bacteria (e.g., sulphate reducing

bacteria), methanogenic and acetogenic bacteria [200].

Natural background levels of CO range between 0.01 and 0.23 mg/m^3 (0.01-0.20 ppm). Concentrations in urban areas depend on weather and traffic density as well as time and distance from the sources. Although 8-hour mean concentrations are generally less than 20 mg/m^3 (17 ppm), maximum 8-hour mean concentrations of up to 60 mg/m^3 (53 ppm) have been occasionally reported [2].

Trend analysis shows that CO emissions have generally decreased in many, but not all OECD countries since about 1970, reflecting decreased use of solid fuels in domestic heating and small industries as well as the increasing use of catalytic converters in automobiles which change most of the CO to carbon dioxide [11,12,20]. A catalytic converter can reduce emissions of VOCs and CO by about 85% and NOx by about 60% over the life of a car [11,165]. Such controls have resulted in substantially lowered ambient CO concentrations in many cities in the industrial world. For example, in the U.S., CO levels fell 28% between 1980 and 1989 in spite of a 39% increase in vehicle miles traveled [11,201], while in Japan, ambient CO levels fell approximately 50% between 1973 and 1984 [11,160]. However, it must be noted that in most of the developing world the concentrations of CO are increasing as the number of vehicles and the amount of traffic congestion rise. WHO estimates indicate that unhealthy CO concentrations may currently exist in approx. half of the world's cities [11,201].

Peroxyacyl Nitrates

Photochemical reactions of hydrocarbons and NOx may contribute to the formation of ozone, peroxyacyl nitrates and other chemical species in the urban environment [2-5,202]. Peroxyacyl nitrates, e.g., peroxyacetyl nitrate (PAN) and higher homologues of PAN, including peroxypropionyl-, peroxy-n-butyryl-, peroxyisobutyryl-, peroxyglutaryl-, and peroxybenzyl nitrates have no known direct sources and are therefore excellent indicators of photochemical pollution [203,204].

The peroxyacyl nitrates serve as vehicles ("reservoirs") for the long-range transport of reactive nitrogen over regional and continental scales [2-5,202,204,205]. Peroxyacetyl nitrate (PAN), which is the most abundant of the peroxyacyl nitrates, is formed by the photochemical reactions of acetaldehyde in the presence of nitrogen dioxide [2-5]. Other aldehydes present in the atmosphere may also react to form peroxyacyl nitrates. For example, peroxypropionyl nitrate (PPN), peroxybutyryl nitrate (PBN) and peroxybenzyl nitrate are all produced by analogous photochemical reactions of nitrogen dioxide with the respective aldehyde [2-5,204].

It has been suggested that in the atmosphere, peroxyglutaryl nitrate (PGN) may be formed by the reaction of OH with the dialdehyde glutaraldehyde in the presence of nitrogen dioxide. Glutaraldehyde is one of the most abundant dialdehydes in urban atmospheres found at concentrations up to 0.3 µg/m^3 (0.1 ppb), and is the product of the photochemical degradation of cyclopentene [206]. Peroxyacetyl nitrate concentrations have been reported to reach maximum values of 80 µg/m^3 in the U.S. and 90 µg/m^3 in the Netherlands where an increase in this oxidant's concentrations in the last decade has been noted [2].

Peroxyacyl nitrates (which have been characterised in the Los Angeles, California area more than anywhere else in the world) are ubiquitous, though they have been found at somewhat lower levels in all urban areas worldwide [207].

A number of studies have reported PAN and PPN ratios at urban [208] as well as mountain sites [204]. Factors that may influence PPN/PAN ratio include: their relative thermal stability, variations in the concentrations of their precursor hydrocarbons and their relative removal by deposition and by reaction with radicals and compounds, e.g., OH, ozone and nitrate [204].

Additionally, highly reactive biogenic hydrocarbons including isoprene and terpenes (as well as their respective oxidation products methylvinyl ketone and methacrolein) may serve as precursors to the formation of PAN and PPN [204,209]. The phytotoxicity of the peroxyacyl nitrates, particularly PAN, is well documented [203].

Carbonyl Compounds

Carbonyl compounds, primarily aldehydes and ketones, are found in urban and industrial atmospheres as primary pollutants. A wide variety of aldehydes have been detected in the troposphere and are believed to be principally products of atmospheric photochemical reactions [206,210-219]. Carbonyl compounds (except formaldehyde) are the direct precursors of peroxyacyl nitrates in the atmosphere.

Carbonyl compounds, principally formaldehyde, are via their photolysis promoters of free radicals whose importance is preponderant in moderately or highly polluted atmospheres; they are formed in all emission sources [214].

Formaldehyde and acetaldehyde are the most abundant of the aldehydes formed from tropospheric photochemical reactions. Their concentrations range from sub-ppbv levels in remote locations [210,211,213] to up to tens of ppbv in urban environments [2,3,210-220]. However, significant fractions of total carbonyls (about 10%) may be present in the troposhere as acetone, acrolein, propanal, butanal, methylethyl ketone and benzaldehyde.

Aldehydes are formed via photolysis reactions of methane and isoprene and other biogenic and anthropogenic hydrocarbons. In industrial countries, aldehydes and ketones are also emitted into the atmosphere during manufacturing processes and via losses during transportation.

In general, the lifetimes of aldehydes in the atmosphere are in the order of hours, with the principal gas phase loss routes by photolysis and reaction with OH radicals estimated to cause a daily loss rate of about 80% of atmospheric acetaldehyde emissions [3-5,208].

Formaldehyde

As an outdoor pollutant, formaldehyde is directly emitted by mobile and stationary sources. It is produced industrially in large quantities and used in many applications [2,210,211,213]. Other important man-made sources are automobile exhaust from engines without catalytic converters, and residues, emissions or wastes produced during the manufacture of formaldehyde or materials derived from or treated with it, petroleum refineries, power plant combustion or incinerators [210,211,213].

As noted earlier, formaldehyde is also formed in the troposphere by photochemical reactions involving virtually all classes of hydrocarbon pollutants [2,3,210-219]. During smog episodes, *in situ* production of formaldehyde may be larger than direct emissions, e.g., 500 tons vs 30-70 tons/day in southern California [218,219]. It has been calculated that the average rate of global production of formaldehyde from methane in the troposphere is of the order of 4×10^{11} kg/year, while the total industrial production of formaldehyde in recent years has been about 3.5×10^4 kg/year [210]. Formaldehyde is emitted as a product of the incomplete combustion by internal combustion engines which greatly depends on the grade of fuel and the operating conditions. Motor vehicles are by far the most important source of formaldehyde emissions. The use of exhaust catalytic converters can reduce the emissions to less than one-tenth. The emissions of formaldehyde have not been quantifiable on a global basis [213]. Automotive exhaust itself contains formaldehyde at concentrations of 29-48 ppm (35.7-52.9 mg/m^3) and this source has been reported to account for much of the formaldehyde present in the atmosphere [2,3,21,210,213]. The natural background concentration of formaldehyde is a few $\mu g/m^3$.

In urban air, the annual average concentration of formaldehyde is approximately 0.005-0.01 mg/m^3, with higher levels in the vicinity of industrial processes [2,3,210,213]. Concentrations of formaldehyde are about one order of magnitude greater during short-term peaks occuring during peak traffic periods in built-up urban areas or under photochemical smog conditions [2,3,210,213]. Ambient levels of formaldehyde in the range of 5-60 ppbv have typically been reported in polluted atmospheres in the U.S. (in contrast, acetaldehyde levels are in the order of 60% of formaldehyde levels) [208].

However, it should be noted that formaldehyde levels of up to 150 ppbv have been measured in southern California in the 1960s and data from the late 1970s to the present time indicate lower concentrations, with maxima of up to 30-80 ppbv measured in samples of short duration, e.g., 1 hour [218].

The use of ethanol-based fuels as a constituent in gasahol (20% v/v in normal usage) and in pure form as a fuel in a smaller portion (10-15%) of vehicles with engines designed to burn hydrated ethanol and with no catalytic controls (as utilised in Brazil), has led to increased primary emissions and high ambient levels of formaldehyde and acetaldehyde and other higher aldehydes in polluted air.

The proposed use of methanol-based fuel, either as pure methanol (M-100) or with 15% petrol (M-85 v/v), in specially designed vehicles in the U.S. has been shown to lead to at least 35% less smog producing hydrocarbons (e.g., less "indirect" formaldehyde formed in the atmosphere from the transformation of reactive hydrocarbon emissions) but can cause the emisssion of 3 to 5 times more formaldehyde *per se* than that of petrol engines of equivalent technology [194].

Formaldehyde is removed from the atmosphere by photolysis, by reaction with the hydroxyl radical, and by wet and dry deposition [3,117,220]. It should also be noted that in-cloud oxidation of formaldehyde plays a major role in controlling the concentration of formic acid [218,221], which is the major contributor to acid rain in the natural tropical ecosystems [221].

Acetaldehyde

Acetaldehyde occurs in air as a result of natural and anthropogenic sources, with the latter being by far the greatest source. The annual U.S. atmospheric emissions of acetaldehyde in 1978 were initially reported to range from 2.2-12.2 million kg/year. A more detailed estimation of 52 million kg in 1978 from all sources (80% of which was due to wood burning in residences) was later reported [212]. The major processing and manufacturing sources for the emission of acetaldehyde included coffee roasting, acetic acid, vinyl acetate, ethanol, acrylonitrile and crotonaldehyde.

Air monitoring data between 1975 and 1978 showed mean ambient concentrations of 5-124 $\mu g/m^3$ acetaldehyde in ambient air in southern California under conditions of moderate to severe photochemical pollution at levels of 5.4-62 $\mu g/m^3$ and in air near and in refuse-reclamation areas in Japan at levels of 5.4-13.7 $\mu g/m^3$ [212].

Photolysis of acetaldehyde in the atmosphere leads to the formation of HO_2 radicals, CO and methyl peroxyl radicals, and by the reaction with OH to the peroxyacetyl radical and peroxyacetyl nitrate (PAN). In polluted urban air, daytime decomposition of acetaldehyde via reaction with OH is expected to be a major route of PAN formation, especially away from the immediate vicinity of NO emission sources [208].

Hydrogen Peroxide

Hydrogen peroxide, together with ozone and the OH radical, constitute the principal oxidants in the lower atmosphere [5,117]. Both hydrogen peroxide and the OH radical are by-products of ozone photodissociation and each of the principal oxidants interact with each other and with other key trace gases in a variety of ways. Hydrogen peroxide which forms in gaseous and condensed phases is subject to washout by precipitation [117,222]. Hydrogen peroxide also contributes to acid precipitation because it is the oxidant that converts sulphur dioxide to sulphuric acid in clouds and rain droplets at low pH [223].

Recent measurements have shown that hydrogen peroxide is present over the northeastern U.S. at concentrations of up to 4 ppbv in autumn, approximately one-tenth of typical ozone concentrations. Atmospheric concentrations of hydrogen peroxide in other regions of the U.S. are in the range of 1 ppbv to about 50 ppbv, with an uncertainty of about one order of magnitude depending on the data input used in modelling [224].

Thompson [117] has attempted to model the probable past and future concentrations of the principal atmospheric oxidants. Predictions of future concentrations of hydrogen peroxide are sensitive to assumed nitrogen oxide distributions. Increases in methane, carbon dioxide and non-methane hydrocarbon (NMHC) emissions convert OH to HO_2 and hydrogen peroxide, except when NOx concentrations increase rapidly enough for nitric acid formation to compete with hydrogen peroxide formation.

Depletion of stratospheric ozone and a warmer, moister climate favour hydrogen peroxide formation at the expense of tropospheric OH and ozone, but if cloud and precipitation enrichment were to remove the additional hydrogen peroxide, concentrations of hydrogen peroxide could be increasing at even greater rates than tropospheric ozone. However, increases of NOx emissions tend to counteract increases of atmospheric hydrogen peroxide [117]. Recent increases in hydrogen peroxide concentration in Greenland ice cores suggest that increases in methane and CO concentrations will add to the atmospheric burden of hydrogen peroxide [117].

Hydrochloric Acid

The 2 major sources of atmospheric HCl are fossil fuel combustion and the incineration of domestic and industrial waste [225-227]. The fossil fuel of principal concern is coal and the amount of HCl generated depends on its chlorine content. In the United Kingdom, coal is the largest single source of HCl emissions. The mean chloride content of British coal is 0.23% and it has been estimated that 99% of this is most probably emitted as HCl in stack gases during combustion. The total annual HCl emission in the U.K. is estimated to be 240 ktons, based on coal delivery in the U.K. of 1.12×10^5 kt in 1983. The estimated total emission of HCl from 12 other west European countries is about 380 ktons/year [225].

Other sources of HCl to the atmosphere include the incineration of domestic and industrial waste, where HCl arises from chlorides in material such as vegetable matter, paper, polyvinyl chloride (PVC) plastic, dry cell batteries and salt. It is estimated that waste incineration accounts for about 16 ktons/year HCl to the atmosphere, of which approx. 8 ktons arise from HCl emissions from PVC waste in municipal incinerators. In the U.K. coal burning and waste incineration account for about 99% of all HCl emissions [225].

Industrial sources of HCL emission are relatively small compared with emissions from coal burning and waste incineration and include: glass manufacture, production of steel (steel pickling acid and regeneration). In the Federal Republic of Germany, power stations and industrial furnaces produced 81.4% of HCl emissions, waste incineration produced 17.5% and other sources only 1.1% [228].

Another potential anthropogenic source of atmospheric HCl arises from the production and use of chlorinated hydrocarbons which are released into the atmosphere as solvents, refrigerants, etc., and which react very slowly in the atmosphere to yield HCl. In the U.K. the chlorinated hydrocarbons represent a potential HCl source of about 400 ktons/year. However, it should be noted that the atmospheric reactions of chlorinated hydrocarbons with OH radicals to produce HCl are so slow that the acidity produced as HCl is well dispersed over the Northern Hemisphere and is considered not distinguishable from the background acidity of the atmosphere.

Natural sources may be an additional important source of atmospheric HCl. For example, HCl is emitted from volcanoes and the world emission from this source, although very uncertain, has been estimated to range from 750-7600 ktons/year. Another source of HCl in the atmosphere is methylchloride which is produced in the sea by marine plants or micro-organisms and also on land via the combustion of vegetation. Methylchloride in the atmosphere reacts with OH radicals and the chloride content is eventually converted to HCl. Globally it has been estimated that natural sources produce 5600 ktons of methyl chloride per year, which is equivalent to about 400 ktons of HCl.

There are insufficient definitive data to determine how concentrations of HCl vary with time of day, season, source or area characteristics, e.g., urban versus rural setting [227].

It has recently been suggested that the observed depletion of ozone over Antarctica could in some measure be accounted for by the reaction between atmospheric HCl and chlorine nitrate, which is greatly enhanced in the presence of ice particles. This reaction has two important effects: it promotes the formation of nitric acid, with the corresponding depression of NO_2, and it generates Cl_2, which photolyses rapidly to produce catalytically active free radicals that may rapidly destroy ozone in the absence of high NO levels [41,42,229].

Ammonia and Ammonium

Ammonia and ammonium are important atmospheric components. Ammonia is the primary neutralising agent for atmospheric acids and is a ubiquitous component of the atmospheric aerosol [230,231]. The main sources of NH_3 are emissions from livestock wastes and to a lesser degree from fertiliser application. Fertiliser factories also yield localised emissions and other small contributions arise from traffic and coal combustion. Natural ecosystems are generally believed to be sinks for ammonia, since uptake from growing plants is well documented and NH_3 volatilised from agricultural sources has been implicated in the decline of European forests and heathlands [230].

The spatial distribution of annual emissions of ammonia in England and Wales summed over different sources amounts to approximately 70 ktons/year. Studies of longer time trends imply a 50% increase in NH_3 emissions over Europe between 1950 and 1980 [231]. Ammonia is suggested to be the only significant gaseous atmospheric trace species capable of neutralising airborne acidity. In this process, it converts strong acids to relatively neutral ammonium salt aerosols.

Atmospheric concentrations of ammonia and ammonium are typically in the order of a few $\mu g/m^3$ and may be subject to seasonal and rapid temporal variations [230-233]. Large emissions of NH_3 can lead to high concentrations of ammonium nitrate (e.g., as found over the east Los Angeles basin). Hence ammonia can play an important role in altering oxidation and pollutant deposition systematically on a regional basis and is involved in the acid rain problem [231,232].

Organochlorine Pesticides and Polychlorinated Biphenyls

The global spread of air pollution has been recognised over the last several decades as a major global atmospheric issue. Atmospheric transport of toxic organic compounds from source regions and subsequent deposition to receptors such as land and water is the most important pathway for distribution of anthropogenic organic compounds globally [60].

The major industrial nations and the main portion of the global population are concentrated in the Northern Hemisphere. Their discharge of persistent man-made organic chemicals (xenobiotics) into the atmosphere can be traced to applications of agrochemicals, to energy production, traffic and waste disposal. In the Southern Hemisphere, direct discharge of xenobiotics into the environment is mainly a result of pesticide use for crop protection and for insect disease vector control programmes for humans and animals. It is less well correlated with industrial production and all its aspects [60].

The organochlorine pesticides and polychlorinated biphenyls (PCBs) are two classes of important semi-volatile anthropogenic compounds that are of primary concern because of their global transport, toxicity and, in the case of the PCBs, their persistence [234-240]. A broad spectrum of halogenated hydrocarbons representing predominantly organochlorine pesticides are emitted into the atmosphere via direct industrial, commercial, agricultural or residential emissions, evaporation from contaminated waters, soils or vegetative surfaces or re-enter the atmosphere by processes such as volatisation and resuspension [60,234-240].

In urban and rural locations, hexachlorobenzene (HCB) concentrations are reported to be within the range of 0.2-0.3 nanograms/m^3 while lindane concentrations are in the range of 0.02-7 ng/m^3.

Background concentrations in remote marine atmospheres are reported to be within a range of 0.03-0.23 ng/m^3 for HCB and 0.01-5 ng/m^3 for lindane [235].

The atmospheric transport of the chlorinated pesticides and PCBs is regarded as an important pathway for the input of these contaminants to fresh water bodies such as the Great Lakes in the U.S. and remote locations as diverse as the Canadian and Scandinavian high Arctic, the Antarctic, the Indian and the Pacific Oceans [60,234-242]. Samples of peat, bogs and Arctic snow attest to the atmospheric transport and subsequent deposition of halogenated organic compounds (primarily organochlorine pesticides) such as hexachlorocyclohexanes (HCH), lindane, alpha and gamma chlordane, heptachlor, DDT, toxaphene, HCB, the cyclodienes dieldrin and endrin and the PCBs [236,237].

In a study of peat cores in the mid-latitudes of North America, the input (source functions) derived from peat profiles was consistent with production and use information in the U.S. for PCBs, HCB, hexachlorocyclohexanes, DDT and toxaphene [237,242].

In one study of organochlorine pesticides and PCBs in Canadian snow, Gregor and Gummer [241] found that hexachlorocyclohexanes (HCHs), consisting of lindane (gamma HCH) (0.20-4.08 ng/litre) and the alpha isomer of HCH (0.43-8.74 ng/litre), usually made up more than 75% of the total organochlorine pesticides measured. These were followed in abundance by alpha-endosulphan and dieldrin at levels generally ranging between 0.5 and 1.0 ng/litre and alpha and gamma chlordane and heptachlor at concentrations less than 0.5 ng/litre. PCB concentrations ranged from 0.02 to 1.76 ng/litre with most of the samples having concentrations less than 1.0 ng/litre [241].

It is estimated that 9×10^8 g per year of PCBs cycle through the U.S. atmosphere [242], which is less than 1% of the total PCBs in the environment. It has been estimated that the atmospheric pathway contributes 60-90% of the PCB input into the Great Lakes and Lake Superior receives more than 78% of its PCB burden from the atmosphere [237]. Recent studies suggest that PCBs, chlordanes and alpha-HCH concentrations are decreasing in air [238,239,244]. Other chemicals which have not been controlled, such as DDT, polychlorinated camphenes and dieldrin, are not decreasing in air at a noticable rate [238].

Air concentrations of lower chlorinated PCBs in rural England have decreased by up to a factor of 50 between 1965-1969 and 1985-1989; however, high molecular weight PCBs, while decreasing, did not decrease in concentration to such a great extent [244].

The distribution of atmospheric PCBs between vapour phase, aerosols and rain was elaborated by Duinker and Bouchertall [245], who separated PCB congeners in filtered air, in particulates and in rain collected simultaneously in an urban area in the former Federal Republic of Germany. The PCB mixture was dominated by congeners with a low degree of chlorination in the filtered air, by congeners with a high degree of chlorination in the aerosols and in rain. The vapour phase represented up to 99% of total atmospheric concentrations for the most volatile congeners. Particle scavenging was the most dominant source of PCBs in rain, despite the small contribution (only 1 or 2%) of particulate PCBs to the total atmospheric concentration. Little data is available concerning the chemical reactivity of the organochlorine pesticides and PCBs under tropospheric conditions. The major chemical reaction for many of these compounds in the troposphere appears to be with hydroxyl radicals.

Polychlorinated Dibenzodioxins and Polychlorianted Dibenzofurans

Polychlorinated dibenzo-p-dioxins (PCDDs) and polychlorinated dibenzofurans (PCDFs), which do not occur naturally nor are they intentionally released, are of increasing toxicological and environmental concern. This is a consequence of their ubiquity in the environment and the reported carcinogenicity of specific isomers of these two important classes of chlorinated derivatives. There are 75 isomers of the PCDDs and 135 PCDF isomers of which 2,3,7,8-tetrachlorodibenzo-p-dioxin (TCDD) is by far the most toxic. Toxicities can vary by a factor of 1,000 to 10,000 for isomers as closely related as 2,3,7,8- and 1,2,3,4-TCDD and 1,2,4,7,8-pentachlorodibenzodioxin [246-249].

The principal sources of emission of the PCDDs and PCDFs into the atmosphere are the incineration of municipal, hazardous and hospital wastes and of sewage sludge which contain PCDDs and PCDFs as unintentional by-products or trace impurities. Other sources include: overheating and emissions from fires and explosions involving PCBs; chemical plant accidents (e.g., near Seveso, Italy in 1976); fossil fuel combustion; automobile operation and the improper disposal of contaminated production waste [246-253].

Recent studies have shown the presence of numerous PCDD/PCDF congeners in Swedish, Danish and Canadian incinerator wastes with virtually all the congeners present [247-251]. The 2,3,7,8-TCDD congener was always present as a minor constituent, whereas in all samples 1,2,3,7,8-penta-CDD was a peak of "medium" size. The toxic hexa-CDDs and hexa-CDFs were always medium or major components. A striking similarity in the pattern of PCDDs and PCDFs was found between the samples from different incinerators. Hutzinger et al. [252] suggested that about 3-4% of the total PCDD stack emissions near municipal incinerators may be tetrachloro isomers of which about 5% could be 2,3,7,8-TCDD.

PCDDs and PCDFs emitted from a variety of combustion processes can undergo long-distance transport and can enter ultimate environmental sinks such as soils, sediments, oceans or lakes through wet and dry deposition and vapour uptake [242,246-248,251, 254]. These components are either absorbed to particulate matter of different size ranges formed during combustion processes when emitted from the source or are present in the vapour phase. PCDDs and PCDFs during the course of time can undergo association with aerosols as they are transported [255] and certain congeners are extremely stable substances which, once released, are persistent in the environment [246-253].

About 20% of atmospheric TCDD exists in the vapour phase [254,256]. Air-to-vegetation transfer of atmospheric TCDD accounts for about 66% of TCDD in forage that beef and dairy cattle consume [13].

Ambient air in urban industrialised areas contains 0.01 to 10 picograms/m^3 PCDD and PCDF levels which are 5 to 10 times higher than those found in rural areas. The isomer profiles closely resemble those found in emissions from incineration plants and traffic [248,252,257].

Polycyclic Aromatic Hydrocarbons

Polycyclic aromatic hydrocarbons (PAHs) are widespread environmental contaminants that are formed from both natural (forest and prairie fires) and principally anthropogenic sources such as the incomplete combustion of almost any fuel, e.g., fossil, wood and biomass. The urban atmosphere contains many PAHs which are primarily related to incomplete fuel combustion in domestic heating, industrial plants and vehicular traffic [2,3,24,258-263]. A large number of PAHs ranging from naphthalene to 5- and 6-ring and higher PAHs, their alkyl substituted analogues and their oxygen- and nitrogen-containing derivatives are emitted from motor vehicle sources. In addition, heterocyclic analogues containing ring O-, S-, and N-atoms are combustion source emissions [3].

More than 100 PAH compounds have been identified in the organic fraction of urban atmospheric particulate of which more than half have been confirmed by comparison with reference substances [262,263]. Although PAHs in air are associated with both the gas phase and particulate matter, the more extensive studies have been performed on PAH in the particulate phase [3,262,263]. The ratio of PAHs in the vapour and particulate phase of urban and rural samples in ambient air vary considerably with the season and the scavenging effects of rain and snow. In temperate climates, the 2- to 4-ring PAHs are found primarily in the gas phase and under mid-continental wintertime temperatures (in the U.S.) the distribution shifts markedly toward the particulate phase [3].

Air emission from various combustion sources can transport PAHs long distances before they are deposited on land and water surfaces through dry and wet deposition [255]. Atmospheric transformations of PAHs depend to a great extent on the phase with which they are associated. For PAHs present in the gas phase, reactions primarily with the hydroxyl radical and to a lesser extent with N_2O_5 lead to atmospheric PAH lifetimes of a few hours or less [3]. The daytime decay of PAHs on atmospheric particles is influenced by humidity, sunlight and temperature. Occurring reactions, including photolysis, are strongly dependent on the nature of the absorbent species [3,264].

There is increasing evidence that a number of PAHs can react with atmospheric oxidants, e.g., peroxyacetyl nitrate, nitric acid and nitrous acid, to form various nitroarenes whose toxicity (primarily mutagenicity) is often greater than that of the parent compound [266].

Recent studies from Scandinavia and the U.S. have shown that 2-nitropyrene and 2-nitrofluoranthene, nitro-PAHs not observed directly from combustion processes, are the major nitro-PAHs of ambient particulate matter [3,265].

Pitts [266] demonstrated that in gas phase reactions, several PAHs which are abundant in urban atmospheres react with OH radical in the presence of NOx during the daytime and with N_2O_5 at night to produce nitroarenes such as 2-nitrofluoranthene, 1-nitropyrene and 2-nitropyrene. It should also be noted that a number of nitroarenes have been found in primary emissions of diesel soot, e.g.,1-nitropyrene, 3-nitrofluoranthene and 8-nitrofluoranthene [266-268].

Arey et al. [269] reported that in ambient atmospheres the nitro derivatives of the 2-ring PAH may be significantly more abundant than the particle-associated nitrofluoranthenes and nitropyrenes. It was shown that the majority of nitroarenes present in ambient air are formed from the gas phase reactions of N_2O_5 and/or the OH radical in the presence of NOx. Helmig et al. [270] recently reported the formation of mutagenic nitrobenzopyranones from the OH radical-initiated reaction of phenanthrenes in the presence of NOx and showed that these and probably other nitropolycyclic lactones are present in ambient air particles.

Many uncertainties remain regarding the persistence of PAHs, their chemical transformation and their transport and fate in the atmosphere [3,258,259,264]. For example, there are reports that PAHs degrade rapidly in the atmosphere with lifetimes as short as several hours. In contrast, a number of studies suggest that PAHs degrade slowly, if at all, in the atmosphere and eventually deposit on soil or water. This is supported by studies of marine sediments, the ultimate sinks of the PAHs. These studies have shown that the relative abundance of PAHs, even at the most remote locations, is similar to the level in combustion sources, suggesting that PAHs are stable in the atmosphere.

The measurement of PAHs over the last 40 years has undergone dramatic changes primarily reflecting the advances in analytical methodology. From the first investigations in the 1950s until the mid 1970s, the concentrations of few PAHs were measured, most commonly benzo(a)pyrene (BaP), which served as an indicator for the PAH class [258,259,261-263].

The general conclusions which could be drawn from early studies [261,271-273] from the 1950s until the mid 1960s that primarily measured atmospheric BaP in Europe and the U.S. include: BaP levels in Europe were generally about 5-100 ng/m^3 in winter with some higher concentrations of up to 610 ng/m^3 found; in the summer the levels of BaP were generally much lower, averaging a few ng/m^3; lower levels of BaP were measured in U.S. towns, with 2-3 ng/m^3 the average levels found in 32 towns during the period of 1966-1970; levels of 0.03-3.5 ng/m^3 were found in Los Angeles (1971-1972).

A few data concerning PAHs other than BaP were measured during the period 1958-1968 in a small number of European, U.S. and Australian towns [261,274].

The development of high resolution gas chromatography and HPLC since the 1970s has permitted the determination of a broader range of PAHs (generally 10-15) to be determined in atmospheric samples. Typical average BaP levels were found in the range of about 1-20 ng/m^3 in Europe and about 1 ng/m^3 in the U.S. For other PAHs, individual average levels were generally measured in the ranges of about 1-50 ng/m^3 in Europe, 0.1-1 in North and South America and in Australia, 1-10 in Japan and as maximum values 10-100 ng/m^3 in Calcutta [261]. The highest values of PAH with relativly high vapour pressure (3- and 4-ring compounds) were obtained in studies where vapour phase PAHs were also collected, apart from particulate matter. A variety of factors contributed to the variations in PAH levels found during recent decades. Vehicle fuels and domestic heating are commonly indicated as the principal sources of PAH pollution in urban air [2,3,261,275]. Additional major sources of PAH pollution in urban air may be industrial emissions such as those from coke ovens.

Mitigating factors that can result in the lowering of PAH emissions include: decreased coal burning for residential heating, greater utilisation of gas or oil for home heating, introduction of anti-smoke regulations concerning industrial emissions, solid waste incineration, open fires and the greater utilisation of catalytic converters for cars in some countries. Counter-balancing these factors are the increased traffic found in almost all developed and many developing countries [11,12,261].

The total annual release of PAHs from mobile sources in the U.S. has been estimated. In the case of benzo(a)pyrene, all mobile sources produced about 43 metric tons in 1979, including 27 tons from motor vehicles; 63% and 37% of the BaP emissions from motor vehicles occurred in urban and rural areas, respectively. It was projected that the total motor vehicle BaP emissions in the U.S. will decrease by the year 2000 to 24 metric tons, of which only about 40% will be in urban areas [258]. On the basis of motor vehicle emission values for 1979, the average daily BaP concentration in the urban atmosphere in the U.S. was calculated to be 1.3 ng/m^3 [124]. United States annual BaP atmospheric emission from all combustion sources, including both mobile and stationary sources, was estimated at between 300 and 1,300 metric tons [258].

The emissions of BaP in the atmosphere from several sources in the Federal Republic of Germany in 1981 were estimated to amount to 18 tonnes, of which 56% was caused by heating with coal, 30% by coal production, 13% by motor vehicles and less than 0.5% by heating with oil and coal-fired power generation [2]. Earlier BaP emissions resulting from the use of hard coal briquettes for heating purposes were much higher since such briquettes were made employing a binder with 7% pitch which contained 1% BaP [2].

While PAH levels have progressively decreased in the last few decades primarily in the OECD countries [11,12], it should be re-stressed that the situation in central and eastern Europe and the former Soviet Union is quite different due to their former heavy reliance on the combustion of brown coal and lignite for domestic heating and power generation and industrial uses, as well as the widespread use of inefficient 2-stroke vehicles as noted earlier [11,12,87-91]. Hence PAH emissions could be expected to be much higher than those found in western Europe, the U.S. and Japan until major structural and remedial steps are undertaken in those regions [11,12,87-91].

In one study involving the continuous monitoring of air over the highly industrialised region of Upper Silesia in southern Poland in 1987, over 100 PAHs were found in extracts from airborne particulates [271]. Fifteen major PAHs were evaluated quantitatively at 20 measuring stations during the summer and winter periods. The direct mutagenic activity was higher in winter samples than in the summer samples although the summer samples showed high mutagenic activity after metabolic activation. Besides industrial pollution, heavy automobile traffic and combustion of coal for cooking and heating of residential houses contributed to air pollution especially in the winter [276].

An additional recent source of significant quantities of PAH emission (as well as sulphur dioxide, carbon dioxide, CO, soot and other particulate matter) has been the Kuwait oil fires [72-77] in which 4.6 million barrels of oil were burning daily. In one recent study in which inhalable air particulate matter (APM) was collected in Bahrain from July 31, 1991 to August 4, 1991 during the burning of the Kuwaiti oil fields, a total of 32 PAHs were measured with concentrations ranging from 3.1 to 9.1 ng/m^3 and averaging 5.3 ng/m^3. The highest individual PAH levels were benzo(ghi)perylene, benzo(b)fluoranthene, benzo(a)pyrene and indeno(1,2,3-cd)pyrene [277].

Suspended Particulate Matter

The generic classification "atmospheric particulates" includes smoke, soot, dust, ash, liquid droplets and aerosols encompassing an enormous variety of inorganic and organic substances that can be generated from both natural and man-made sources. Hence individual particles can be composed of different chemicals, and can be homogeneous or heterogeneous in structure and vary in size and shape. Particle size has been principally employed as the single most important parameter in specifying the composition of airborne particulate matter. Because of the complexity of particulate matter, multiple terms such as suspended particulate matter, total suspended particulates, black smoke as well as terms referring to the site of deposition in the respirable tract are often used [2].

Mass and composition of particulate matter can be divided into two principal groups: coarse particles larger than 2.5 μm in aerodynamic diameter and fine particles smaller than 2.5 μm in aerodynamic diameter. The natural sources of particulate matter include volcanoes and dust storms while the more widespread and important anthropogenic sources are vehicular traffic, domestic coal burning, power plants, agricultural practices, industrial processes and incinerators [2,4,5,8,11,12,35-37].

The combustion of fuels is the largest source of particulates in most OECD countries; in the European Community it is estimated to be responsible for 95% of man-made particulates [12]. Condensation of gases such as sulphur dioxide and VOCs is also a significant source of particulates. Roughly half of all human-caused particulates arise from the conversion of sulphur dioxide to sulphate particles in the atmosphere [11].

Carbonaceous materials account for a significant fraction of urban and rural aerosols which can be categorised into organic and elemental classes. Elemental carbon, also called black or graphite carbon, is predominantly emitted into the atmosphere in particulate form whereas organic aerosol can be emitted directly in particulate form (primary aerosol) or found in the atmosphere from products of gas-phase photochemical reactions (secondary aerosol) [267].

Since the early 1980s there has been an increased utilisation of diesel engines in both light and heavy duty motor vehicles and of coal for power generation in many countries. This has resulted in the increasingly heavy burden of atmospheric fine particulates as well as gaseous NOx and sulphur dioxide in major urban areas throughout the world [35-37,268,278].

Organic compounds absorbed in the particulate phase of petrol and diesel exhausts have been studied extensively. Diesel particulate organic matter (POM) is emitted in the sub-micron respiratory range (<0.5μm) and, comparable to most combustion-generated particulates, contains a number of promutagenic and carcinogenic PAHs as well as other unidentified mutagens that exhibit strong direct activity in the Ames Salmonella/mammalian microsomal assay [35-37,268,279,280].

The characterisation of organic particulate mixtures is extremely difficult. Urban air particles contain extractable organic matter that has been shown in many instances to possess mutagenic and carcinogenic activity. The concentrations of PAHs in the particulate phase of ambient air have been studied extensively [35-37]. The ratio of PAHs in the vapour and particulate phases of the samples monitored has been shown to vary considerably with the traffic, season and meteorological conditions [18]. A large number of PAHs have been isolated from pariculates emitted in diesel exhausts. These include: phenanthrene, fluoranthene, pyrene, benzo(ghi)fluoranthene, cyclopenteno(cd)pyrene, benzo(a)anthracene, chrysene, benzo(a)pyrene, benzo(e)pyrene, indeno(1,2,3-ed)pyrene, benzo(ghi)pyrene and coronene [281,282].

The nitro-PAHs that have been found in diesel particulates include: nitrofluorenes, nitroanthracenes, nitrophenanthrenes, nitrofluoranthenes, nitropyrene and methylnitropyrene and methylnitrofluoranthenes which are believed to account for a major portion of the direct acting TA-98 Ames mutagenicity of diesel particulates [268,282]. Many mutagenic fractions of diesel particulate extracts have been found to contain oxygenated PAH derivatives including compounds with hydroxy, ketone, quinone, carboxaldehyde, acid anhydride, dihydroxy and acid substituents on the parent PAH [282].

Chemical and physical transformation may occur in the presence of sunlight and oxygen and covers a spectrum of co-pollutants such as HONO, $HONO_2$, PAN and the nitrate radical during transport of wood smoke and diesel particulate organic matter and NOx in the atmosphere over periods of hours, days or even weeks.

Another major source of atmospheric particulates derives from metallic elements in fuel combustion products. Of some 80 elements that are considered as metals, about 50 have been reported to be present in coal, 35 in crude oil, 30 in fuel oil and about 20 in petrol. As a result of combustion, these elements are mobilised and may be emitted into the atmosphere primarily as constituents of particulate matter containing a mixture of inorganic and organic substances [282]. The composition and structure of these particulate emissions depend on the fuel and the combustion processes employed. Combustion of fossil fuels in electric power plants, commercial boilers and furnaces for space heating, as well as in motor vehicle exhausts is the principal anthropogenic source of metallic elements in the atmosphere.

Metallic elements mobilised by coal combustion are partitioned between the slag or bottom ash and fly ash, with some metals temporarily remaining in the gaseous state. During combustion the chalcophile elements (those which readily form sulphides) are volatilised and later condensed onto the surface of fly ash particles. Since the surface area per unit mass increases with decreasing particle size, the concentration of metallic elements increases in the submicron (respirable) range of particle size [283]. The levels of suspended particulate matter are increasing in the urban atmosphere of developing countries [284].

National trends in emissions and urban ambient concentrations of particulates are mixed. In general, western industrialised countries have made significant progress since 1970 in reducing urban particulates as well as national emissions of particulates. However, many developing countries with growing urban vehicle numbers or expanding industrial sectors have had increases in particulate levels (as well as sulphur dioxide and NOx) [11,12].

The United Nations-sponsored Global Environmental Monitoring System estimated in 1987 that 70% of the world's urban population lived in cities where the level of suspended particulates exceeded WHO guidelines [11,160].

As noted earlier, there has been, and to a large extent still is, extensive air pollution in many areas of central and eastern Europe and the former Soviet Union, principally due to the heavy reliance on domestic lignite or brown coal for residential heating, power generation and industrial heating and processes [11,12,87-91]. In addition to the massive amounts of sulphur dioxide generated from these uses, large quantities of particulates are emitted into the atmosphere. For example, in 1985 East Germany (DDR) emitted between 5 and 6 million metric tons of particulate matter, whereas Sweden had an estimated annual emission rate in 1982-1984 of 40,000 metric tons [12].

It should also be noted that due to the recent Kuwait oil fires [72-77] in which 4.6 million barrels of oil were burning daily from over 600 ignited wells, the emission of soot (elemental carbon) amounted to approx. 3400 metric tons per day [72]; this absorbed approx. 75-80% of the sun's radiation in regions of the Persian Gulf. However, the smoke was believed to have minimal global effects since the particle emissions (including soot) averaged 12,000 metric tons per day, which was less than that expected. Additionally, the smoke was not carried high into the atmosphere (about 6 km), i.e., below the base of the stratosphere in the region (about 13 km). As a result of scavenging by clouds and precipitation, the average residence time of these particles in the atmosphere was estimated to be relatively short (days) [72].

Metals and Metalloids

The toxicologically important metals and metalloids such as mercury, cadmium, chromium, lead, nickel, arsenic and selenium are found in significant amounts in the atmosphere as a result of both natural and anthropogenic activities. Particularly since the industrial revolution, a number of metals have become widespread in the environment. They appear in metallic form in pipes, solders, structures, electrical supplies, they are part of inorganic and organic compounds, and have been widely used in paints and pigments, fuel additives and pesticides. It is well established that many trace elements are mobilised in association with airborne particles derived from high-temperature combustion sources such as fossil-fueled power plants, blast furnaces, metallurgical smelters, municipal incinerators and vehicle exhaust [2,6,285-293].

Combustion of hard coal, lignites and brown coal in electrical power plants, commercial and residential burners is the major source of airborne Hg, Mo and Se and a very significant source of As, Cd, Cr, Mn, Pb, Sb and Tl, while the combustion of oil for the same purposes is the most important source of V and Ni and is an important contributor of Sn. The non-ferrous metal industry accounts for the largest fraction of As, Cd, Cu, Zn and Pb (in addition to petrol) emitted [6,92,285,286].

Chemical, physical and biological effects of airborne metals are a direct function of particle size, concentration and composition. The major parameter governing the significance of both natural and anthropogenic emissions of environmentally and toxicologically important metals is particle size. Many elements, notably Pb, Cd, Cr, Ni, Mn, Zn, V, anc Cu, are found at the highest concentration in the smallest particles collected from ambient air [285-289].

Stationary sources are the principal contributors of most of the environmentally significant metals in air. The trend for the immediate future in many developed and developing countries appears to be for greater emission of metals such as As, Be, Cd, Cr, Hg, Mn, Pb, Se, Sb, V and Zn, not only as a result of increased usage patterns but also because of prospective enhanced use of fossil fuels for space heating and electricity generation (whether from conventional coal-fired power plants or new coal technologies such as *in-situ* gasification, coal pyrolysis, or chemical precleaning) particularly in the U.S. For example, in 1973 coal use for electrical power generation in the U.S. produced 3.6 million tons of fly ash, 26% of the total U.S. particulate emissions [290]. With the addition of 241 new coal-fired power plants, coal consumption by U.S. electrical utilities expanded from 446 million tons in 1976 to more than 840 million tons, further increasing the amount of fly ash emitted to the atmosphere with concomitant entrained toxic metals.

Global inventories indicate that coal combustion is an important atmospheric source of mercury and arsenic [286,291,292], while iron and steel production is a significant source of airborne lead. Lead emissions from refuse incineration - although considerable - are small compared with Pb emissions from motor vehicles using leaded-petrol [293].

The major stationary emission sources for Be, Cd, Cr, Mn, Ni, Pb, Ti and Cu are from smelter metallurgical processing and coal and oil combustion. Emissions from incineration are greatly dependent on the composition of the waste material burned [286,294,295]. Many of the metals found in higher concentrations from incinerator atmospheric emissions such as Cr, Pb, Sn and Zn are metals that are used in surface coatings, galvanising solders and similar surface applications where high temperatures could cause flaking and volatilisation from bulk metal scrap [294].

During incineration up to 35% of metals in a hazardous waste stream can be emitted into the atmosphere. The stack emissions can include As, Cd, Hg, Pb and Ni [295]. Refuse incineration is a major source of atmospheric cadmium in the U.S. and the United Kingdom [296,297]. The incineration of 3.15×10^6 tons/year of refuse in the U.K. has been suggested to yield annual emissions of 6 tons of atmospheric cadmium and 115 tons of lead. In the U.S. the incineration of urban refuse may be responsible for the major fractions of Co, Zn, Sb and possibly Sn, In and Ag found in aerosols in many cities [294].

Nriagu [298] described a global inventory of anthropogenic emissions of Cd, Cu, Ni, Pb and Zn to the atmosphere in 1975. A more recent report of Nriagu and Pacryna [6] provides a revision of the earlier data [299] and extends the calculations to many more trace elements.

The following world-wide anthropogenic emissions (median values x 10^3 kg/yr) were reported of elements in 1983 [6]: arsenic: 18,820; cadmium: 7570; chromium: 30,480; mercury: 3,560; nickel: 55,650; lead: 332,350 and selenium: 3,790 (this figure is for particulate Se only, because volatile Se accounts for about 40% of the Se released, the total Se emission was estimated to be 6,320 tonnes/year). The anthropogenic source categories included: coal and oil combustion (electric utilities, industry and domestic), pyrometallurgical (non-ferrous metal production, mining, Pb, Cu-Ni and Zn-Cd production), secondary non-ferrous production, steel and iron production, refuse incineration (municipal, sewage waste), phosphate fertilisers, cement production, wood combustion and mobile sources (petrol-fueled).

Mean global emissions from natural sources have recently been estimated to be (in tonnes/yr): As, 7800; Cd, 1000; Ni, 2600; Pb, 66,000 and Hg, 6000. Approximately 6,000-13,000 times as much Se is annually released into the atmosphere from natural sources, with 60-80% of the total Se emission arising from marine biogenic origins. On average the anthropogenic emissions to the atmosphere of arsenic, cadmium, copper, nickel and zinc exceed the natural inputs of these elements by a factor of 2 or more, while in the case of lead the ratio of anthropogenic to natural emission rates is about 17 [6].

The impact of acidification (acid rain) on the changing chemical speciation and mobilisation of metal, which is particularly enhanced for mercury, aluminum, lead and selenium, should also be noted.

Arsenic

Aside from arsenic trioxide from volcanic activity, only human activities produce significant air concentrations of this metalloid. Hot metallurgical processes, particularly primary and secondary non-ferrous smelters (e.g., copper, lead, zinc and their alloys), are the major source of high occupational and local community exposure to arsenic trioxide and cadmium oxide. Large total amounts of both arsenic and cadmium may be released via coal combustion and municipal incineration. The arsenic concentrations in coal range from 0.34 to 130 µg/g and can reach 1,500 µg/g in some Czechoslovakian lignites [2,286]. Such coals with very high As levels are used locally and should be considered in estimating the local or even national emission levels [6]. For example, in Prague, airborne arsenic concentrations were found to be 450 ng/m^3 on average in winter and 70 ng/m^3 in summer [2].

Additional emissions of arsenic can result from the combustion of wood-containing preservatives, glass enamel production, use of arsenical pesticides, production of high-purity arsenic metal, semi-conductor alloys, lead shot and some lead and copper alloys.

Trivalent arsenic is oxidised to pentavalent arsenic in the outdoor environment; as a result, some smelter emissions deposited near plant sites have As (V) levels. Background levels of arsenic (in particulate form as inorganic arsenic) generally range from 1-10 ng/m^3 in rural areas but can reach several hundred ng/m^3 in some cities and exceed 1000 ng/m^3 near non-ferrous metal smelters and some power plants, depending on the levels of arsenic in the combusted coal [2,286].

Cadmium

Cadmium in particulate urban air pollution arises predominantly as the oxide from hot-metal operations and combustion of products containing trace amounts of cadmium such as cadmium pigments, additives to rubber and plastic, metal from plating and alloys. Refuse incineration is a major source of atmospheric cadmium release at the global level. In Europe, other major sources of atmospheric cadmium are the steel and zinc production industries [2,286].

The yearly means of cadmium in air range from <1 to 5 ng/m^3 in rural areas, 5-15 ng/m^3 in urban areas and 15-50 ng/m^3 in industrialised areas. A compilation of Cd levels for member states of the European Community gave ranges of 0/1-1 ng/m^3 for remote areas, 1-50 ng/m^3 for urban areas and 1-100 ng/m^3 for industrialised areas [2].

In Czechoslovakia, the main source of air pollution by cadmium is from power plants burning coal (predominantly lignite). The average Cd content in lignite is about 13 g/ton. The average emissions of Cd from this source in power plants are about 0.01 mg/m^3, with considerable enrichment with oxides of Cd occurring on the surface of particles <2 µm in diameter. The average concentration of Cd in atmospheric precipitation in Czechoslovakia is 0.2-5.0 g/litre [92].

Some general air pollution (24-hour exposure) levels have been reported for arsenic and cadmium. The levels for arsenic (25-40% deposition and absorption depending on particle size and chemical form) are 0.02-0.07 µg/m^3 or a daily pulmonary dose of 0.08-0.28 µg. For cadmium (25-90% deposition and absorption depending on particle size and compound) 0.002-0.05 µg/m^3 or a daily dose of 0.008-0.2 µg [300].

Mercury

Mercury is emitted into the atmosphere from both natural and man-made sources. The natural sources include: volcanic, crustal degassing, oceans, geysers and forest fires. The principal man-made sources include: coal and oil combustion, incineration of municipal solid waste (including Hg volatilised from discarded batteries) and smelting and reforming processes for the production of copper and zinc. Other anthropogenic sources include: chlor-alkali plants, cement manufacturing, paint production and use [6,286,301-304]. About 65% of anthropogenic emissions of Hg into the atmosphere are from coal burning and another 25% are due to waste incineration; a relatively small amount is due to ore refining [304].

Emission measurements and mass balance calculations performed at coal-burning power stations suggest that 80-100% of the mercury in coal escapes into the atmosphere as elemental mercury vapour rather than in particulate form. Mercury appears to be a highly anomalous metal, existing in ambient air primarily as the reduced elemental form since the atmospheric processes are well known to be oxidising (e.g., production of photochemical smog and oxidation of acid-rain precursors such as sulphur dioxide and nitrogen dioxide). Additionally, most metals exist in ambient air as oxides or other compounds with chemical oxidation states greater than zero (e.g., metal sulphates, nitrates or chlorides) [2,6,301,302].

On a global basis, current anthropogenic emissions of mercury to the troposphere are estimated to be of a similar order of magnitude as pre-industrial emissions from natural sources. It is expected that increased fossil fuel consumption for industrial, commercial or domestic purposes will further increase the anthropogenic mercury [305]. In Europe, anthropogenic emissions of mercury in 1985 were projected to be approx. 2630 tonnes, of which 765 tonnes would be emitted into the atmosphere, while natural emissions would amount to about 570 tonnes, nearly all (527 tonnes) being emitted into the atmosphere [2]. The total global amount and release of mercury due to human activities has been estimated to be approx. 3,000 tonnes/year, while the natural emissions are of the order of 2700-6000 tonnes per year [302,303]. Since the beginning of the 19th century the global deposition of atmospheric mercury may have increased by a factor ranging from 0.5 to 5.1 [304]. The atmospheric concentrations of mercury (total gaseous mercury, of which more than 92% of background consists of elemental Hg) have increased by 1.46±0.17% per year in the Northern Hemisphere and by 1.17±0.16% per year in the Southern Hemisphere. These rates of increase were consistent with the results of soil, peat bog and lake sediment analyses and suggest that human rather than natural sources are at present more important in the mercury cycle [304]. World-wide coal production increased at an annual rate of 2.1% between 1965 and 1987 and about 90% of coal was burned in the Northern Hemisphere [304].

An apparent increasing source of atmospheric mercury in the Southern Hemisphere should be noted. For example, mercury emissions from the Amazon region of South America, where mercury is used in the recovery of gold and silver, accounts for about 2% (70 tons/yr) of total global atmospheric mercury emissions [13].

Background levels of mercury in the troposphere of the Northern Hemisphere are estimated at 2 ng/m^3. In areas of Europe remote from industrial activity, mean concentrations of total Hg in the atmosphere are normally in the range of 2-3 ng/m^3 in the summer and 3-4 ng/m^3 in the winter [2]. Concentrations of atmospheric mercury reported in the member states of the European Community range from 0.001-6 ng/m^3 in remote areas, 0.1-5 ng/m^3 in urban areas to 0.5-20 ng/m^3 in industrial areas [2,306].

The atmospheric residence time for mercury vapour is between 0.4 and 3 years whereas soluble forms of mercury have a residence time of only a few weeks [301,302]. The relatively long residence time for mercury vapour suggests that its emissions from both natural and man-made sources are readily mixed intra-hemispherically and can be transferred inter-hemispherically. Thus mercury emissions from the Northern Hemisphere will be transported to the atmosphere of the Southern Hemisphere [301].

There is a well recognised global cycle for mercury whereby emitted mercury vapor is converted to soluble forms (e.g., divalent mercury) and deposited by rain to soil and water.

The current geographical broad pattern (e.g., U.S., Canada and Sweden) of elevated mercury levels in fish, even in watersheds far removed from anthropogenic sources, suggests that increases in atmospheric mercury deposition are occurring on a hemispheric scale. Atmospheric transport of mercury from the continents should be most pronounced in the Atlantic Ocean because of the proximity to terrestrial sources to the ocean atmosphere [301].

Lead

Airborne lead is derived from both natural and man-made sources [6,286,307-312]. Global emissions from natural sources have been estimated at 66,000 tonnes/yr [6]. Natural concentrations of lead result from airborne dust containing on the average 10-15 µg/g lead, and from gases diffusing from the earth's crust [6,310-312]. The concentration of lead in air from natural origins is about 0.0006 µg/m^3 [308].

Anthropogenic emissions of lead to the atmosphere are derived primarily from combustion of leaded petrol and to a lesser degree from the combustion of coal, metal smelters and the incineration of municipal solid wastes (MSW) [6,13,286,307-312].

In the U.S. about 39,000 tons of lead are emitted to the atmosphere each year, including 35,000 tons as petrol additives (alkyl leads) [13,307]. Although emissions from leaded petrol combustion have declined with the decrease in petrol lead content (from about 0.8 to 0.15 g/litre), leaded petrol consumption in vehicles still accounted for 90% of the total anthropogenic input into the U.S. atmosphere in 1984 [13]. The remaining 10% was from stationary sources, i.e., 5% from the metallurgy industry, 4% from waste combustion and energy production and 1% from miscellaneous sources [13,307].

The major contributors of lead to discards in municipal solid waste in the U.S. in 1986 were lead-acid batteries (accounting for 60% of lead), glass and ceramic products, solder and pigments. It has also been suggested that the uncontrolled burning of used motor oil is the largest industrial source of airborne lead pollution. More than 90% of the oil collected for recycling, almost 800 million gallons annually in the U.S., is claimed to be burned in residential and industrial boilers, resulting in the emission of 25,000 kg of lead into the air [313].

A variety of alkyl lead species may be present in the atmosphere as a result of tetraalkyl lead emissions arising from the use of leaded petrol in motor vehicles. In the atmosphere, tetraalkyl lead compounds are decomposed to trialkyl, and dialkyl lead as well as inorganic Pb, principally via reaction with OH radicals. Half-lives of 5-10 hours for tetramethyl lead and 0-2 hours for tetraethyl lead were estimated for the summer months. Trialkyl lead species also react with the OH radical but the reaction rates are slower than for the tetraalkyl lead compounds. Trimethyl lead has a half-life of 5 days, suggesting that trialkyl lead compounds are fairly persistent intermediates in the atmospheric decomposition of tetraalkyl lead additives for petrol.

Vapour phase alkyl lead compounds have also been measured in atmospheric particulate matter at levels of picograms Pb/m^3 [314]. Most of the lead in the air is in the form of fine particles with a mass median equivalent diameter of one micron. The organic level fraction that escaped combustion is generally below 10% of the total atmospheric lead, with over 90% of lead from leaded petrol emitted as inorganic particles, e.g., PbBrCl [2].

Ambient urban air concentrations of organic lead measured in the U.S. have been found to vary from 0.006-0.3 µg/m^3, while levels varied in Stockholm from 0.4-3.337 µg/m^3 with daily levels of tetraalkyl lead ranging from 0.22-0.59 µg/m^3 [310].

Lead emissions have been reduced in most OECD countries particularly from the mid and late 1980s, largely as a result of regulatory legislation limiting the use of lead additives in petrol and the greater use of catalytic exhaust emission controls. Atmospheric emissions of lead decreased most sharply in North America by over 50% between the mid 1970s and the mid 1980s. In Europe, reduction of lead emissions have been more modest starting later (e.g., mainly in the late 1980s) and the reductions ranged from 45% in the Netherlands to 60% in the U.K. [12]. Currently in most European cities urban lead levels are in the range of 0.5 to 3.0 µg/m^3 (annual means) [2]. In rural areas levels of lead range from 0.1 to 0.3 µg/m^3 [2].

In spite of much progress in lowering the lead levels in petrol with the commensurate reduction in airborne lead, lead contamination continues to be a sizable problem in that as many as one-third of the world's cities have air lead levels exceeding the WHO lead standard. Many of these cities are in developing countries where traffic chokes some urban areas, lead levels in petrol are often high and conversion to unleaded fuel is not yet underway [11].

It should be added that the combustion of lignite in many cenral and eastern European countries has greatly exacerbated environmental lead pollution. For example, in Czechoslovakia, although the main source of lead pollution is from road traffic, power plants and residences burning fossil fuels also produce significant amounts of atmospheric lead. The average lead content of Czechoslovakian lignite is 134 grams/tonne, and average emissions of Pb from the combustion of lignite in power stations are about 0.17 mg Pb/m^3. While the average annual lead concentrations in the air of urban and rural areas are 0.5-10.0 and 0.1 µg/m^3, respectively, in the centre of Prague the concentrations of lead in air can reach 20 µg/m^3 for short periods [92].

Chromium

Chromium in air can arise from natural (such as wind erosion of shales, clays and many kinds of soils) and anthropogenic sources. The latter include: chromite mining, metallurgical processes, the combustion of coal, cement producing plants, wearing of break-linings, and catalytic emission control systems in vehicles [2,286,310,312,315-317]. Chromium is generally associated with particulates (mass median diameters ranging from 1.5-1.9 microns) in ambient air at concentrations of 0.001-0.1 µg/m^3 [306,315,317].

During the period of 1960-1969, approx. 200 urban stations in the U.S. had annual mean concentrations of 0.01-0.03 µg/m^3 [310]. During the period 1977-1980 many urban and rural areas in the U.S. had chromium concentrations in the range of 5.2 ng/m^3 (24-hour background level) to 156.8 ng/m^3 (urban annual average) [316].

A recent survey of member states of the European Community reported chromium air levels as follows: "remote areas": 0-3 ng/m^3; urban areas: 4-70 ng/m^3 and industrial areas: 5-200 ng/m^3 [306]. In addition, chromium ranges in air of 1-140 ng/m^3 in continental Europe, 45-67 ng/m^3 in Hawaii and 20-70 ng/m^3 in Japan have been reported [2,318].

Nickel

Analogous to other metals, nickel is emitted into the environment from both natural and man-made sources. The major anthropogenic sources (which far exceed natural sources) include: the combustion of coal, residual and fuel oils, incineration of municipal wastes and nickel mining and refining [2,6,286,312, 315,317-321].

Coal and oil combustion are the principal sources of atmospheric nickel in the U.S., with the combustion of oil accounting for 60-98% [2,320]. Atmospheric nickel is considered to exist mainly in the form of aerosols, with different nickel concentrations in particles depending on the type of emitting source [319]. Nickel containing particles released from oil combustion in the California urban area were in the fine size fractions below 1 micron while in coal-fired plants, nickel enrichment occurred in the smaller particulate fraction (<1 micron) [2,289]. Nickel sulphate is the major nickel species in air [2].

The total annual nickel global emission from anthropogenic sources is 43.1x10^6 kg/yr compared to 8.5x10^6 kg/yr derived from natural sources [2,315,321]. The average particulate concentration for nickel has been reported to range from 0-0.6 ng/m^3 in remote areas, 9-50 ng/m^3 in semi-remote areas and 60-300 ng/m^3 in urban areas [2]. Nickel concentration ranges for member states of the European Community were 0.1-0.7 ng/m^3 in remote areas, 3-100 ng/m^3 in urban and 8-200 ng/m^3 in industrial areas [2,306]. Nickel concentrations of particulate matter as high as 3310 µg/m^3 have been found in the ambient air of nickel-processing centres [2]. Particle size measurements of nickel in both urban and remote areas showed mass median aerodynamic diameters of 0.83-1.67µm (U.S. urban), 1.2 µm (Toronto urban) and 0.6 µm (England rural). At least 50% of airborne nickel is in fine particles of <2-3 µm diameter [2,323].

Asbestos

Asbestos is the generic name for a group of naturally occurring mineral silicate fibres of serpentine and amphibole series. The principal varieties of asbestos are chrysotile, crocidolite, amosite, anthophyllite, tremolite and actinolite. Although chrysotile is a reasonably well defined mineral, the 5 amphibole asbestiform fibres possess variable chemical composition. The asbestos fibres are bundles of thinner fibres made up of fibrils which in the case of chrysotile have a diameter of 20-25 nm [2,324,325].

Emissions of asbestos result from natural weathering as well as mining and milling, manufacture of products, construction activities, transport and use of asbestos-containing products, demolition, removal and disposal. Additional sources of asbestos emission arise from processing, rain acidity (which can corrode asbestos-cement sheets) and from the wear of vehicle brake linings [2,324-333].

Asbestos fibres of respirable size form part of a range of fibrous aerosols in the lower atmosphere. Other fibres include man-made mineral fibres [334,335], fibrous silica and aluminium oxide, fibrous gypsum etc. Asbestos fibres may travel considerable distances in the atmosphere because of their aerodynamic properties and since no chemical decomposition of the fibres occurs, the only cleaning mechanism is via washout by rain or snow [2,324,325,327].

The general levels of asbestos found in urban areas vary from 100-1000 fibres (F)/m^3 [2,325,327] and are below 100 F/m^3 in rural areas remote from asbestos emission sources [2,324]. Although levels of asbestos fibres in occupational settings are often higher by orders of magnitude than those found in environmental settings, e.g., 10^5 F/m^3 to more than 10^8 F/m^3, they are now being reduced to below 2×10^6 F/m^3 in most countries and to 0.2-0.5×10^6 F/m^3 in some countries [2,329].

Although the use of spray-on asbestos as a fire-proofing material or insulation has been banned in the U.S. as well as in several European countries, asbestos is incorporated into cement materials such as roofing, shingles, cement pipes, jointing and gaskets, asphalt coats and sealants. As a result of these applications, an estimated 20% of buildings, including hospitals, schools and other public and private structures, contain asbestos-containing materials (ACM) [330,331]. Asbestos in buildings does not spontaneously shed fibres, but physical damage to ACMs by decay, renovation or demolition can cause the release of airborne fibres [326].

Average concentrations of asbestos in urban ambient air are typically less than 1 ng/m^3 and rarely exceed 5 ng/m^3. Concentrations of 100 ng/m^3 to 1000 ng/m^3 have been measured in ambient air near specific asbestos emission sources and in schools and office buildings containing damaged or deteriorating friable asbestos materials. Buildings with intact ACMs seldom show increased concentrations of airborne asbestos over ambient levels [2,326-333]. However, indoor asbestos fibre concentrations can be considerably higher than those found outside [2,332].

Man-Made Mineral Fibres

Man-made mineral fibres (MMMF), also known as man-made vitreous fibres (MMVF), is a generic term which denotes fibrous inorganic substances made primarily from glass, rock or clay. They are generally classified into three groups: glass fibres (comprising glass wool and glass filaments); rockwool and slagwool, and ceramic fibres [324-326]. The term "mineral wool" has also been used to describe "rockwool" and "glasswool". The chemical composition of MMMFs will vary with the source materials, their mechanical properties and durability in the products prepared.

Durable man-made fibres can also be produced from chemicals (e.g., DuPont developed Fybex (potassium octatitinate and Kevlar, an aramid) [324-326]. Most commercial fibrous glass products have mean fibre diameters of about 7.5 μm, which results in mean aerodynamic diameters >22μm. In comparison, slag and rockwool fibres have smaller diameters, typically 3-8 μm [324-326]. Ceramic fibres are typically made of alumina, silica and other metal oxides or non-oxide materials such as silicon carbide [324,325]. Ceramic refractory fibres are smaller and shorter than ceramic textile fibres with average diameters of 2.2-5.0 μm and lengths varying from 40-250 mm [324,325].

The global production of man-made mineral fibres has been estimated at 6 million tonnes in 1985 [325]. In the U.S. fibrous glass accounts for 80% of the MMMF production [325]. In contrast to the considerable data reported for asbestos in ambient air [324-329], there is a paucity of data relating to MMMF in other than occupational settings [324-326]. For example, concentrations ranging from 4×10^{-5} to 1.7×10^{-3} fibres/cm have been measured in ambient air [325]. Few data are available concerning concentrations of MMMF present in the general environment. Concentrations ranging from 4×10^{-5} to 1.7×10^{-3} fibres/cm have been reported in a small number of ambient air sites in California and Germany [324,325].

REFERENCES

1. Graedel TE, Hawkins DT, Claxton LD: Atmospheric compounds: Merging the chemical and bioassay data. In: Graedel TE, Hawkins DT and Claxton LD (eds) Atmospheric Chemical Compounds. Academic Press, Orlando, FL 1986 pp1-42
2. WHO: Air Quality Guidelines For Europe. European Series No 23. Regional Office for Europe, World Health Organization, Copenhagen 1987 p 410
3. Seinfeld TH: Urban air pollution: State of the science. Science 1989 (243):745-752
4. Ember LR, Layman PL, Lepkowski W, Zurer PS: Tending to global commons. Chem Eng News 1986 (Nov 24):14-64
5. McElroy MB, Salawitch RJ: Changing composition of the global stratosphere. Science 1989 (243):763-770
6. Nriagu JO, Pacyna JM: Quantitative assessment of worldwide contamination of air, water and soil by trace metals. Nature 1988 (333):134-139
7. Lloy PJ, Daisey JM: Airborne toxic elements and organic substances. Environ Sci Technol 1985 (20):8-14
8. Shah JJ, Sing HB: Distribution of volatile organic chemicals in outdoor and indoor air. Environ Sci Technol 1988 (22):1383-1388
9. Graham JD, Green LC, Roberts MJ: In Search of Safety - Chemicals and Cancer Risk. Harvard Univ Press, Cambridge MA 1988
10. Schroeder WH, Lane DA: The fate of toxic airborne pollutants. Environ Sci Technol 1988 (22):240-246
11. The World Resources Institute: World Resources 1992-1993. Oxford Univ Press, New York 1992
12. OECD: The State of the Environment. Organization For Economic Co-Operation and Development, Paris 1991
13. Travis CC, Hester ST: Global chemical pollution. Environ Sci Technol 1991 (25):814-819
14. Spengler JD, Sexton K: Indoor air pollution: A public health perspective. Science 1983 (221):9-17
15. National Research Council: Indoor Pollutants. National Academy of Science Press, Washington, DC 1981
16. Lebowitz MD: Health effects of indoor pollutants. Am Rev Publ Hlth 1983 (4):203-210
17. Lewtas J: Toxicology of complex mixtures of indoor air pollutants. Ann Rev Pharmacol Toxicol 1989 (29):415-429
18. Yocum JE: Indoor-outdoor air quality relationships - A critical review. J Am Pollut Control Assoc 1982 (32):500-508
19. Fishbein L, Henry CJ: Introduction: Workshop on the methodology for assessing health risks from complex mixtures in indoor air. Environ Hlth Persp 1991 (95):3-5
20. Fishbein L: Indoor environments: The role of metals. In: Merian E (ed) Metals and their Compounds in the Environment. VCH, Weinheim 1991 pp 287-309
21. Greim H, Sterzyl H, Lilienblum W, Mücke W: Indoor air pollution - A review. Toxicol Env Chem 1989 (23):191-206
22. Berry MA: Indoor air quality: Assessing health impacts and risks. Toxicol Ind Hlth 1991 (7):179-186
23. Wallace LA: The Total Exposure - Assessment Methodology (TEAM) study: An analysis of exposures, sources and risks associated with four volatile organic chemicals. J Am Coll Toxicol 1989 (8):883-895
24. Wallace LA: Comparison of risks from outdoor and indoor exposure to toxic chemicals. Environ Hlth Persp 1991 (95):7-13
25. Goldstein BD: Predicting the risks of indoor air pollutants. Toxicol Ind Hlth 1991 (7):195-201
26. Stolwijk JAJ: Assessment of population exposure and carcinogenic risk posed by volatile organic compounds in indoor air. Risk Anal 1990 (10):49-57
27. U.S. EPA: Indoor Air Assessment. Indoor Concentrations of Environmental Carcinogens. U.S. Environmental Protection Agency, Research Triangle Park, NC 1991 EPA/600-8-90/042
28. Stolwijk JAJ: Sick building syndrome. Environ Hlth Persp 1991 (95):99-101
29. WHO: Health Aspects Related to Indoor Air Quality. Report on a WHO Working Group. EURP. Reports and Studies. No 211. WHO Regional Office, Copenhagen 1979
30. Hileman G: Multiple chemical sensitivity. Chem Eng News 1991 (July 22):26-42
31. Ashford NA, Miller CS: Chemical Exposures: Low Levels and High Stakes. Van Nostrand, New York 1991 p 214
32. U.S. EPA: Report to Congress on Air Quality. Vol II. Assessment and Control of Indoor Air Pollution. U.S. Environmental Protection Agency, Washington, DC 1989 EPA/400/1-89/001c
33. Crutzen PJ, Andrae MO: Biomass burning in the tropics: Impact on atmospheric and biogeochemical cycles. Science 1990 (250):1669-1678
34. Setzer AW, Pereira MC: Amazonia biomass burnings in 1987. An estimate of their tropospheric emissions. Ambio 1001 (20):19-22
35. Lewtas J: Combustion emissions: Characterization and comparison of their mutagenic and carcinogenic activity. In: Stich H (ed) Carcinogens and Mutagens in the Environment. Vol 5. CRC Press, Boca Raton, Fl 1985 pp 60-74
36. Lewtas J: Genotoxicity of complex mixtures: Strategies for the identification and comparative assessment of airborne mutagens and carcinogens from combustion sources. Fund Appl Toxicol 1988 (10):571-589
37. Lewtas J, Gallagher J: Complex mixtures of urban air pollution: Identification and comparative assessment of mutagenic and tumorigenic chemicals and emission sources. In: Vainio H, Sorsa M, McMichael AJ (eds) Complex Mixtures and Cancer Risk. International Agency for Research on Cancer, Lyon 1990 pp 252-260
38. Anderson JG, Toohey DW, Brune WH: Free radicals within the Antarctic vortex: The role of the CFCs in Antarctic ozone loss. Science 1991 (251):39-46
39. Stolarski R, Bojkov R, Bishop L, Zerefos C, Staehlin J, Zawodny J: Measured trends in stratospheric ozone. Science 1992 (256):342-349

40 Brune WH, Anderson JG, Toohey DW, Fahey DW: The potential for ozone depletion in the Polar stratosphere. Science 1991 (252):1260-1266
41 Toon OB, Turco RP: Polar stratospheric clouds and ozone depletion. Sci Amer 1991 (264):68-74
42 Solomon S: Progress towards a quantitative understanding of Antarctic ozone depletion. Nature 1990 (347):347-354
43 Solomon S, Albritton DL: Time-dependent ozone depletion potentials for short- and long-term forecasts. Nature 1992 (357):33-37
44 National Academy of Sciences: Ozone Depletion, Greenhouse Gases and Climate Change. National Academy Press, Washington, DC 1990
45 National Academy of Sciences: Policy Implication of Greenhouse Warming. National Academy Press, Washington, DC 1991
46 Dickinson RE, Cicerone RJ: Future global warming from atmospheric trace gases. Nature 1986 (319):109-115
47 Schneider SH: The greenhouse effect: Science and policy. Science 1989 (243):771-781
48 Schneider SH, Rosenberg N: The greenhouse effect: Its causes, possible impacts and associated uncertainties. In: Rosenberg N (ed) Greenhouse Warming: Abatement and Adaptation. Resources for the Future, Washington, DC 1989 pp7-34
49 Rosswall T: Greenhouse gases and global change: International collaboration. Environ Sci Technol 1991 (25):567-573
50 Hileman B: Global warming. Chem Eng News 1989 (March 13):25-44
51 Hileman B: Web of interactions makes it difficult to untangle global warming data. Chem Eng News 1992 (April 27):7-19
52 UNEP/WHO: Climate Change and World Agriculture. Geneva 1991
53 UNEP: Intergovernmental Panel on Climate Change. UN Environmental Programme, Geneva 1990
54 Boyden S, Dover S: Natural-resource consumption and its environmental impacts in the Western World: Impacts of increasing per capita consumption. Ambio 1992 (21):63-69
55 Swisher J, Masters G: A Mechanism to reconcile equity and efficiency in global climate protection: International carbon emission offsets. Ambio 1992 (21);154-159
56 Philips VD: Living in a terrarium. Environ Sci Technol 1990 (25):574-578
57 Cline WR: Global Warming: The Economic Stakes. Institute for International Economics, Washington, DC 1992
58 Piver WT: Global atmospheric changes. Environ Hlth Persp 1991 (96):131-137
59 Arrhenius E: Population, development and environmental disruption - An issue on efficient natural resource management. Ambio 1992 (21):9-13
60 Ballschmitter K: Global distribution of organic compounds. Environ Carcinogen Ecotox Revs 1991 (C9):1-46
61 Oehme M: Further evidence for long-range air transport of polychlorinated aromates and pesticides: North America and Eurasia to the Arctic. Ambio 1992 (20):293-297
62 Schwartz SE: Acid deposition: Unravelling a regional phenomenon. Science 1989 (243):753-763
63 Dunmore J: Acid rain in Europe. In: DocTer Institute for Environmental Studies-European Environmental Yearbook 1987. DocTer International, London 1987 pp 665-666
64 Hordijk L: Use of rains model. Environ Sci Technol 1991 (25):596-603
65 Streets DG: A Review of Acid Rain Models For Europe. Report - Task Force on Integrated Assessment Modeling. Economic Commission for Europe, United Nations, Geneva 1988
66 Eriksson E, Karltun E, Lundmark JE: Acidification of forest soils in Sweden. Ambio 1992 (21):150-154
67 Kamari J (ed): Impact Models to Assess Regional Acidification. Kluwer, Dordrecht 1990
68 Saenger J (ed): The State of the Earth. Unwin Hyman, London 1990
69 Hileman B: Volcanic emissions may cause global cooling. Chem Eng News 1992 (May 25):5-6
70 Powell CS: Greenhouse gusher. Sci Amer 1991 (265):20
71 Gerlach T: Etna's greenhouse pump. Nature 1991 (351):352-353
72 Hobbs PV, Radke LF: Airborne studies of the smoke from the Kuwait oil fires. Science 1992 (256):987-991
73 Johnson DW, Kilsby CG, McKenna DS, Saunders RW, Jenkins GJ, Smith FB, Foot JS: Airborne observations of the physical and chemical characteristics of the Kuwait oil smoke plume. Nature 1991 (353):617-621
74 Browning KA, Allam RJ, Ballatd SP, Barnes RTH, Bennetts DA, Maryon RH: Environmental effects from burning oil wells in Kuwait. Nature 1991 (351):363-367
75 Hahn J: Environmental effects of the Kuwait oil field fires. Environ Sci Technol 1991 (25):1530-1532
76 Evliya H: Rain in Turkey: Possible effect of the Gulf War. Environ Sci Technol 1992 (26):873-875
77 Thompson AM: The oxidizing capacity of the Earth's atmosphere: Probable past and future changes. Science 1992 (256):1157-1165
78 Rogge WF, Hildemann LM, Mazurek MA, Cass GR, Simoneit BRT: Sources of fine organic aerosols. 1. Charbroilers and meat cooking operations. Environ Sci Technol 1991 (25):1112-1125
79 Anon: Tougher laws on toxic emissions urged. Chem Eng News 1989 (April 3):23-24
80 U.S. House of Representatives: The National Toxic Release Inventory-Preliminary Air Toxic Data. Subcommittee on Health and the Environment, Committee on Energy and Commerce. Washington, D.C. 1989 (March 22) p78
81 WHO/UNEP: Global Environmental Monitoring System. Yale Press, London 1987 pp 4-7
82 Moldan B, Schnoor JL: Czechoslovakia: Examining a critically ill environment. Environ Sci Technol 1992 (26):14-21
83 Czech Federal Government: Statistical Year Book of the C.S.S.R. 1987. SNTL and ALFA Publishing, Prague 1988

84. Czech Federal Government: Joint Environmental Study. Czech Ministry of the Environment, Prague 1991
85. Frumkin H, Levy BS, Levenstein C: Occupational and environmental health in Eastern Europe: Challenges and opportunities. Am J Ind Hlth 1991 (20):265-270
86. French HE: Green Revolutions: Environmental Reconstruction in Eastern Europe and the Soviet Union. World Watch Paper No 99. World Watch Institute, Washington, D.C. 1990
87. Kabala SJ: The environmental crisis in central Europe: A developing perspective. In: Proceedings of the Conference on Public Health and the Environmental Crisis in Central Europe. Woodrow Wilson School for Scholars, Washington, D.C. 1990
88. Burger G: East Germany's environmental health hazards: Their current and future impact. In: Proceedings of the Conference on Public Health and the Environmental Crisis in Eastern Europe. Woodrow Wilson International School for Scholars, Washington, D.C. 1990
89. Revich BA: Quality of air in industrial cities of the U.S.S.R. and child health. Sci Total Environ 1992 (119):121-132
90. Feshbach M, Friendly A Jr: Ecocide in the U.S.S.R. Basic Books, Washington,D.C. 1992
91. Pope V: Toxic Waste Land. U.S.News World Report 1992 (April 13):40-51
92. Kral R, Mejstrik V, Velicka J: Concentrations of cadmium, lead and copper in atmospheric precipitation in Czechoslovakia. Sci Total Environ 1992 (111):125-133
93. Barry JM: Wroclaw, Poland: Efforts toward a sustainable future. J Environ Hlth 1992 (54):8-13
94. Goldemburg J, Johansson TB, Reddy AKN, Williams RH: Energy for Development. World Resources Institute, Washington, D.C. 1987
95. Boden TA: Trends 90-A Compendium of Data on Global Change. Carbon Dioxide Information Analysis. Oak Ridge National Laboratory, Oak Ridge, TN 1990
96. Sarmiento Jl, Sundquist ET: Revised budget for the oceanic uptake of anthropogenic carbon dioxide. Nature 1992 (356):589-591
97. Hileman B: The role of global warming continues to perplex scientists. Chem Eng News 1992 (Feb 10):26-28
98. Khahil MAK, Rasmussen RA: Atmospheric methane: Recent global trends. Environ Sci Technol 1990 (24):549-553
99. Cicerone RJ, Oremland RS: Biochemical aspects of atmospheric methane. Global Biochem Cycles 1988 (2):297-327
100. Robertson K: Emissions of N_2O in Sweden - Natural and anthropogenic sources. Ambio 1991 (20):151-153
101. IPCC: Climate Change. Intergovernmental Panel on Climate Change. Cambridge University Press, Cambridge 1990
102. Rodhe H, Eriksson H, Robertson K, Svensson L: Sources and sinks of greenhouse gases in Sweden: A case study. Ambio 1992 (20):143-145
103. Prinn R, Cunnold D, Rasmussen R, Simmonds P, Alyea F, Crawford A: Atmospheric emissions and trends of nitrous oxide deduced from ice-gage data. J Geophys Res 1990 (96):18369-18385
104. Cicerone RJ: Analysis of sources and sinks of atmospheric nitrous oxide. J Geophys Res 1989 (94):18265-18271
105. Yokoyama T, Nishinomiya S, Matsuda H: Nitrous oxide emissions from fossil fuel fired power plants. Environ Sci Technol 1991 (25):347-348
106. Manzer LE: The CFC-ozone issue: Progress on the development of alternatives to CFCs. Science 1990 (249):31-35
107. Zurer PS: Industry consumers prepare for compliance with pending CFC ban. Chem Eng News 1992 (June 22):7-13
108. Molina MJ, Rowland FS: Stratospheric sink for chlorofluoromethanes: Chlorine atom-catalyzed destruction of ozone. Nature 1974 (249):810-812
109. Anders MW: Metabolism and toxicity of hydrofluorocarbons: Current knowledge and needs for the future. Environ Hlth Persp 1991 (96):185-191
110. Charles D: EPA's plans for cooling the global greenhouse. Science 1989 (243):1542-1543
111. Abrahamson D: Aluminum and global warming. Nature 1992 (356):484
112. Fabian P, Borchers R, Kruger BC, Lal S: CF_4 and C_2F_6 in the atmosphere. J Geophys Res 1987 (92):9831-9835
113. Lashof DA, Ahuja DR: Relative contribution of greenhouse emissions to global warming. Nature 1990 (344):529-531
114. Hisham MWM, Grosjean D: Methyl chloroform and tetrachloroethylene in Southern California, 1987-1990. Environ Sci Technol 1991 (25):1930-1936
115. Zurer P: U.S. seeks tighter rules on ozone protection. Chem Eng News 1989 (May 1):8-9
116. Talukdar R, Mellouki A, Gierczak T, Burkholder JB, McKeen SA, Ravishankar AR: Atmospheric lifetime of CHF_2Br, a proposed substitute for halons. Science 1991 (252):693-695
117. Rowland FS, Isaksen ISA (eds): The Changing Atmosphere: Report of the Dahlem Workshop On the Changing Atmosphere. Wiley-Interscience, New York 1988 pp141-158
118. Lippmann M: Health effects of tropospheric ozone. Environ Sci Technol 1991 (25):1954-1956
119. Penkett SA: Changing ozone: Evidence for a perturbed atmosphere. Environ Sci Technol 1991 (25):631-635
120. Scheere KL: Modeling ozone concentrations. Environ Sci Technol 1988 (22):488-495
121. Killus JP, Whitten GZ: Isoprene: A photochemical kinetic mechanism. Environ Sci Technol 1984 (18):142-148
122. U.S. Congress Office of Technology Assessment: Catching Our Breath: Next Steps For Reducing Urban Ozone. U.S. Government Printing Office, Washington, D.C. 1989 pp106-107
123. Walcek CJ: A threshold estimate of ozone and hydrogen peroxide dry deposition over the North East United States. Atmos Environ 1987 (21):2649-2659
124. Hartkamp H, Bachhawsen P: A method for the determination of hydrogen peroxide in air. Atmos Environ 1987 (21):2207-2213

125 Rowland EF: Stratospheric ozone in the 21st century: The chlorofluorocarbon problem. Environ Sci Technol 1992 (25):622-629
126 Farman JC, Gardiner BG, Shanklin JD: Large losses of total ozone in Antarctica reveal seasonal ClOx/NOx interactions. Nature 1985 (315):207-210
127 Kerr RA: Ozone destruction worsens. Science 1992 (252):204
128 Zurer P: Ozone depletion: Arctic hole geared, sulfate aerosol blamed. Chem Eng News 1992 (Feb 10):4-5
129 World Meteorological Organization: Scientific Assessment of Stratospheric Ozone. Rept No 20, Vol 1, Geneva 1990
130 Solomons S, Garcia RR, Rowland FS, Wuebbles DJ: On the depletion of Antarctic ozone. Nature 1986 (321):755-758
131 McElroy MP, Salawitch RJ, Wofsy SC, Logan JA: Reductions of Antarctic ozone due to synergistic actions of chlorine and bromine. Nature 1986 (321):759-762
132 Fisher DA, Hales CH, Filkin DL, Koo MKW, Sze ND et al: Model calculations of the relative effects of CFCs and their replacements on stratospheric ozone. Nature 1990 (344):508-512
133 Fisher DA, Hales CH, Wang WC, KO MKW, Sze ND: Model calculations of the relative effects of CFCs and their replacements on global warming. Nature 1990 (344):513-516
134 Solomon S, Tuck A: Evaluating ozone depletion potentials. Nature 1990 (348):203-204
135 Fisher DA, Ko MKW, Wuebbles D, Isaksen I: Evaluating ozone depletion potentials. Nature 1990 (348):203-204
136 Brown AC, Canosa-Mas CE, Parr AD, Rothwell K, Wayne RP: Tropospheric lifetimes of three compounds for possible replacements of CFCs and halons. Nature 1990 (347):541-543
137 Wigley TML, Raper SCB: Implications for climate and sea level of revised IPCC emission scenarios. Nature 1992 (357):293-300
138 Kerr RA: Greenhouse science survives sceptics. Science 1992 (256):1138-1140
139 Moffat AS: Does global change threaten the world food supply? Science 1992 (256):1140-1141
140 Norby RJ, Gunderson CA, Wullschleger SO, O'Neill EG, McCracken MK: Productivity and compensatory responses of yellow poplar trees in elevated carbon dioxide. Nature 1992 (357):322-324
141 Kerr RA: Greenhouse skeptic out in the cold. Science 1989 (246):1118-1119
142 Penner JE, Dickinson RE, O'Neill CA: Effects of aerosol from biomass burning on the global radiation budget. Science 1992 (256):1432-1434
143 Hammitt JK, Lempert RJ, Schlesinger ME: A sequential-decision strategy for abating climate change. Nature 1992 (357):315-318
144 Haugen PM, Drange H: Sequestration of carbon dioxide in the deep ocean by shallow injection. Nature 1992 (357):318-322
145 Houghton JT, Jenkins GJ, Ephraums JJ (eds): Climate Change. The IPCC Scientific Assessment. Cambridge University Press, Cambridge 1990
146 Houghton JT, Callander BA, Varney SK (eds): Climate Change-1992. The Supplementary Report to the IPCC Scientific Assessment. Cambridge University Press, Cambridge 1992
147 Hatfield CB: Will we reach the greenhouse? Nature 1991 (351):355
148 Bierbaum R, Friedman RM: The road to reduced carbon emissions. Issues Sci Technol 1992 (8):58-65
149 Warrick RA, Barrow EM, Wigley TML: The Greenhouse Effect and its Implications for the European Community. Commission of the European Communities, Brussels 1990
150 Hanson JE, Lacis AA: Sun and dust versus greenhouse gases: An assessment of their relative roles in global climate change. Nature 1990 (346):713-719
151 Wigley TML, Raper SCB: Natural variability of the climate system and detection of the greenhouse effect. Nature 1990 (344):324-327
152 Ramaswamy V, Schwartzkopf MD, Shine KP: Radiative forcing of climate from halocarbon-induced global stratosphere ozone loss. Nature 1992 (355):810-812
153 Charney J: Carbon Dioxide and Climate. National Academy of Sciences, National Academy Press, Washington, D.C. 1979
154 Dickinson RE: The Greenhouse Effect Climatic Change and Ecosystems. Wiley, New York 1986 pp 206-270
155 U.S. EPA: Air Quality Criteria For Particulate Matter and Sulfur Oxides. Vols I-II (EPA-600/8-82-029a, b, c). U.S. Environmental Protection Agency, Research Triangle Park, N.C. 1982
156 WHO: Sulfur Oxides and Suspended Particulate Matter. Environmental Health Criteria No 8. World Health Organization, Geneva 1979
157 Amdur MO, Sarofim AF, Neville M, Quann PJ, McCarthy JF: Coal combustion aerosols and SO_2: An interdisciplinary analysis. Environ Sci Technol 1986 (20):138-145
158 Gordon GE: Airborne particles. Environ Sci Technol 1991 (25): 1822-1829
159 Anon: California, Indiana, Ohio and Texas allegedly are the highest emitters of acid rain precursors. Environ Sci Technol 1989 (23):375
160 UNEP/WHO: Assessment of Urban Air Quality. Global Monitoring System. United Nations, London 1988 p 25
161 Jackson CI: A tenth anniversary review of the ECE convention on long-range transboundary air pollution. Internat Environ Affairs 1990 (2):222-225
162 McCormick J: Acid Earth: The Global Threat of Acid Pollution. Earth Scan Publ, London 1989 pp 15,21
163 U.S. EPA: The Clean Air Act Amendments of 1990: Summary Materials. U.S. Environmental Protection Agency, Washington, D.C. 1990 p 15
164 Anon: ES&T currents. Environ Sci Technol 1991 (25):811
165 Cortese AD: Clearing the air. Environ Sci Technol 1990 (24):444
166 WuDunn S: Difficult algebra for China: Coal = Growth = Pollution. New York Times 1992 (May 26):1,5

167 Last JA; Global atmospheric change: Potential health effects of acid aerosol and oxidant gas mixtures. Environ Hlth Persp 1991 (96):151-157
168 Lioy PJ, Lippmann M: Measurements of exposure to acid sulfur aerosols. In: Lee SD (ed) Aerosols. Lewis, Chelsea, MI 1986
169 Singh SB, Salas LJ, Smith AJ, Shigeishi H: Measurements of some potentially hazardous organic chemicals in urban environments. Atmos Environ 1981 (15):601-612
170 Janssen LH, van Wakeren JH, van Duuren H, Elshout AJ: A classification of NO oxidation rates in power plant plumes based on atmospheric conditions. Atmos Environ 1988 (22):45-53
171 U.S. EPA: Air Quality for Oxides of Nitrogen. Rept No EPA-600/82-026F. U.S. Environmental Protection Agency, Research Triangle Park, N.C. 1982
172 Anon: ES&T currents. Environ Sci Technol 1991 (25):357
173 Rodhe H: Acidification in a global perspective. Ambio 1989 (18):156
174 Galloway JN, Zhao D, Xiong J, Likens GE: Acid rain: A comparison of China, United States and remote areas. Science 1987 (236):1559-1562
175 Rodhe H, Galloway J, Dianwu Z: Acidification in Southeast Asia - Prospects for the coming decades. Ambio 1992 (21):148-150
176 Mellanby K (ed): Air Pollution, Acid Rain and the Environment. Elsevier, London 1988
177 Blank LW, Crane AJ, Skeffington RA: The long term ecological effects of pollutants. Sci Total Environ 1992 (116):145-158
178 Tyler PE: On Norway's border, Russian Arctic in crisis. New York Times 1992 (May 10):17
179 Kamari J, Forsius M, Kortelainen P, Mannio J, Verta M: Finnish lake survey: Present status of acidification. Ambio 1991 (20):23-27
180 Graedel TE: Hydrocarbons. In: Graedel TE, Hawkins DT, Claxton LD (eds) Atmospheric Chemical Compounds. Academic Press, Orlando 1986 pp 11-298
181 Löfgren L, Petersson G: Butenes and butadiene in urban air. Sci Total Environ 1992 (116):195-201
182 Kliendienst TE, Shepson PB, Edney EO, Cupitt LT, Claxton LD: The mutagenic activity of propylene photooxidation. Environ Sci Technol 1985 (19):620-627
183 IARC: IARC Monographs on the Evaluation of the Carcinogenic Risk of Chemicals to Humans. Vol 19. Some Monomers, Plastics and Synthetic Elastomers and Acrolein. International Agency For Research on Cancer, Lyon 1979
184 Mullins JA: Industrial emissions of 1,3-butadiene. Environ Hlth Persp 1990 (86):8-10
185 Fajen JM, Roberts DR, Ungers LJ, Krishnan ER: Occupational exposure to 1,3-butadiene. Environ Hlth Persp 1990 (86):11-19
186 IARC: IARC Monographs on the Evaluation of the Carcinogenic Risk of Chemicals to Humans. Vol 39. Some Chemicals Used in Plastics and Elastomers. International Agency For Research on Cancer, Lyon 1986 pp155-179
187 Merian E, Zander M: Volatile aromatics. In: Hutzinger O (ed) Handbook on Environmental Chemistry. Vol 3, Part B. Anthropogenic Compounds. Springer-Verlag, Berlin 1982 pp 117-161
188 Hanson DJ: Benzene emissions ordered cut by 90%. Chem Eng News 1989 (Sept 4):5-6
189 Adler MM, Carey PM. Presented at the Air & Waste Management Association Meeting. Anaheim, CA 1989 June; Paper 89-34 A.6
190 Dasch JM, Williams RL: Benzene exhaust emissions from in-use General Motors vehicles. Environ Sci Technol 1991 (25):853-857
191 U.S. EPA: Ambient Air, Water Quality Criteria for Benzene. EPA Rept 440/5-8-018. U.S. Environmental Protection Agency, Washington, D.C. 1980 pp C1-C8, C16-C35, C-68-C100
192 Korte F, Klein W: Degradation of benzene in the environment. Ecotox Environ Safety 1982 (6):311-327
193 U.S. EPA: The Report of the Strategic Options Sub-Committee: Relative Risk Reduction Project. Rept EPA SAB-90-021C. U.S. Environmental Protection Agency, Washington, D.C. 1990 pp 70-73
194 Machiele PA: A health and safety assessment of methanol as an alternative fuel. In: Kohl WL (ed) Methanol as an Alternative Fuel Choice: An Assessment. Johns Hopkins Foreign Policy Institute, Paul H Nitze School of Advanced International Studies, Washington, D.C. 1990 pp 217-239
195 U.S. EPA: Analysis of the Economic and Environmental Effects of Methanol as an Alternate Fuel. U.S. Environmental Protection Agency Office of Mobile Sources, Washington, D.C. 1989 (Special Report)
196 IARC: IARC Monographs on the Evaluation of the Carcinogenic Risk of Chemicals to Humans. Vol 41. Some Halogenated Hydrocarbons and Pesticide Exposures. International Agency for the Research on Cancer, Lyon 1986 pp 161-186
197 Edwards PR, Campbell I, Milne GS: The impact of chloromethanes on the environment. Part 2. Methyl chloride and methylene chloride. Chem Ind 1982 (17):619-622
198 WHO: Tetrachloroethylene. Environmental Criteria No 31. World Health Organization, Geneva 1984
199 U.S. EPA: Health Assessment Document for Tetrachloroethylene (Perchloroethylene). Final Rept No EPA-600/8-82-005F. U.S. Environmental Protection Agency, Washington, D.C. 1985
200 Conrad R, Schultz H, Seller W: Emission of carbon monoxide from submerged rice fields into the atmosphere. Atmos Environ 1988 (2):821-823
201 U.S. EPA: National Air Quality and Emission Trends. Report 1989. U.S. Environmental Protection Agency, Washington, D.C. 1991
202 Singh HB, Hanst PL: Peroxyacyl nitrate (PAN) in the unpolluted atmosphere: An important reservoir for nitrogen oxides. Geophys Res Lett 1981 (8):941-946
203 Singh HB, Salas LJ, Ridley BA, Shetter JD: Relationship between peroxyacetyl nitrate and nitrogen oxides in the clean troposphere. Nature 1985 (318):347

204 Williams EL, Grosjean D: Peroxypropionyl nitrate at a Southern California mountain forest site. Environ Sci Technol 1991 (25):653-659
205 Singh HB: Reactive nitrogen in the troposphere. Environ Sci Technol 1987 (21):320-327
206 Rogers JD, Rhead LA: Peroxyglutaryl nitrate formation and infrared spectrum. Atmos Environ 1987 (21):2519-2522
207 Hisham MWM, Grosjean D: Air pollution in Southern California museums: Indoor and outdoor levels of nitrogen dioxide, peroxyacetyl nitrate, nitric acid and chlorinated hydrocarbons. Environ Sci Technol 1991 (25):857-862
208 Tanner RL, Miguel AH, de Andrade JB, Gaffney JS, Streit GE: Atmospheric chemistry of aldehydes: Enhanced peroxyacetyl nitrate formation from ethanol-fueled vehicular emissions. Environ Sci Technol 1988 (22):1026-1034
209 Mudd JB: Peroxyacyl nitrates. In: Mudd JB, Kozlowski TT (eds) Responses of Plants to Air Pollution. Academic Press, New York 1975 pp 97-119
210 WHO: Formaldehyde. Environmental Criteria No 89. International Programme on Chemical Safety, World Health Organization, Geneva 1989
211 IARC: Monographs on the Evaluation of the Carcinogenic Risk of Chemicals to Humans. Vol 29. Some Industrial Chemicals and Dyestuffs. International Agency for Research on Cancer, Lyon 1982 pp 345-390
212 IARC: Monographs on the Evaluation of the Carcinogenic Risk of Chemicals to Humans. Vol 36. Allyl Compounds, Aldehydes, Epoxides and Peroxides. International Agency for Research on Cancer, Lyon 1985 pp 101-132
213 National Research Council: Formaldehyde and Other Aldehydes. National Academy Press, Washington, D.C. 1981
214 Grosjean D: Formaldehyde and other carbonyls in Los Angeles ambient air. Environ Sci Technol 1982 (16):254-262
215 Tanner RL, Meng Z: Seasonal variations in ambient atmospheric levels of formaldehyde and acetaldehyde. Environ Sci Technol 1984 (18):713-726
216 Zhou X, Mopper K: Measurement of sub-parts-per-billion levels of carbonyl compounds in marine air by a single trapping procedure followed by liquid chromatography. Environ Sci Technol 1990 (24)1482-1485
217 Kalabokas P, Carlier P, Fresnet P, Mouvier G, Toupance G: Field studies of aldehyde chemistry in the Paris area. Atmos Environ 1988 (22):147-155
218 Grosjean D: Ambient levels of formaldehyde and formic acid in Southern California: Results of a one-year base line study. Environ Sci Technol 1991 (25):710-715
219 Grosjean D, Swanson RD, Ellis C: Carbonyls In Los Angeles air - Contribution of direct emissions and photochemistry. Sci Total Environ 1983 (29):65-85
220 Seinfeld JH: Atmospheric Chemistry and Physics of Air Pollution. Wiley, New York 1986
221 Sanhueza E, Ferrer Z, Romero J, Santana M: HCHO and HCOOH in tropical rains. Ambio 1991 (20):115-118

222 Walcek CJ: A Theoretical estimate of ozone and hydrogen peroxide over the northeast United States. Atmos Environ 1987 (21):2649-2659
223 Penkett SA, Jones BMR, Brice KA, Eggleton AEJ: Importance of atmospheric ozone and H_2O_2 in oxidizing SO_2 in cloud and rain water. Atmos Environ 1979 (13):123-137
224 Hartkamph L, Bachawsen P: A method for the determination of hydrogen peroxide in air. Atmos Environ 1987 (21):2207-2213
225 Lightowlers PJ, Cape JN: Sources and fate of atmospheric HCl in the U.K. and Western Europe. Atmos Environ 1988 (22):7-15
226 Sturges WT, Harrison RM: The use of nylon filters to collect HCl: Efficiencies, interferences and ambient concentrations. Atmos Environ 1989 (23):1987-1996
227 Kamrin MA: Workshop on the health effects of HCl in ambient air. Regul Toxicol Pharmacol 1992 (15):73-82
228 Matthes T: Die Novellierung der TALuft-Stellungnahme zu den für Abfallverbrennungs-anlagen beabsichtigten Änderungen. In: Müllverbrennung 1984. Vortrage der VGB Konferenz vom 28./29. November 1984. Technische Vereinigung der Großkraftwerksbetreiber, Essen, Germany 1984
229 Molina MJ, Tso TI, Molina LT, Wang FC: Antarctic stratospheric chemistry of chlorine mitrate, hydrogen chloride and ice: Release of active chlorine. Science 1987 (238):1253-1257
230 Langford AO, Fehsenfeld FC: Natural vegetation as a source or sink for atmospheric ammonia: A case study. Science 1992 (255):581-583
231 Apsimon HM, Kruse M, Bell JNB: Ammonia emissions and their role in acid deposition. Atmos Environ 1987 (21):1939-1946
232 Asman WAH, Drukker B, Janssen AJ: Modelled historical concentration and depositions of ammonia and ammonium in Europe. Atmos Environ 1988 (22):725-735
233 Harrison RM, McCartney HA: Ambient air-quality at a coastal site in rural Northwest England. Atmos Environ 1980 (14):233-244
234 IARC: IARC Monographs on the Evaluation of the Carcinogenic Risk of Chemicals to Humans. Vol 20. Some Halogenated Hydrocarbons. International Agency for Research on Cancer, Lyon 1979 pp 45-55
235 Lane DA, Johnson ND, Barton SC, Thomas GHS, Schroeder WH: Development and evaluation of a novel gas and particle sampler for semi-volatile chlorinated organic compounds in ambient air. Environ Sci Technol 1989 (22):941-947
236 Gregor DJ, Gummer WD: Evidence of atmospheric transport and deposition of organochlorine pesticides and polychlorinated biphenyls in Canadian Artic snow. Environ Sci Technol 1989 (23):561-565
237 Rapoport RA, Eisenreich SJ: Historical inputs of high molecular weight chlorinated hydrocarbons to Eastern North America. Environ Sci Technol 1988 (22):931-941
238 Hoff RM, Muir DCG, Grift NP: Annual cycle of polychlorinated biphenyls and organohalogen

pesticides in air in southern Ontario. 1. Air concentration data. Environ Sci Technol 1992 (26):266-275
239 Hoff RM, Muir DCG, Grift NP: Annual cycle of polychlorinated biphenyls and organohalogen pesticides in air in Southern Ontario. 2. Atmospheric transport and sources. Environ Sci Technol 1992 (26):276-283
240 Oehme M: Further evidence for long-range air transport of polychlorinated aromates and pesticides: North America and Eurasia to the Artic. Ambio 1991 (20):293-297
241 Gregor DJ, Gummer WD: Evidence of atmospheric transport and deposition of organochlorine pesticides and polychlorinated biphenyls In Canadian Arctic snow. Environ Sci Technol 1989 (23):561-565
242 Eisenreich SJ, Looney BB, Thornton JD: Airborne organic contaminants in the Great Lakes ecosystem. Environ Sci Technol 1981 (15):30-38
243 Murphy TJ, Formanski LJ, Brownawell B, Meyer JA: Polychlorinated biphenyl emissions to the atmosphere in the Great Lakes region municipal landfills and incinerators. Environ Sci Technol 1985 (19):942-946
244 Jones KC, Sanders G, Wild SR, Burnett V, Johnston AE: Evidence for a decline of PCBs and PAHs in rural vegetation and air in the United Kingdom. Nature 1992 (356):137-139
245 Duinker JC, Bouchertall F: On the distribution of atmospheric polychlorinated biphenyl congeners between vapor phase, aerosol and rain. Environ Sci Technol 1989 (23):57-62
246 WHO: Polychlorinated Dibenzo-p-Dioxins and Dibenzofurans. Environmental Health Criteria No 88. World Health Organization, Geneva 1989
247 Fiedler H, Hutzinger O, Timms CW: Dioxins: Sources of environmental load and human exposure. Toxicol Environ Chem 1990 (29):134-157
248 Vainio H, Hess A, Jappinen P: Chlorinated dioxins and benzofurans in the environment - A hazard to public health? Scand Work Environ Hlth 1989 (15):377-382
249 Jones KC, Bennett W: Human exposure to environmental polychlorinated dibenzo-p-dioxins and dibenzofurans: An exposure committment assessment for 2,3,7,8-TCDD. Sci Total Environ 1989 (78):99-116
250 Erickson MD, Swanson SE, Flura JD, Hinshaw GD: Polychlorinated dibezofurans and other thermal combustion products from dielectric fluids containing polychlorinated biphenyls. Environ Sci Technol 1989 (23):462-470
251 Rappe C, Bergquist PA, Hansson M: Chemistry and analysis of polychlorinated dioxins and dibenzofurans in biological samples. Banbury Rept. No 18: Biological Mechanisms Of Dioxin Action. Cold Springs Harbor Laboratory, Cold Springs Harbor, N.Y. 1984 pp 17-25
252 Hutzinger O, Blumich MJ, Berg MV, Olie K: Sources and fate of PCDDs and PCDFs: An overview. Chemosphere 1984 (14):551-560
253 Oehme M, Mano S, Mikalsten A, Kerschmer P: Quantitative method for the determination of femtogram amounts of polychlorinated dibenzo-p-dioxins and dibenzofurans in outdoor air. Chemosphere 1986 (6):455-470
254 Bidleman TF: Atmospheric processes. Environ Sci Technol (22):361-367
255 Broman D, Naf C, Zebuhr Y: Long-term high- and low-volume air sampling of polychlorinated dibenzo-p-dioxins and dibenzofurans and polycyclic aromatic hydrocarbons along a transect from urban to remote areas on the Swedish Baltic coast. Environ Sci Technol 1991 (25):1841-1850
256 Hunt GT, Maisel BE: Atmospheric PCDDs and PCDFs in wintertime in a northeastern United States urban coastal environment. Chemosphere 1990 (20):1455-1462
257 Rappe C, Andersson R, Bergquist PA: Overview on environmental fate of chlorinated dioxins and dibenzofurans: Sources, levels and isomeric patterns in various materials. Chemosphere 1987 (16):1603-1618
258 National Academy Of Sciences: Polycyclic Aromatic Hydrocarbons: Evaluation of Sources and Effects. National Academy Press, Washington, D.C. 1982
259 IARC: IARC Monographs on the Carcinogenic Risk of Chemicals to Humans. Vol 12. Polynuclear Aromatic Compounds. Part 1. Chemical, Environmental and Experimental Data. International Agency for Research on Cancer, Lyon 1983
260 Ahlen E: Air pollution and cancer: Investigation of hazardous constituents from various emission sources for their carcinogenic impact. Münchener Med Wochenschr 1985 (127):218-221
261 Menichini E: Urban air pollution by polcyclic aromatic hydrocarbons: Levels and sources of variability. Sci Total Environ 1992 (116):109-135
262 Baek SO, Goldstone ME, Kirk PWW, Lester JN, Perry R: Concentrations of particulate and gaseous polycyclic aromatic hydrocarbons in London air following a reduction in the lead content of petrol in the United Kingdom. Sci Total Environ 1992 (111):169-199
263 Baek SO, Field RA, Goldstone ME, Kirk PWW, Lester JN, Perry R: Polycyclic aromatic hydrocarbons: Sources, fate and behavior. Water Air Soil Pollut 1991 (60):279-300
264 Behymer TD, Hites RA: Photolysis of polycyclic aromatic hydrocarbons absorbed on fly ash. Environ Sci Technol 1988 (22):1311-1319
265 Ramdahl K, Zielinska B, Arey J, Atkinson R, Winer AM, Pitts JN Jr: Ubiquitous occurrence of 2-nitrofluoranthene and 2-nitropyrene in air. Nature 1986 (321):425-427
266 Pitts JN Jr: Nitration of gaseous polyaromatic hydrocarbons in simulated and ambient urban atmospheres: A source of mutagenic nitroarenes. Atmos Environ 1987 (21):2531-2547
267 Turpin BJ, Huntzinger JJ, Larson SM, Cass GR: Los Angeles summer midday particulate carbon: Primary and secondary aerosol. Environ Sci Technol 1991 (25):1788-1793
268 Pitts JN Jr.: Formation and fate of gaseous and particulate mutagens and carcinogens in real and simulated atmospheres. Environ Hlth Persp 1983 (47):115-140

269 Pitts JN Jr, Van Cawenberghe KA, Grosjean D, Schmid JP: Atmospheric reaction of PAH: Facile formation of mutagenic nitro derivatives. Science 1978 (202):515-521
270 Arey J, Atkinson R, Zielinska B, McElroy PA: Diurnal concentrations of volatile polycyclic aromatic hydrocarbons and nitroarenes during a photochemical air pollution episode in Glendora, California. Environ Sci Technol 1989 (23):321-327
271 Helmig D, Arey J, Harger WP, Atkinson R, Lopez-Cancio J: Formation of mutagenic nitrodibenzopyranones and their occurrence in ambient air. Environ Sci Technol 1992 (26):622-624
272 Sawicki E: Analysis of atmospheric carcinogens and their cofactors. In: Environmental Pollution and Carcinogenic Risks. Inserm Symposia Series, Vol 52. IARC Scientific Publications No 13. International Agency for Research on Cancer, Lyon 1976 pp 297-354
273 Sawicki E, Hauser TR, Elbert WC, Fox FJ, Mekker JE: Polynuclear hydrocarbon composition of the atmosphere in some large American cities. Am Ind Hyg Assoc J 1962 (23):137-142
274 Pott F: Environmental contamination by PAH: Air. In: Grimmer G (ed) Environmental Carcinogens: Polycyclic Aromatic Hydrocarbons. CRC Press, Boca Raton, FL, 1983 pp 84-101
275 Hoffman D, Wynder EL: Environmental respiratory carcinogenesis. In: Searle CE (ed) Chemical Carcinogens. ACS Monograph No 173. American Chemical Society, Washington, D.C., 1976 pp 324-365
276 Motykiewicz, G, Cimander B, Szeliga J, Tkocz A, Chorazy M: Mutagenic activity of complex air pollutants in Silesia. In: Vainio H, Sorsa M, McMichael AJ (eds) Complex Mixtures and Cancer Risk. International Agency for Research on Cancer, Lyon 1990 pp 261-268
277 Madany IM, Raveendran E: Polycyclic aromatic hydrocarbons, nickel, vanadium in air particulate matter in Bahrain during the burning of oil fields in Kuwait. Sci Total Environ 1992 (116):281-289
278 OECD: Air Report. ENV/AIR 81.18. 2nd Review. Organization of European Communities Development, Paris 1984 p 21
279 Nishioka, MG, Howard CC, Contos DA, Ball LM, Lewtas J: Detection of hydroxylated nitro aromatic and hydroxylated nitropoycyclic aromatic compounds in an ambient air particulate extract using bioassay-directed fractionation. Environ Sci Technol 1988 (22):908-915
280 Lewtas J: Evaluation of the mutagenicity and carcinogenicity of motor vehicle emissions in short term bioassays. Environ Hlth Persp 1983 (47):141-152
281 Stendberg U, Alsberg T, Westerholm R: Emission of carcinogenic components from automobile exhausts. Environ Hlth Persp 1983 (47):53-63
282 Schuetzle D: Sampling of vehicle emissions for chemical analysis and biological testing. Environ Hlth Persp 1983 (47):65-80
283 Vouk VB, Piver WT: Metallic elements in fossil fuel combustion products: Amounts and form of emissions and evaluation of carcinogenicity and mutagenicity. Environ Hlth Persp 1983 (47):201-225
284 UNEP: Environmental Data Report. 1989-1990. Basic Blackwood, Oxford 1989
285 Merian E: Introduction on environmental chemistry and global cycles of chromium, nickel, cobalt, beryllium, arsenic, cadmium and selenium and their derivatives. Toxicol Environ Chem 1984 (8):9-38
286 Merian E (ed) Metals and their Compounds in the Environment. VCH, Weinheim 1991
287 Lee RE, Von Lehmden DJ: Trace metal pollution and the environment. J Air Pollut Control Assoc 1973 (73):853-862
288 Lee RE, Duffield FV: Some Sources of Environmentally Important Metals In the Atmosphere. Adv Chem Series. No 170, American Chemical Society, Washington, D.C. 1977
289 Natusch DFS, Wallace JR, Evans CA: Toxic trace elements: Preferential concentration in respirable particles. Science 1974 (183):202-209
290 U.S. EPA: National Emissions Report. EPA-450/2-76-007. U.S. Environmental Protection Agency, Research Triangle Park, N.C. May, 1973
291 Chadwick MJ, Highton NN, Lindman K: Environmental impacts of coal mining and utilization. Pergamon Press, Oxford 1978 pp 197-199
292 Chilvers DC, Peterson PJ: Global cycling of arsenic. In: Hitchinson TC, Meema RM (eds) Lead, Mercury, Cadmium and Arsenic in the Environment. John Wiley, Chichester, U.K. 1987 pp 279-302
293 Hutton M, Wadge A, Mulligan PH: Environmental levels of cadmium and lead in the vicinity of a major refuse incinerator. Atmos Environ 1988 (22):411-416
294 Greenberg RR, Zoller WH, Gordon GE: Composition and size distribution of particles released in refuse incineration. Environ Sci Technol 1978 (12):560-569
295 Fishbein L: Potential metal toxicity from hazardous waste incineration. Toxicol Environ Chem 1989 (18):287-309
296 Wadge AM, Hutton M: The cadmium and lead content of suspended particulate matter emitted from a U.K. refuse incinerator. Sci Total Environ 1987 (67):91-98
297 Lantzy RJ, Mackenzie FT: Atmospheric trace metals: Global cycles and assessment of man's impact. Geochim Cosmochim Acta 1979 (43):511-525
298 Nriagu JO: Global inventory of natural and anthropogenic emissions of trace metals in the atmosphere. Nature 1979 (279):409-411
299 Pacyna JM: Anthropogenic emissions of metals. In: Hutchinson TC, Meema KM (eds) Lead, Mercury, Cadmium and Arsenic in the Environment. John Wiley, Chichester, U.K. 1987 pp 69-87
300 Peters JM, Thomas D, Falk H, Oberdoster G, Smith TJ: Contribution of metals to respiratory cancer. Environ Hlth Persp 1986 (70):71-83
301 Fitzgerald WF, Clarkson TW: Mercury and monomethylmercury: Present and future concerns. Environ Hlth Persp 1991 (96):159-166
302 WHO: Inorganic Mercury. Environmental Health Criteria No 118. International Programme for

Chemical Safety. World Health Organization, Geneva 1991
303. WHO: Methyl Mercury. Environmental Health Criteria No 101. International Programme for Chemical Safety. World Health Organization, Geneva 1990
304. Slemr F, Langer E: Increase in global atmospheric concentrations of mercury inferred from measurements over the Atlantic Ocean. Nature 1992 (355):434-436
305. Zacharewski, TR, Cherniak EA, Schroeder WH: FTIR investigation of the heterogenous reaction of HgO with sulfur dioxide at ambient temperature. Atmos Environ 1987 (21):2327-2332
306. Lahmen E: Heavy Metals: Identification of Air Quality and Environmental Problems in the European Community. Vols 1 and 2 (Report No EUR 10678 EN/I and EUR 10678 En/II). Commission of the European Communities, Luxembourg
307. EPA: Air Quality Criteria for Lead. EPA-600/8-83/028df. U S. Environmental Protection Agency, Washington, D.C. 1986
308. WHO: Lead - Environmental Aspects. Environmental Health Criteria No 85. International Programme on Chemical Safety. World Health Organization, Geneva 1989
309. Nriagu JO: Global metal pollution: Poisoning the biosphere. Environment 1990 (32):7-33
310. IARC: IARC Monographs on the Evaluation of the Carcinogenic Risk of Chemicals to Humans. Vol 23. Some Metals and Metallic Compounds. International Agency for Research on Cancer, Lyon 1980 pp 242, 243, 344-346
311. Nriagu JO: Lead in the atmosphere. In: Nriagu JO (ed) The Biogeochemistry of lead in the Environment. Elsevier-North Holland, Amsterdam, 1978 (Part A) pp 137-184
312. Fishbein L: Environmental metallic carcinogens: An overview of exposure levels. J Toxicol Env Hlth 1976 (2):77-109
313. Anon: ES & T currents. Environ Sci Technol 1992 (26):223
314. Hewitt CN, Harrison RM: Atmospheric concentrations and chemistry of alkyl lead compounds and environmental alkylation of lead. Environ Sci Technol 1987 (21):360-366
315. IARC: IARC Monographs on the Evaluation of the Carcinogenic Risk of Chemicals to Humans. Vol 49. Chromium, Nickel and Welding. International Agency for Research on Cancer, Lyon 1990
316. U.S. EPA: Health Assessment Document for Chromium. Final Report (EPA-600/8-83-014F). U.S. Environmental Protection Agency, Research Triangle Park, N.C. 1984
317. O'Neill I.K, Schuller P, Fishbein L (eds) Environmental Carcinogens - Selected Methods of Analysis. Vol 8. Some Metals: As, Be, Cd, Cr, Ni, Pb, Se and Zn. IARC Sci Publ No 71, International Agency for Research on Cancer, Lyon 1986
318. Bowen HJM: Environmental Chemistry of the Elements. Academic Press, London 1984
319. WHO: Nickel. Environmental Health Criteria No 108. International Programme on Chemical Safety. World Health Organization, Geneva 1991
320. U.S. EPA: Health Assessment Document for Nickel and Nickel Compounds. U.S. Environmental Protection Agency, Washington, D.D. 1986 pp 1-83
321. Sunderman FW Jr (ed) Nickel in the Human Environment. IARC Sci Publ No 53. International Agency for Reaearch on Cancer, Lyon 1984 pp 487-495
322. Schmidt JA, Andren AW: The atmospheric chemistry of nickel. In: Nriagu JO (ed) Nickel in the Environment. Wiley, New York 1980 pp 93-135
323. National Research Council of Canada: Effects of Nickel in the Canadian Environment. Report No 18568. Ottawa 1981
324. IARC: IARC Monographs on the Evaluation of Carcinogenic Risks of Chemicals to Man. Vol 14. Asbestos. International Agency for Research on Cancer, Lyon 1977 p 104
325. WHO: Asbestos and Other Natural Mineral Fibres. Environmental Health Criteria No 77. World Health Organization, Geneva 1988
326. Mossman BT, Bignon J, Corn M, Seaton A, Gee JBL: Asbestos: Scientific developments and Implications for Public Policy. Science 1990 (247):294-301
327. Commins BT: The Significance of Asbestos and Other Mineral Fibres on Environmental Ambient Air. Commins Association, Maidenhead, U.K. 1985
328. OECD: Air Report. ENV/Air 81.18. 2nd Revision. Organization for European Communities, Paris 1984 p 21
329. Nicholson WJ: Asbestos and inorganic fibres. Arbete Och Halsa 1981 (17):17
330. U.S. EPA: Assessing Asbestos in Public Buildings. EPA Report 60/j-88-002. U.S. Environmental Protection Agency, Washington, D.C. 1988
331. Chesson J, Haffield J, Schulte B, Dutrow E, Blake J: Airborne asbestos in public buildings. Environ Res 1990 (51):100-107
332. U.S. EPA: Preliminary Air Pollution Information Assessment. EPA Report No.600/8-87-014. U.S. Environmental Protection Agency, Research Triangle Park, N.C. 1987
333. U.S. EPA: Report to Congress. Study of Asbestos Containing Materials in Public Buildings. U.S. Environmental Protection Agency, Washington, D.C. 1988 pp 8
334. IARC: IARC Monographs on the Evaluation of Carcinogenic Risks to Humans. Vol 43. Man-Made Mineral Fibres and Radon. International Agency for Research on Cancer, Lyon 1988

Sources, Nature and Levels of Indoor Air Pollutants

Lawrence Fishbein [1] and Kari Hemminki [2]

1 Office of Toxicology Sciences, Center for Food Safety and Nutrition, Food and Drug Administration, Washington, D.C. 20204, U.S.A.
2 Centre for Nutrition and Toxicology, CNT Novum, S-141 57 Huddinge, Sweden

There is increasing recognition that the indoor air environment may play a critical role in regard to the scope of exposure of an individual to a broad spectrum of constituents (chemical, physical and microbial), a number of which, either individually or in complex mixtures, are carcinogenic (e.g., radon-222, asbestos, formaldehyde, environmental tobacco smoke) or may have other toxicological significance [1-27]. This facet is underscored by summaries of human activity pattern studies which indicate that, over the last 2 decades, individuals spend the majority of their time indoors. In the modern industrialised societies, employed individuals spend approximately 60% of their day at home, 30% at work and 5% in transit [10,11]. Typical figures of time spent indoors range from 60-75% [8,10-13], to nearly 90% for employed men and 95% for homemakers [1,2,4,8-10,14]. Although there are many different micro-environments such as offices, public buildings, schools, private vehicles and public transport, approximately 75% of the time spent indoors is spent at home [4,8].

Additionally, it is important to note that susceptible populations such as the very young, the very old and the chronically ill, who are expected to spend the greatest percentage of their time indoors (perhaps in excess of 95%) [8,10], may be at greater potential risk to exposure to deleterious indoor environments [1-14].

Indoor air pollution is not confined to developed countries. The pernicious effects of fumes from the combustion of wood, fossil fuels and biomass for cooking and heating in homes with poor or no ventilation has been well documented in developing countries [5,7,22]. It should be noted that roughly two-thirds of the world's households cook with wood, crop residues or animal dung used in simple stoves made of rock or clay. Most of these households are in rural areas of South America, Africa and Asia [5,7,22,28]. Additional potential sources of higher exposure to toxicants are provided in those parts of the world where there are cottage industries in which solvents such as benzene are used in buildings that also serve as home and workplace [22].

Indoor air concentrations of total suspended particles and respirable particulates often exceed outdoor concentrations and the level of contaminants in a dwelling is profoundly influenced by the exchange between indoor and outdoor air [1,4,5-10,15-18] as well as by life styles, the usage patterns of unvented or improperly vented combustion appliances or usages, by air infiltration and ventilation, by chemical reactions and by adsorption or absorption of the constituents or particulate elements on indoor surfaces [1-27].

Indoor micro-environments with proximity to industrial sites such as power plants, smelters, municipal and hazardous waste disposal areas, airports, busy roadways and parking centres and garages without effective air cleaning systems will often contain pollutant concentrations that will not differ appreciably from concentrations measured in the outdoor environments [10].

The broad spectrum of chemical pollutants plus bioeffluents from humans and animals, infectious or allergenic microorganisms (bacteria, viruses, fungi, protozoa) and other contamination such as toxins from moulds, all can significantly pollute indoor air [1-10,19-27].

Cumulative exposure to these contaminants depends on the rates of accumulation of these substances in different rooms of a house or building and the amount of time a person spends in a particular room. Rates of accumulation depend on a number of factors including release rates of contaminants from materials of construction, infiltration of outside air and the ventilation of air within buildings.

In addition, there is increasing evidence that a significant number of cases of poor indoor air quality are the result of energy saving practices (primarily in developed countries) implemented since the 1970s, coupled with inadequate design, operation and maintenance of ventilation and filtration. Significant levels of both chemical and biological contaminants have been frequently associated with the cleanliness of the heating, ventilation and air conditioning systems [19-33].

Exposure to indoor air environments has been reported to cause in some cases specific illnesses but more commonly the broad spectrum of complaints which constitute the "sick-building" syndrome [19,23,29-33] and indeed the term has already become part of the everyday lexicon in many quarters. The World Health Organisation [33] in 1983 defined the sick-building syndrome as being characterised by a high frequency of irritative sympoms of the eyes, throat and lower airways, skin reactions, non-specific hypersensitivity, mental fatigue, headache, nausea and dizziness among individuals staying in a particular building.

Multiple chemical sensitivity (MCS) [6,22,34-36] is also being given wide currency, although clinical manifestations and diagnoses have not been agreed upon.

A number of agents often found in indoor environments are mostly known to be hazardous in high concentrations, but the lower limits of their dose-response relationships are poorly defined. Additive, potentiating and/or synergistic toxicological relationships are believed to occur as a result of exposure to the myriad of indoor pollutants [10,22], e.g., radon and asbestos, cigarette smoking and asbestos and cigarette smoking and radon [37].

Air pollution problems which can lead to the sick-building syndrome are believed to affect approximately 30% of the large buildings in the U.S. [30,38]. Stolwijk [39] reported that the following factors were largely responsible for a number of episodes of sick-building syndrome in the U.S.: ventilation adequacy - 52%; indoor air quality - 17%; outdoor air quality - 11%; microbial contamination - 5%.

Sources and Nature of Indoor Toxicants

It is broadly acknowledged that most pollutant sources do not emit a single pollutant but generate complex mixtures. Many hundreds of specific airborne pollutants which can be generated both intermittently or continuously from a broad array of sources (both from the outside as well as the inside of structures and dwellings) have been detected in indoor environments [1,2,4-11,15-27,40-43]. Many individual pollutants such as carbon monoxide, nitrogen dioxide and formaldehyde found indoors are also found outdoors.

External sources include soil, water supplies and the ambient air from diverse micro-environments as noted earlier. Internal sources include but are not limited to: combustion sources (unvented heaters and gas stoves, gas furnaces and water heaters, wood stoves, fire places and kerosene heaters), a broad variety of personal activities (e.g., smoking, use of household chemicals, home-care and personal-care products, hobbies), use of solvents, paints, pesticides and a variety of building materials, furniture, furnishings, other fittings and metabolic and waste products of humans and animals [1,2,4-11,13-27,40-43]. Table 1 illustrates the 9 major classes of indoor air pollutants which include carcinogenic and non-carcinogenic agents (radon, asbestos, volatile organic chemicals (VOCs), pesticides, formaldehyde, polycyclic aromatic hydrocarbons (PAHs), inorganics, respirable particles and environmental tobacco smoke (ETS)) arising from 14 major sources [21]. Identical mixtures from different sampling sites are rarely, if ever, encountered in indoor air. Although similar mixtures may be found in a variety of indoor environments, the concentrations of individual components may differ drastically (e.g., composition and concentration of ETS) [21].

Table 1. Sources of indoor air pollutants [21]

Sources	Radon	Asbestos	Volatile organic compounds	Pesticides	Formaldehyde	Polycyclic aromatic hydrocarbons	Inorganics	Respirable particles	Environmental tobacco smoke
Air-conditioning systems								X	X
Building materials	X	X	X	X	X			X	
Copying machines			X						
Earth or ground	X		X	X		X	X	X	
Furnishings			X		X				
Gas stoves			X				X		
Household products			X	X	X			X	
Insulation		X						X	
Heaters, gas			X			X	X	X	
Heaters, kerosene			X			X	X	X	
Tobacco smoking			X			X	X	X	X
Vehicle exhaust			X		X	X	X	X	
Woodstoves			X	X		X	X	X	

Table 2 illustrates order of magnitude values of the concentration ranges of 9 pollutant gases and 3 classes of inert and biological particles found inside buildings, and their indoor/outdoor concentration ratios [19]. For almost all the pollutants the concentrations are usually greater inside the building than outside.

Table 3 depicts the indoor/outdoor concentrations of some substances in randomly selected dwellings and further illustrates the greater indoor concentrations of indoor pollutants contrasted to outdoor levels [9]. The level of contaminants in a dwelling is profoundly influenced by the exchange between indoor and outdoor air [4-8,10,15-20].

The indoor pollutants of most concern are those that originate indoors; since the indoor air dilution is small and ventilation in the home is generally less than one change per hour, the concentrations are higher than would be found outdoors [4].

Of the many hundreds of specific airborne pollutants which have been detected in varying concentrations in indoor environments, 10 classes are generally considered to be of greatest toxicological concern. These are: environmental tobacco smoke, radon, asbestos, volatile organic compounds, formaldehyde, PAHs, combustion gases, particulate matter, pesticides and biological contaminants [1-27,37-43].

Table 2. Order of magnitude values for indoor pollution

Pollutant	Concentration range
A) Gases	
Radon and related substances	10-3000 Bq/m^3
CO	1-100 mg/m^3
NO$_2$	0.05-1 mg/m^3
SO$_2$	0.02-1 mg/m^3
CO$_2$	600-9000 mg/m^3
O$_3$	0.04-0.4 mg/m^3
Formaldehyde	0.05-2 mg/m^3
Organic compounds	?
B) Particles (inert and biological)	
Breathable particles	0.05-0.7 mg/m^3
Asbestos	<10^4 fibres/m^3
Microorganisms	?

from [19]

Table 3. Indoor/outdoor concentrations ratio of some substances, for randomly selected dwellings [9]

Substance/group of substances	Ratio of concentrations indoors outdoors	Remarks
Sulphur dioxide	~ 0.5	
Nitrogen dioxide	≤ 1	
	2-5	NO_2 source indoors
Carbon dioxide	1-10	
Carbon monoxide	≤ 1	
	1-5	CO source indoors
Suspended particles	0.5 - 1	excluding tobacco smoke
	2-10	including tobacco smoke
Formaldehyde	≤ 10	
Higher aliphatic hydrocarbons	2-5	
Aromatic hydrocarbons	1-3	
Volatile halogenated hydrocarbons	10-50	
Polychlorinated biphenyls	5-10	
Radon	up to 100	living rooms
	up to 1000	basements
N-nitrosodimethylamine	≤ 1	excluding tobacco smoke
	< 1	including tobacco smoke

Environmental Tobacco Smoke

Environmental tobacco smoke (ETS) is a complex mixture of particles, aerosols and gases (often in photochemically altered forms) and is the sum of the sidestream smoke and that part of the mainstream smoke which the smoker exhales [27,44-54]. Mainstream smoke (MS) is produced at the burning end of the cigarette at temperatures of about 800-900° C drawn through the cigarette and inhaled by the smoker. Sidestream smoke (SS) is formed at the burning end of the cigarette at a temperature of about 600° C. ETS is a mixture of approximately 15-20% of the exhaled mainstream smoke and 80-85% of sidestream smoke [49]. The size of the SS particles is smaller and more readily inhalable than MS particles due to dilution of the smoke. Approximately 4000 compounds have been identified in tobacco mainstream smoke and about 10% of these compounds have been quantified in both sidestream and mainstream smoke in a number of investigations [44-49].

ETS is a major indoor source pollutant and a large number of individuals can be exposed to ETS since about 25-35% of the adult population in many countries smoke tobacco and most smoking is performed indoors [50]. Repace and Lowrey [53] calculated that the total tonnage of tobacco consumed in the U.S. in 1986 was 471,480 tonnes (438,000 tonnes of tobacco from cigarettes, plus 11,078 tonnes from pipes, plus 22,000 tonnes from cigars). Since the average person spends about 90% of their time indoors [52,53], it was suggested that an estimated 424,330 tonnes of ETS are emitted into U.S. indoor micro-environments each year from tobacco smoking at 1986 consumption rates [53].

In 1988, 5.2 trillion cigarettes were produced: 1.2 trillion (23%) in China; 1 trillion (21.3%) in the Americas; 700 billion (13.4%) in western Europe; 730 billion (14%) in Asian countries other than China and 700 billion (14%) in eastern Europe (55,56). It was estimated that 1 billion people smoked 5.2 trillion cigarettes worldwide in 1988 and during the same year 3 million died from diseases caused by smoking [57]. While most of these deaths occurred in the developed world (where smoking rates are declining by 1.5% per year, rates in developing countries are rising at the rate of 2.1%/year) (see also chapter one). There appears to be a significant decrease in the total U.S. cigarette consumption and per capita consumption in adults aged 18 years and older: from 1984, when 600.4 billion cigarettes were consumed with a per capita consumption of 3446 cigarettes, to 1987 when 574.0 billion cigarettes were consumed with a per capita consumption of 3197 cigarettes [58]. In 1991 the estimated per capita cigarette consumption in the U.S. was 2713 cigarettes.

Combustion of tobacco indoors is said to contaminate indoor air with approximately 4000-5000 chemicals [27,53], 43 of which are carcinogenic with "sufficient evidence" by IARC criteria [48]. Tobacco-specific components of ETS include nicotine, some N-nitrosamines, some aromatic amines and N-heterocyclic hydrocarbons.

Sidestream smoke is often emitted into relatively small indoor environments with relatively low ventilation rates. Hence most sidestream components, particles, nitrogen oxides, alkenes, PAHs and nitrosamines are suggested to be present at concentrations well above those found in non-smoking but still polluted areas (e.g., outdoor areas in urban centres) [45].

Some of the main substances present in the gaseous phase and in the particulate matter of mainstream (MS) and sidestream (SS) smoke and in smoke-polluted air are listed in Table 4 [49]. For almost all particulate matter, sidestream smoke contains more carcinogens than mainstream smoke [48,59].

Except for nicotine and tobacco-specific nitrosamines which occur in tobacco smoke only, all of these substances are ubiquitous (e.g., CO and respirable suspended particles) in the indoor and outdoor environments and originate from various sources. The indoor concentrations of the compounds increase generally in proportion to the number of cigarettes, cigars or pipes smoked and in relation to the room's dimensions and ventilation rate [49].

Although several ETS components such as CO, nicotine, nitrogen oxides, aromatic hydrocarbons, acrolein, acetone, nitroso compounds, benzo(a)pyrene and respirable suspended particles (RSP) have been measured as potential markers of the combustion of tobacco in indoor air pollution, no single compound, with the possible exception of nicotine, has been found to represent ETS exposure reliably or to provide an estimate of the disease-causing potential of ETS [27].

Table 4. Relevant substances in the gaseous phase and in the particulate matter of mainstream smoke (MS) and sidestream smoke of cigarettes (SS), and in room air [49]

	Range/cigarette		Concentration range in room air
	MS	SS	
Carbon monoxide (CO)	2 - 20 mg	46 - 61 mg	3 - 20 ppm
Nitrogen oxide (NO)	0.07 - 0.17 mg	1.6 - 3 mg	50 - 200 ppb
Nitrogen dioxide (NO_2)	n.n.	0.16 mg	10 - 70 ppb
Ammonia (NH_3)	50 µg	5,300 - 8,500 µg	100 - 450 µg/m^3
Hydrogen cyanide (HCN)	150 - 550 µg	100 - 250 µg	10 - 120 µg/m^3
Formaldehyde	20 - 90 µg	450 - 1,500 µg	20 - 100 µg/m^3
Acetic aldehyde	18 - 1,400 µg	2,400 µg	400 - 500 µg/m^3
Acrolein	25 - 140 µg	925 µg	15 - 25 µg/m^3
Benzene	10 - 100 µg	488 µg	5 - 16 µg/m^3
Volatile Nitrosamines:			
NDMA	0.2 - 20 ng	155 - 398 ng	5 - 70 ng/m^3
Nicotine*	[0.5 - 2 mg]	3 - 4 mg	20 - 100 µg/m^3
Particles (TPM)	5 - 30 mg	20 - 50 mg	0.1 - 0.5 mg/m^3
Phenol	10 - 130 µg	270 - 320 µg	<1 - 20 µg/m^3
Tobacco-specific Nitrosamines:			
NNN	0.2 - 5.5 µg	0.15 - 6 µg	<1 - 6 ng/m^3
NNK	0.1 - 4.2 µg	0.2 - 0.8 µg	<2 - 11 ng/m^3
Benzo(a)pyrene	10 - 50 ng	25 - 103 ng	3 - 25 ng/m^3
Cadmium	100 ng	430 - 720 ng	9 - 31 ng/m^3

* nicotine is a constituent of particulate matter in mainstream smoke and of the gaseous phase in sidestream smoke and in room air

Nornicotine levels in body fluids has been proposed as an indicator of exposure to tobacco smoke. In a series collected by Jarvis et al. [60], nornicotine plasma levels of individuals inhaling smoke passively were 0.7% of those of active smokers. In persons without apparent inhalation of passive (sidestream) smoke, the percentage was 0.3.

The overall contribution of ETS to indoor air pollution in residences has been assessed primarily by site and personal monitoring for RSP [27,61-65] as well as by more recent monitoring for fine particles (effective aerodynamic diameter < 2.5 μm) [64,65]. In all of these studies, significant increases in RSP and fine particle concentrations have been measured in homes with smokers [63-65].

Radon

Radon-222 is a member of the radioactive decay chain of uranium-238, and radon is a member of the decay chain of thorium-232. The half-life of radon-222 is 3.8 days, and it decays into short-lived isotopes of polonium, lead, bismuth and thallium which are referred to as radon daughters. In closed spaces, radon and its daughters are in equilibrium: for one unit of radon there are 0.3-0.5 units of its daughters. Uranium and radium occur abundantly in the earth's crust. The average concentration of radon gas in the atmosphere at ground level is about 3 Bq/m^3, with a range of 0.1 (over oceans) to 10 Bq/m^3 (1Bq=27 pCi). The concentration of radon varies widely in different parts of the world. High concentrations of radon have been noted especially in areas where terrestial gamma radiation is high [66].

Radon and its short-lived decay products in indoor air are the greatest contributors to the total dose burden from natural radioactivity [10,26,27]. The alpha-emitting polonium-218 and polonium-214 decay products (radon daughters) are of most concern. Indoor radon concentrations are generally higher than outdoor concentrations [67]. The instantaneous rate of radon entry into any given building may be highly variable, causing indoor radon concentrations to fluctuate markedly [67].

Radon enters houses and buildings in the air that is drawn from the underlying soil (via cracks or other openings in basements or crawl spaces) by small differences in air pressure between indoors and outdoors. Only a small part of infiltrating air actually comes from the soil, but that is what causes the radon to enter into houses [26]. The entry rate depends on the permeability of the soil to air flow, along with geologic, meteorological and structural factors [26,27].

The chemical form and concentration of radon's decay products (isotopes of polonium, lead and bismuth) also depend on the amount of airborne particles and the pattern of air movement in a particular building or residence.

In the U.S., concentrations of radon in single-family residences vary over 4 orders of magnitude from a few bequerels/m^3 of air to more than 10,000 Bq/m^3 with an average level of about 50 Bq/m^3 [27,67-69]. In 2 large U.S. monitoring programmes on indoor air radon, concentration mean levels between 55 and 160 Bq/m^3 were recorded [70,77].

The U.S. Environmental Protection Agency (EPA) estimates that 7% of American homes (approximately 4 million) contain radon above the EPA action level of 4 pCi/litre (150 Bq/m^3) with 1-3% of the homes exceeding 8 pCi/l. Other workers claim that the average radon levels in American homes, measured over the long term, are about 1.5 pCi/l, with only 2% of the homes in the U.S. having radon concentrations at or above 8 pCi/l [26,67,72,73].

In Finland (population of 5 million), some 40,000 radon measurements have been carried out in houses and apartments. The mean radon measurements in room air are shown in Figure 1 [74]. It can be seen that extensive local differences exist. However, at any particular locality there may be houses differing in radon concentrations by a factor of 10.

In attached houses, the mean radon levels are around 150 Bq/m^3 while in apartment houses the levels of radon are 50-70 Bq/m^3 in Finland. The source of radon in apartment houses is the building material. In Scandinavia the radon levels in homes are approximately at the levels noted in Finland.

A geographical clustering of high concentrations is observed on a regional scale [27,69].

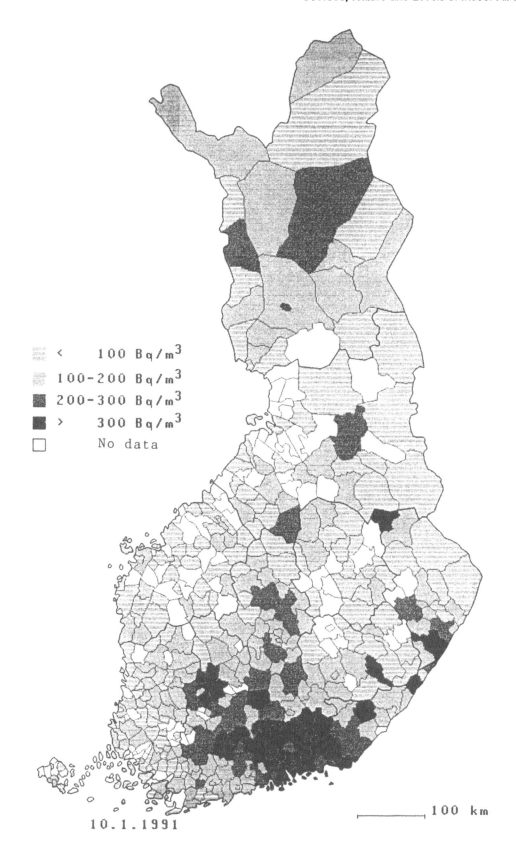

Fig. 1. Radon levels in 23,000 attached homes in Finland measured by the Finnish Radiation Protection Board [74]

Table 5. Distribution of radon daughter EER concentrations in different countries [71]

Country	Arithmetic mean (Bq/m^3)	Percentage of dwellings exceeding		
		100 Bq/m^3	200 Bq/m^3	400 Bq/m^3
Sweden) Finland) Norway)	50	10	3	1
United States	27	5	1	0.1
Canada	25	3	1	0.2
United Kingdom	10	< 0.1	-	-
Fed. Rep. of Germany	25	0.7	0.1	-

Typically, radon levels are high in basements where the concentrations are often 2-3 times higher than in the rest of the home. The source of radon and its daughters in the air of dwellings is predominantly the underlying soil. Building materials, ground water and utility natural gas can also be contaminated with radon. As uranium-containing rock is the main source of radon, ground water may contain particularly high concentrations of radon. Many homes in Finland use water from drilled wells where radon concentrations on average are around 1000 Bq/l, and extremes exist [75]. In the U.S., water from granite aquifers contains radon levels of 100 Bq/l or higher [70,76].

Table 5 shows the mean concentrations and relative frequencies of radon daughter equilibrium radon (EER) concentrations exceeding 100, 200 and 400 Bq/m^3 in dwellings in Sweden, Finland, Norway, the U.S., Canada, the United Kingdom and Germany [62]. A small fraction of dwellings in each country have concentrations 10 times higher than the national average of that country. In Europe and North America, the mean radon daughter concentrations range between 10 and 50 Bq/m^3.

Asbestos, Other Mineral Fibres and Man-Made Mineral Fibres

Asbestos dust consists of inorganic mineral fibres that range from 0.5 to 200 microns in length and less than 3 microns in diameter (see also the chapter by L. Fishbein, p. 56). Two major types of asbestos are common: a) chrysotile asbestos (fibres less than 3 microns in length), which comprises about 95% of all asbestos used in buildings; b) amphibole asbestos (fibres over 5 microns in length), which, although having limited commercial use *per se*, is often found as a contaminant of chrysotile asbestos.

The pathology of different forms of asbestos varies, with long, thin amphibole fibres being the most pathogenic, particularly in the induction of mesothelioma [77,78].

An estimated 20% of buildings including hospitals, schools and other public and private structures contain asbestos-containing materials (ACM) [79,80]. Asbestos in buildings does not spontaneously shed fibres, but physical damage to ACM by decay, renovation or demolition can cause release of airborne fibres [77].

Average concentrations of asbestos in urban ambient air are typically less than 1 ng/m^3 and rarely exceed 5 ng/m^3. Concentrations of 100 ng/m^3 to 1000 ng/m^3 have been measured in ambient air near specific asbestos emission sources and in schools and office buildings containing damaged or deteriorating friable asbestos materials. Buildings with intact asbestos containing materials seldom show increased concentrations of airborne asbestos over ambient levels [27,77-82].

Data regarding the presence of inplace ACM and the potential for exposure to asbestos were recently collected in 886 buildings from 16 different building categories in New York City [83]. Overall, 68% of the buildings in New York City contain ACM. The estimated total amount of ACM in the city was 323 million square feet, most of which is in thermal insulation. Overall, 16% of all ACM had greater than 10% of its surface damaged and another 68% of ACM had some, but less than 10% of its surface damaged. About half of all ACM is in mechanical spaces within buildings.

Indoor asbestos fibre and other mineral fibre concentrations can be considerably higher than outdoor concentrations [27,78,81,84]. For example, in the Cappadocian region in Turkey, erionite-containing rock has been used traditionally as building and insulation material, and indoor air samples in such conditions also contain up to 10,000 fibres/m^3. In Cappadocian villages, even outdoor fibre concentrations may be as high as 3,000 fibres/m^3 [84].

Several potential sources of indoor airborne asbestos exist other than friable surfacing and insulation materials. These include weathering and entrainment asbestos cement wall and roofing materials, and wearing of vinyl asbestos tiles. Concentrations ranging from 20 ng/m^3 to 4,500 ng/m^3 and as high as 5 fibres/l for fibres > 5 microns long have been measured in a variety of enclosed spaces (e.g., schools, buildings and subways) [27,81]. The greatest potential source of fibre release inside buildings is the friable sprayed asbestos used as insulating fireproofing or for decoration or acoustic purposes. Nevertheless, on rare occasions, nonfriable material such as vinyl-asbestos floor tile may be implicated in indoor asbestos contamination [78-82,85,86].

In buildings without specific asbestos sources, concentrations are generally below 1000 fibres/m^3, while in buildings with friable asbestos, concentrations vary irregularly; usually less than 1000 fibres/m^3 are found but in some cases exposures can reach 10,000 fibres/m^3 (as counted with an optical microscope) [78,87].

It is important to cite another potential source of elevated indoor asbestos concentrations. In a recent limited study, Hardy et al. [88] suggested that indoor asbestos concentrations exceeding the ambient background asbestos level may occur if an ultrasonic humidifier charged with asbestos-contaminated water is operated under single-room conditions. Asbestos in drinking water supplies results from its natural occurrence in raw waters, industrial processes, abrasion-induced accumulation from asbestos cement pipe (ACP) and ACP leaching from "aggresive" soft or acidic waters. Health care professionals have historically recommended home humidifiers to alleviate symptoms associated with some chronic and/or acute pulmonary diseases. Portable humidifiers have become an increasingly popular means for maintaining comfortable indoor humidity levels in office and other indoor environments.

In contrast to asbestos and other natural mineral fibres, very much less data are available concerning indoor air levels and exposures to man-made mineral fibres [37]. Concern was expressed in the U.S. in the late 1960s over health problems associated with possible erosion of fibrous glass used to line ventilation and heating ducts. Glass fibres were found in settled dust and walls and permanent structures in some buildings [89]. However, in some cases there was a decrease in fibre concentration after fibre-containing outdoor air had passed through the air-transmission system [90].

Extensive measurements of concentrations of man-made mineral fibres in schools and office buildings in Denmark were reported by Schneider [91] and Rindel et al. [92]. Although a random sample of mechanically ventilated schools which had man-made mineral fibre noise baffles or linings in ducts showed concentrations of undetectable-0.0001 fibre/cm^3, under special circumstances, e.g., after water damage or faulty construction, high concentrtions were found e.g., 0.084 fibre/cm^3 in a nursery school in which ceilings were covered with man-made mineral fibre boards containing water-soluble binder [37,91,92].

Volatile Organic Chemicals

Volatile organic chemicals (VOCs) (also known as gas phase organics), of which more than 900 have been found throughout indoor environments, constitute an extremely broad category of compounds of varying reactivities and physical properties [1-27,41,42,93-101]. The release of many VOCs into the ambient environment is a direct consequence of their use [41,42]. The major sources of the VOCs include: paints, solvents, cleaners, adhesives, caulks, cleansers, pesticides, building materials and furnishings (new carpets, PVC materials and their additives), particle board, personal activities (e.g., smoking), home-care and personal-care products (room air deodorizers), hobbies etc. Additionally, VOCs such as chloroform arise from showering, dish washing and clothes washing [1-30].

Many VOCS have been measured indoors at concentrations greater than that in ambient air where the concentrations of many of them are regulated [1,2,4,10,15-18,27,41,42]. Aliphatic hydrocarbons were the compounds found most frequently, followed by aromatic hydrocarbons and chlorinated hydrocarbons.

A number of studies conducted in more than 1500 homes in Europe and the U.S. under widely differing protocols provides a substantial body of data characterising the sources and levels of indoor VOCs in residential environments [15-18,27,41,93-102]. The salient findings include: a) an extremely wide variety of VOCs were found in all indoor residential environments with more than 300 different compounds detected in some studies; b) a number of these VOCs were detected consistently in all studies; c) concentrations of most VOCs varied widely within and among homes (often differing by 2 or more orders of magnitude) and more than 250 VOCs were found at concentrations higher than 1 ppb [81]; d) except in the case of extreme outdoor pollution [15-18,27,41,100], indoor VOCs were higher than outdoor concentrations, with median indoor/outdoor concentration ratios normally ranging between 2 and 5 and occasionally up to several orders of magnitude higher for some compounds, and e) indoor sources varying widely in number and type were most important contributors to VOC concentrations [15-18,27,41,93-102]. In offices the concentrations of VOCs can be higher than those found in dwellings, reaching values of 10-80 times the concentrations found outdoors [82,83].

The EPA's Total Exposure Assessment Methodology (TEAM) studies [15-18,27,100] which have been conducted over the last decade have provided data on personal exposures (including indoor and outdoor concentrations) to volatile organic chemicals for more than 1000 persons representing more than 1 million residents in 10 U.S. cities. These studies involved 12-hour integrated personal exposures and corresponding breath and outdoor concentrations of 11 to 19 target VOCs determined in 650 households at 5 sites. Estimated frequency distributions of personal air exposures, outdoor air concentrations and exhaled breath concentrations were determined for all target VOCs (e.g., benzene, trichloroethylene, tetrachloroethylene, 1,1,1-trichloroethane, chloroform, carbon tetrachloride, p-dichlorobenzene, p-xylene and o-xylene). The TEAM studies showed that the indoor-outdoor or personal monitor-outdoor monitor differences were always higher than unity (the ratios ranged between 2 and 199), depending on the indoor use of the compounds (Tables 6 and 7) [27,84]. Breath concentrations correlated more closely with personal exposures than did outdoor concentrations. Benzene concentrations were found to be significantly higher (30-50%) in homes of smokers than non-smokers [16,18,27].

Major exposures were associated with the use of deodorizers (p-dichlorobenzene), washing clothes and dishes (chloroform), visiting dry-cleaning establishments (1,1,1-trichloroethane, tetrachloroethylene), active and passive smoking (benzene and styrene), painting and using paint removers (n-decane and undecane).

The TEAM studies showed that average benzene levels in personal air were 2 times higher than outside air concentrations. Wallace [15] found that exposure to benzene concentrations indoors was greater than exposure to benzene levels near petrol stations in most cases. Personal air concentrations ranged from 7.5-28 µg/m^3 with a geometric mean concentration of 13.7 µg/m^3, while outdoor air concentrations ranged from 1.9 to 16 µg/m^3 with a geometric mean of 5.6 µg/m^3.

Table 6. Indoor-outdoor relationships: overnight personal air means compared to outdoor means

Compound	Arithmetic mean			Geometric mean		
	Outdoor [a]	Personal [b]	Ratio	Outdoor	Personal	Ratio
Chloroform	1.2[c]	8.7	7	0.55	3.3	6
1,1,1-Trichloroethane	5.4	110	21	3.7	19	5
Benzene	8.6	30	3	4.1	12	3
Carbon Tetrachloride	1.2	14	12	0.8	1.8	2
Trichloroethylene	2.1	7.3	3	1.4	2.6	2
Tetrachloroethylene	3.7	11	3	2.1	6.3	3
Styrene	0.90	2.7	3	0.55	1.5	3
m,p-Dichlorobenzene	1.5	56	37	1.0	5.1	5
Ethylbenzene	3.8	13	3	2.5	6.4	3
o-Xylene	4.0	16	4	2.8	5.3	2
m,p-Xylene	11	55	5	8.3	16	2

[a] N = 86; [b] N = 340; [c] µg/m^3

Table 7. Personal-outdoor air comparisons: daytime mean values and ratios

Compound	Arithmetic mean			Geometric mean		
	Outdoor [a]	Personal [b]	Ratio	Outdoor	Personal	Ratio
Chloroform	1.5[c]	7.4	5	0.58	3.0	5
1,1,1-Trichloroethane	8.6	820	96	3.3	19	6
Benzene	9.5	26	3	3.8	11	3
Carbon Tetrachloride	1.0	4.6	5	0.70	1.3	2
Trichloroethylene	2.4	19	8	1.4	3.0	2
Tetrachloroethylene	8.3	78	9	3.8	9.2	2
Styrene	0.82	15	18	0.61	1.8	3
m,p-Dichlorobenzene	1.9	35	18	0.78	4.7	6
Ethylbenzene	4.3	25	6	2.6	7.3	3
o-Xylene	4.0	17	4	2.6	6.1	2
m,p-Xylene	12	48	4	7.0	18	2

[a] N = 90; [b] N = 344; [c] µg/m^3

Pleil [103] recently compared the presence an amounts of specific compounds such as propane, benzene, chloroform, carbon tetrachloride, trichloroethylene and tetrachloroethylene in summer and winter samples and correlated these to variables including building materials, age of buildings, interior decoration etc. (Table 8). For compounds such as benzene, chloroform and methyl chloroform, the older houses showed higher concentrations which were suggested to arise from buiding materials, the presence of basements and attached garages.

Formaldehyde

Formaldehyde is an ubiquitous contaminant in indoor air, particularly in residential environments where concentrations often exceed outdoor levels by one or more orders of magnitude.

Formaldehyde has been widely employed in the wood products industry where it is principally used in the preparation of phenol-formaldehyde, urea-formaldehyde, melamine-formaldehyde and acetal resins in particle board, plywood insulation and laminates which are commonly used in construction and

Table 8. Presence and amounts of specific compounds as related to various parameters of residential structure or activity [103]

Compounds	Correlation category	Comparison of mean (ppb) levels when detected	
		Summer samples	Winter samples
Propane	Gas heat installed vs electric	30 vs 0	40 vs 4
Benzene	House vs apartment	8.6 vs 1.2	5 vs 5
	Age > 15 years vs younger	17 vs 1.5	4.6 vs 4.8
	Brick vs wood frame	11.7 vs 1.5	3.4 vs 5
	Basement vs other foundation	24 vs 1.7	2 vs 4
	Gas heat installed vs electric	17 vs 1.2	3.9 vs 2.8
	Garage: attached or under vs not	24 vs 1.5	8 vs 2.9
	Storage of volatiles: inside vs not	13 vs 1.8	7 vs 2
	Heat on: woodstove vs average	NA	1.5 vs 4.8
	gas vs average	NA	4.7 vs 4.8
	kerosene vs average	NA	16.2 vs 4.8
	electric vs average	NA	3.2 vs 4.8
Chloroform	Apartment vs house	2.6 vs 1.7	3.8 vs 1.7
	Age > 5 years vs less	1.9 vs 0	2.7 vs 1.5
	Brick vs wood frame	2 vs 1.6	2.6 vs 1.5
Methyl chloroform	Age > 15 years vs less	2.5 vs 1.3	1 vs 0.7
	Brick vs wood frame	2.4 vs 0.9	0.8 vs 0.7
	Gas heat installed vs electric	2.5 vs 1.4	0.9 vs 0.6
Carbon tetrachloride	No particular correlations found		
Trichloroethylene	Apartment vs house	1.8 vs 1.6	2.8 vs 1.6
	Volatiles storage inside vs not	1.7 vs 1.6	2.6 vs 1.0
	heat on: woodstove vs average	NA	1.2 vs 1.6
	gas vs average	NA	2.4 vs 1.6
	kerosene vs average	NA	1 vs 1.6
	electric vs average	NA	2.2 vs 1.6
Tetrachloroethylene	Wall-to-wall carpet vs other floor coverings	0.9 vs 0.6	1.5 vs 0.2
	Volatiles storage inside vs not	1.2 vs 0.5	2.5 vs 0.2

NA = not analysed

are the major sources of formaldehyde in mobile and conventional homes [27,104-114].

In homes, most formaldehyde exposure is from pressed wood products made with urea-formaldehyde (UF) resin adhesives. Other sources of formaldehyde in residences include: tobacco smoke, household products, urea-formaldehyde foam insulation, unvented gas heaters, permanent-press cloth, adhesives and paint preservatives [109-114].

Mobile homes, because of their air-tight structures, extensive use of pressed wood products and relatively small volumes, are more likely to exhibit elevated formaldehyde concentrations than conventional homes [106-108]. Since 1985, the U.S. has limited formaldehyde emissions from plywood and particle board used in manufactured housing such as mobile homes.

Numerous monitoring studies have been conducted to measure the concentrations of formaldehyde in indoor environments in U.S., British, Dutch, Canadian and Swiss homes with and without UFFI (urea-formaldeyde foam insulation) [27,110-112]. Despite the wide variety of conditions under which these residential formaldehyde studies were conducted, results for given types of housing tended to be consistent within certain broad ranges. Indoor residential concentrations of formaldehyde were significantly higher than outdoor concentrations which ranged from 0.002 to 0.006 ppm in remote unpopulated regions to 0.010 to 0.020 ppm and sometimes 0.050 ppm in highly populated areas and industrial air. The range of formaldehyde concentrations measured in complaint homes, mobile homes and homes containing large quantities of particle board or urea-formaldehyde insulation tended to be from 0.02 to 0.80 ppm, with levels as high as 4 ppm in some instances. Older conventional homes tended to have the lowest concentrations of formaldehyde, with values typically less than 0.05 ppm. In newer conventional homes (less than 1 year old), formaldehyde levels generally fell within the range of 0.05 ppm to 0.2 ppm with few measurements exceeding 0.3 ppm. It should be noted that concentrations of 0.1 to 0.8 ppm formaldehyde had been common in earlier homes insulated with UFFI.

In most countries the formaldehyde problem has been succesfully managed where it has been recognised by utilising improved particle board quality and reducing the amount of formaldehyde containing material in other indoor items. From earlier levels as high as 0.05-0.2 mg/m^3 on average (and in earlier extreme cases 10 times higher) [33,66,115], the levels now rarely exceed 0.2 mg/m^3 and are usually below 0.1 mg formaldehyde/m^3.

Polycyclic Aromatic Hydrocarbons and Particulates

Indoor levels of polycyclic aromatic hydrocarbons (PAHs) reflect ambient outdoor air as well as indoor air sources. Exposure to PAHs in air is related to the total amount of PAHs distributed between the gas and aerosol phases as well as the particle size distribution [10,27]. Approximately 50% of indoor particulate concentration of benzo(a)pyrene has been estimated to penetrate indoors [116]. Concentrations of the PAHs can be spatially and temporally variable within homes [116]. Median indoor air levels of PAHs in homes appear to be in the order of 8 nanograms/m^3 with a range of less than 1 ng/m^3 and maximum values in the 30-80 ng/m^3 range [117]. Smoking has the greatest effect on both PAH concentration and mutagenicity [4,27,118-120]. The concentrations of a number of PAHs in tobacco smoke and various smoke-polluted indoor environments (e.g., anthracene, benzo(a)pyrene, benzo(e)pyrene, benzo(a)fluorene, benzo(ghi)perylene, coronene, dibenzo(aj)anthracene and fluoranthene) ranged from 0.1 to 99 ng/m^3 [27, 119].

A more recent evaluation of the effect of smoking on indoor PAH in 8 U.S. homes [121] found additional PAHs (other than those listed above) and a number of nitro-PAHs (e.g., naphthalene, acenaphthalene, phenanthrene, pyrene, chrysene, 9-nitroanthracene, 9-nitrophenanthrene and 2-fluoranthene). Higher levels of those PAHs were found in the homes with smokers compared to homes without smokers. Additionally, levels of the PAHs and nitro-PAHs were generally higher indoors than outdoors. Indoor air levels of PAHs associated with sidestream smoke have been reported to be in the range of 3-29 ng/m^3 [116,117,120].

Another major source of PAHs in indoor environments arises from the daily use of unvented combustion appliances such as wood burning stoves and fireplaces and kerosene heaters, as well as from the use of biomass fuels for cooking and heating. Unvented kerosene heaters are significant sources of carcinogenic PAHs and nitro-PAHs as well as nitric oxide, nitrogen dioxide, sulphur dioxide, carbon monoxide and indoor air particles (PM-10) [120].

About one-half of the world's population is exposed to concentrations of PAHs that are orders of magnitude greater (e.g., 10-10^2 μg/m^3) than those normally found in areas using more advanced forms of combustion with adequate ventilation [5,7,15,28,37,122]. The levels of PAHs in indoor air depend to a large extent on the types of combustion and fuel as well as the ventilation and exhaust systems employed. When no proper chimneys are present, indoor PAH concentrations may reach high levels and, as noted, wood burning stoves and fireplaces tend to result in some leakage of PAHs into indoor air. In non-occupational environments, indoor and outdoor air are believed to be minor (direct) sources of exposure to PAHs in contrast to food, which is the main source.

It has been shown that inhalable particulate matter (IPM) and particulate matter having a mean median diameter of <10 μm (PM-10) concentrations in non-industrial indoor environments can exceed outdoor ambient concentrations [13,123,124]. Residential wood combustion [13], environmental tobacco smoke [125], the improper use of portable ultrasonic humidifiers with tap water [126-128] and kerosene heaters used under unvented conditions [120,129,130] are significant sources of IPM in many indoor environments. In a field study conducted by the WHO in rural Kenya, average particulate levels in houses where wood or crop residues were used for cooking were 20 times higher than the WHO exposure guidelines; levels of aromatic hydrocarbons were also very high [131].

Pesticides

A large variety of pesticides (including insecticides, termiticides, rodenticides, fungicides, herbicides and germicides) are extensively employed in or in close proximity to indoor environments [10,27]. Pesticides, primarily in the vapour phase, are applied in and around buildings and hence can enter indoor spaces through cracks and other openings in foundations or be directly introduced. Numerous investigations in the U.S. [10,27,132-135] indicate that the average U.S. residence contains a number of pesticides that are typically 1 to 2 orders of magnitude higher than ambient outdoor concentrations. In the pilot phase of the Non-Occupational Pesticides Exposure Study (NOPES) [27,134], air concentrations of 31 of the most commonly used pesticides and 2 oxidation products were measured inside 9 residences and compared with corresponding outdoor concentrations and personal exposures. Twenty-four pesticides were detected in the indoor samples at concentrations ranging from 1.7 ng/m^3 to 15.0 ng/m^3. Chlorpyrifos, diazinon, chlordane, proxopur and heptachlor were the most frequently found pesticides in the indoor samples. Their concentrations were generally about 1 order of magnitude higher than those of any other pesticide found in the same sample; mean indoor air concentrations ranged from 0.16 to 2.4 μg/m^3 and were almost always 1 to 2 orders of magnitude higher than outdoor concentrations. Twenty-five pesticides were found in outdoor samples at concentrations ranging from < 1.0 ng/m^3 to 410 ng/m^3 [27,134].

Studies of both military [27,134] and non-military residences [136] in the U.S. have reported detectable levels of chlordane >0.5 μg/m^3. Houses at greatest risk were those constructed over a crawl space with post-construction treatment of chlordane. Air concentrations of the termiticides chlordane and heptachlor were generally significantly higher in basements than in upper floor rooms, often by as much as an order of magnitude [134]. Mean chlordane concentrations of 1 to 10 μg/m^3 have been found in apartments 10 to 15 years after treatment [137].

Metals

The major sources of metals in indoor environments are: cigarette smoking (main and passive), street and soil dusts, house paint, fuel combustion with inadequate ventilation (wood, fossil fuels and biomass), and consumer and household products [2,7,27]. The major elements of consideration in terms of their toxicological potential are lead, nickel, cadmium, mercury, chromium and arsenic.

The dusts found indoors can originate from surface soil contaminated with metals from vehicular traffic, metal fall-out from combustion of fossil fuels, proximity to smelters and municipal solid waste incinerators etc., which can be tracked into the residence or building from deposition of airborne particles originating outdoors [2,7,138].

Concern over the presence of lead in house dust has led to attempts to identify the contributions from the various sources of lead. It is well recognised that in general, the principal sources of house lead are paint-lead, soil lead, auto exhaust lead and road dust lead. What is less obvious is which sources predominate at different scales of urbanisation, in locations close to industrial activity, in areas with differences in local geology and in houses of various ages [139].

Lead is a major source of indoor pollution, especially in older homes where lead-based paints were employed. Lead concentrations as high as 2 μg/m^3 have been measured in residences with wall paints that contain lead compounds or in residences that are near major roads [2].

In the U.S. the Consumer Product Safety Commission banned the use of paints containing more than 0.06% lead in 1977, but many homes built before that time were painted with products containing much higher levels of lead.

While mercury is not normally considered an indoor air pollutant, there is increasing evidence and concern that it may be an important one. Mercury compounds were used as preservatives in 25 to 30% of interior latex paints in the U.S. until 1990. During indoor painting, according to the EPA, exposure to mercury vapour from paints containing 200 ppm mercury may reach 200 µg/m^3. The OSHA threshold limit value for mercury vapour is 50 µg/m^3, with a ceiling value of 100 µg/m^3, (acute exposure standard). Mercury levels in painted homes may remain near the inhalation reference (RfD) level of 0.3 µg/m^3 for months after painting [140].

Cooking-Related Contaminants

There has been increasing concern recently regarding contaminant exposures in indoor environments (e.g., restaurants, kitchens). It has been shown by several groups that grilling of meat or fish can give rise to a number of mutagenic and carcinogenic products in the fried foodstuffs [141,142]. Additionally, epidemiological data suggests that professional cooks may have an increased risk of lung cancer [143,144].

Extensive studies have revealed that grilling and/or frying of fish and meat can give rise to a number of heterocyclic amines which are formed from certain amino acids and tissue components [145,146]. Over 200 volatile compounds have been identified from heat-formed degradation products of fat and fried meat and fish. These include short-chain fatty acids, carbohydrates, aldehydes and ketones, nitrosamines, heterocyclic amines and PAHs. For example, when pork or beef are heated at 210° C, MeIQx (2-amino-3,8-dimethylimidazo[4,5-f]quinoline) and DiMeIQx (2-amino-3,4,5-trimethyl-imidazo [4,5-f]-quinoxaline) were found at levels of 0.04 ng/g and 0.02 ng/g meat grilled; formaldehyde, acrolein and acetaldehyde were produced at levels of 5 ng/g, 40 ng/g and 38 ng/g, respectively. Additionally, grilling of bacon gave rise to air concentrations of 1.4 µg/m^3 of N-nitroso-pyrrolidine [147].

All of these compounds have been identified in workplace (factory, restaurant, grill, kitchen and backery) ambient air (Table 9) [147]. Relatively high acrolein concentrations were found in all types of kitchens with some measurements in restaurant kitchens even exceeding the Finnish 15 minute TLV value of 0.25 mg/m^3 (147). The concentrations of heterocyclic amines were below the limit of detection in all kitchens where measurements were carried out. Readily volatilised PAHs were detected in most cooking facilities (e.g., naphthalene in all and fluorene and phenanthrene in most of them).

Table 9. Air concentrations of suspected carcinogens and fat mist in the cooking environment [103]

Environment (N)	Formaldehyde (mg/m^3)	Acetaldehyde (mg/m^3)	Acrolein (mg/m^3)	Heterocyclic amines (µg/m^3)	Fat mist (mg/m^3)	Benzo(a)-pyrene (µg/m^3)
Factory (N = 1)	0.02	0.03	0.01	<0.007	0.2	n.d.
Restaurant (N=3)	0.05-0.07	0.1-0.2	0.1-0.6	<0.003	2-16	n.d.
Grill kitchen* (N = 2)	0.2-0.7	0.07-0.1	0.06-0.2	<0.016	0.1-1.5	0.4
Bakery (N = 1)	0.03	0.7	0.01	n.m.	<0.01	n.d.

* The grill was gas heated from underneath to 300 °C or more
n.d. = not detected
n.m. = not measured

Conclusions

Humans spend a large proportion of their time indoors, which makes indoor exposure to harmful agents particularly important. Indoor air pollution has two sources, i.e., from indoors and from outdoors. Usually the outdoor contaminants are relatively evenly distributed indoors and outdoors, unless large particles are involved. The normal ventilation systems do not appreciably lower the level of outdoor contaminants. Radon is a unique example of a contaminant leaching from the soil and accumulating indoors.

The contaminants originating indoors are many and relate to construction and interior materials, or to human activities such as smoking, cooking and sanitation. In addition, microbial products may be present. The experiences with formaldehyde, radon and asbestos show that technical measures can vastly reduce the level of indoor air pollution. However, the solutions before rather than after construction or installation tend to be most cost effective and health promoting.

REFERENCES

1. Spengler JD, Sexton K: Indoor air pollution: A public health perspective. Science 1983 (221):9-17
2. National Research Council: Indoor Pollutants. National Academy of Science Press, Washington, DC 1981
3. Lebowitz MD: Health effects of indoor pollutants. Am Rev Publ Hlth 1983 (4):203-210
4. Lewtas J: Toxicology of complex indoor air pollutants. Ann Rev Pharmacol Toxicol 1989 (29):415-439
5. Yocum JE: Indoor-outdoor air quality relationships - A critical review. J Am Pollut Control Assoc 1982 (32):500-508
6. Fishbein L, Henry CJ: Introduction: Workshop on the methodology for assessing health risks from complex mixtures in indoor air. Environ Hlth Persp 1991 (95):3-5
7. Fishbein L: Indoor environments: The role of metals. In: Merian E (ed) Metals and Their Compounds in the Environment. VCH Press Weinheim, Germany 1991 pp287-309
8. Esmen NA: Indoor air pollution. Environ Hlth Persp 1985 (62):259-265
9. Greim H, Sterzl H, Lilienblum W, Mucke W: Indoor air pollution - A review. Toxicol Environ Chem 1989 (23):191-206
10. Berry MA: Indoor air quality: Assessing health impacts and risks. Toxicol Ind Hlth 1991 (7):179-186
11. Ott W: Total human exposure: An emerging science focuses on humans as receptors of environmental pollution. Environ Sci Technol 1985 (19):880-886
12. Szalai A: The use of time-daily activities of urban and suburban populations in twelve countries. Mouton Publ, The Hague 1972
13. Sexton K, Spengler JD, Treitman RD: Effects of residential wood combustion on indoor air quality. Atmos Environ 1984 (18):1371-1387
14. Moschandreas DJ: Exposure to pollutants and daily time budgets of people. Bull NY Acad Med 1981 (57):845-859
15. Wallace LA: The total exposure. Assessment methodology (TEAM) study: An analysis of exposure, sources and risks associated with four volatile organic chemicals. J Am Coll Toxicol 1989 (8):883-895
16. Wallace LA, Pellizzari ED, Hartwell TD, Davis V, Michael LC, Whitmore RW: The influence of personal activities on exposure to volatile organic compounds. Environ Res 1989 (50):37-55
17. Wallace LA: Personal exposure to 25 volatile organic compounds. EPA's 1987 TEAM study in Los Angeles, California. Toxicol Ind Hlth 1991 (7):203-208
18. Wallace LA: Comparison of risks from outdoor and indoor exposure to toxic chemicals. Environ Hlth Persp 1991 (95):7-13
19. Lowenstein JC: Current state of research on air quality inside buildings. In: Bieva CJ, Courtois Y, Govaerts M (eds) Present and Future of Indoor Air Quality. Elsevier Sci Publ BV, Amsterdam 1989 pp 43-50
20. Lioy PJ, Avdenko M, Harkov R, Atherholt T, Daisey JM: A pilot indoor-outdoor study of organic particulate matter and particulate mutagenicity. J Air Pollut Control Assoc 1985 (35):653-657
21. Jayanty RKM, Peterson MR, Naugle DF, Berrt MA: Exposure assessment: methods of analysis for environmental carcinogens. Risk Anal 1990 (10):587-595
22. WHO: Global environmental monitoring system. Assessment of urban air quality. United Nations Environmental Programme (UNEP). World Health Organization, United Nations, London 1988 pp 81-88
23. Stolwijk JAJ: Assessment of population exposure and carcinogenic risk posed by volatile organic compounds in indoor air. Risk Anal 1990 (10):49-57
24. Molhave L, Bach B, Peterson OF: Human reactions to low concentrations of volatile organic compounds. Environ Int 1986 (12):167-175
25. Burrell R: Biological agents as health risks in indoor air. Environ Hlth Persp 1991 (95):29-34
26. Nero AV: Controlling indoor air pollution. Sci Amer 1988 (258):42-48
27. U.S. Environmental Protection Agency: Indoor air assessment. Indoor air concentrations of environmental carcinogens. EPA/600-8-90/042. Research Triangle Park, NC 1991
28. Davidson CI, Lin SN, Osborne JF, Pandey MR, Rasmussen RA, Khalil MAK: Air pollution in the Himalayas. Environ Sci Technol 1986 (20):561-567
29. Norback D, Edling C: Environmental and personal factors related to the prevalence of sick building syndrome in the general population. Br J Ind Med 1991 (48):451-462
30. Woods JE: An engineering approach to the control of indoor air quality. Environ Hlth Persp 1991 (95):15-21
31. Stolwijk JAJ: Sick building syndrome. Environ Hlth Persp 1991 (95):99-100
32. Skov P, Valbjorn O, Pedersen BV: Influence of indoor climate on the sick building syndrome in an office environment. Scand J Work Environ Hlth 1990 (16):363-371
33. World Health Organization: Health aspects related to indoor air quality. Report of a WHO Working Group. EURP. Reports and Studies No 211. WHO Regional Office for Europe, Copenhagen 1979
34. Hileman B: Multiple chemical sensitivity. Chem Eng News 1991 (July 22):26-42
35. Ashford NA, Miller CS: Chemical Exposures: Low Levels and High Stakes. Van Nostrand, New York 1991 p 214
36. Barinaga M: Better data needed on sensitivity syndrome. Science 1990 (251):1558
37. IARC: IARC Monographs on the Evaluation of Carcinogenic Risks to Humans. Vol 43/ Man-Made Mineral Fibres and Radon. International Agency for Research on Cancer, Lyon 1988
38. Smith SC: Controlling "Sick Building Syndrome". J Env Hlth 1990 (53):22-23
39. Stolwijk JAJ: The sick building syndrome. Practical control of indoor air problems. Proceedings of ASHRAE Conference IAQ '87. Arlington, Va, May 18-22, 1988

40. U.S. Environmental Protection Agency: Report to Congress on Indoor Quality. Vol II. Assessment and Control of Indoor Air Pollution. EPA/400/1-89/001C. Washington, DC 1989
41. Ember LR: Survey finds high indoor air levels of volatile organic chemicals. Chem Eng News 1988 (Dec. 5):23-25
42. Shah JJ, Singh HB: Distribution of volatile organic chemicals in outdoor and indoor air. Environ Sci Technol 1988 (22):1383-1388
43. Tancrede M, Wilson R, Zeise L, Crouch EAC: The carcinogenic risk of some organic vapors indoors: A theoretical survey. Atmos Environ 1987 (21):2187-2204
44. O'Neill IK, Brunnemann KD, Dodet B, Hoffman D: Environmental Carcinogens - Methods of Analysis and Exposure Measurement. Vol 9. Passive Smoking. IARC Sci Publ No 81. International Agency for Research on Cancer, Lyon 1987
45. National Research Council: Environmental Tobacco Smoke: Measuring Exposures and Assessing Health Effects. National Academy of Sciences Press, Washington, DC 1986 pp7-1-7-46
46. U.S. Dept. of Health, Education and Welfare: The Health Consequences of Involuntary Smoking. A Report of the Surgeon General. DHHS Publ. No. (CDC) 87-8398; Washington, DC 1986
47. Lofroth G: Environmental tobacco smoke: Overview of chemical composition and genotoxic components. Mutat Res 1989 (222):73-80
48. IARC: IARC Monographs on the Evaluation of the Carcinogenic Risk of Chemicals to Humans. Vol 38. Tobacco Smoking. International Agency for Research on Cancer, Lyon 1986 pp83-126
49. Adlkofer FX, Scherer G, Von Meyerinck L, Von Maltzan C, Jarczyk L: Exposure to ETS and its biological effects: A review. In: Bieva CJ, Courtois Y, Govaerts M (eds) Present and Future of Indoor Air Quality. Elsevier Science BV, Amsterdam 1989 pp183-196
50. Sorsa M, Lofroth G: Genotoxicity of environmental tobacco smoke and passive smoking. Mutat Res 1989 (222):71-73
51. Leaderer BP: Assessing exposures to environmental tobacco smoke. Risk Anal 1990 (10):19-26
52. Repace JL, Lowrey AH: A quantitative estimate of non-smoker's lung cancer risk from passive smoking. Environ Int 1985 (11):2-22
53. Repace Jl, Lowrey AH: Risk assessment methodologies for passive smoking - lung induced cancer. Risk Anal 1990 (10):27-48
54. Vainio H, Partanen T: Population burden of lung cancer due to environmental tobacco smoke. Mutat Res 1989 (222):137-140
55. U.S. Dept. of Agriculture/Foreign Agriculture Service: World Tobacco Situation Report. Publ No FT8-88. U.S. Dept. of Agriculture, Washington, DC, August 1988
56. U.S. Dept. of Agriculture/Foreign Agriculture Service: World Tobacco Situation Report. Publ No FT6-89. U.S. Dept. of Agriculture, Washington, DC, July 1987
57. Chandler WV: Banishing Tobacco. World Watch Paper No 68. World Watch Institute, Washington, DC 1986 pp1-42
58. U.S. Dept. of Health and Human Services: Reducing the Health Consequences of Smoking: 25 Years of Progress. A Report of the Surgeon General. DHHS Publ No (CDC) 89-8411. Centers for Disease Control, Rockville, Md 1989
59. Wynder EL, Kabat GC: Environmental tobacco smoke and lung cancer: A critical assessment. In: Kasuga H (ed) Indoor Air Quality. Springer-Verlag, Berlin 1990 pp5-15
60. Jarvis M, Tunstall-Pedoe H, Feyerabend C, Vesey C, Saloojee Y: Biochemical markers of smoke absorption and self-reported exposure to passive smoking. J Epidemiol Comm Hlth 1984 (38);335-339
61. Sexton K, Spengler JD, Treitman RD: Personal exposure to respirable particles: A case study in Waterbury, Vermont. Atmos Environ 1984 (18):1385-1398
62. Spengler JD, Dockery DW, Turner WA, Wolfson JM, Ferris BG Jr: Long-term measurements of respirable sulfates and particles inside and outside homes. Atmos Environ 1981 (15):23-30
63. Spengler JD, Treitman RD, Tosteson TD, Mage DT, Soczek ML: Personal exposures to respirable particulates and implications for air pollution epidemiology. Environ Sci Technol 1985 (15):23-30
64. Spengler JD, Reed MP, Lebret E, Chang BH, Ware JH, Speizer FE, Ferris BG Jr: Harvard's Indoor Air Pollution/Health Study. Presented at 79th Annual Meeting of the Air Pollution Control Association, Minneapolis, MN, June 1986 Paper No 86-6.6
65. Spengler Jd, Ware J, Speizer FE, Ferris BJ Jr, Dockery D, Lebret E, Brunekreef B: Harvard's Indoor Air Quality Respiratory Health Study 1987. In: Seifert B, Esdorn H, Fischer M, Rueden H, Wegner J (eds) Indoor Air'87; Proceedings of the 4th Int Conf on Indoor Air Quality and Climate. Vol 2. Environmental Tobacco Smoke, Multicomponent Studies, Radon, Sick Buildings, Odour and Irritants, Hyperactivities and Allergies. Institute for Water, Soil and Air Hygiene, Berlin 1987 pp182-187
66. World Health Organization: Air Quality Guidelines for Europe. WHO Regional Publications, European Series No 23. Regional Office for Europe, Copenhagen 1987 pp182-198
67. Nazeroff WN, Teichman K: Indoor radon. Environ Sci Technol 1990 (24):774-782
68. Cohen BL: A national survey of 222-radon in U.S homes and correlating factors. Health Phys 1986 (51):175-183
69. Nero AV: The behavior of radon and the indoor environment.In: Nazeroff W, Nero AV (eds) Radon and Its Decay Products. Wiley, New York 1988
70. Nero AV, Schwehr M, Nazeroff W: Distribution of airborne radon-222 concentrations in U.S. homes. Science 1986 (234):922-927
71. Alter H, Oswald R: Nationwide distribution of indoor radon measurements: A preliminary data base. J Air Pollut Control Assoc 1987 (37):227-231
72. Hanson DJ: Radon tagged as cancer hazard by most study researchers. Chem Eng News 1989 (Feb 6):7-13

73 World Health Organization: Indoor Air Pollution Exposure and Health Effects; Report of a WHO Working Group. Euro Reports and Studies. No 78. WHO Regional Office for Europe, Copenhagen 1983

74 Voutilainen A: Huoneilman radonmittaukset Suomen kunnissa. Ymparisto ja Terveys 1991 (1/91):32-37

75 Pirinen P, Maki-Petays N: Selvitys radonpitoisen porakaivoveden kaytosta talousvetena ja siita aiheutuvan terveysriskin arviointi. Ymparisto ja Terveys 1991 (1/91):48-51

76 Michel J: Sources. In: Cother S, Smith J (eds) Environmental Radon. Plenum Press, New York 1987 pp81-130

77 Mossman BT, Bignon J, Corn M, Seaton A, Gee JBL: Asbestos: Scientific developments and implications for public policy. Science 1990 (247):294-301

78 WHO: Asbestos and Other Natural Mineral Fibres. Environmental Health Criteria No 53. International Programme On Chemical Safety, World Health Organization, Geneva 1986

79 U.S. Environmental Health Protection Agency: Assessing Asbestos in Public Buildings. EPA Rept. 60/J-88-002. Washington, DC 1988

80 Chesson J, Haffield J, Schulte B, Dutrow E, Blake J: Airborne asbestos in public buildings. Environ Res 1990 (51):100-107

81 U.S. Environmental Protection Agency: Preliminary Air Pollution Information Assessment. EPA Rept. 600/8-87-014. Research Triangle Park, NC 1987

82 U.S. Environmental Protection Agency: Report to Congress. Study of Asbestos Containing Materials in Public Buildings. Washington, DC 1988 p5

83 Lundy P, Barer M: Asbestos-containing materials in New York City buildings. Environ Res 1992 (58):15-24

84 Hemminki K: Measurement and monitoring of individual exposures. In: Tomatis L (ed) Air Pollution and Human Cancer. European School of Oncology Monograph Series. Springer-Verlag, Berlin 1990 pp35-45

85 Nicholson WJ: Airborne mineral fibre levels in the non-occupational environment. In: Bignon J, Peto J, Saracci R (eds) Non-Occupational Exposure to Mineral Fibres. IARC Publ No 90. International Agency for Research on Cancer, Lyon 1989 pp239-261

86 Sebastien P, Martin M, Bignon J: Indoor airborne asbestos pollution: From the ceiling and the floor. Science 1982 (216):1410-1413

87 Ontario Ministry of the Attorney General: Report of the Royal Commission on Matters of Health and Safety Arising From the Use of Asbestos in Ontario. Vols 1-3. Toronto 1984

88 Hardy RJ, Highsmith VR, Costa DL, Krewer JA: Indoor asbestos concentrations associated with the use of asbestos-contaminated tap water in portable home humidifiers. Environ Sci Technol 1992 (26):680-689

89 Cholak J, Schafer LJ: Erosion of fibres from installed fibrous-glass ducts. Arch Environ Hlth 1971 (22):220-229

90 Balzer JL: Environmental data: Airborne concentrations found in various operations. In: LeVee WN, Schulte PA (eds) Occupational Exposure to Fibrous Glass. DHEW Publ No NIOSH 76-151; NTIS Publ No PB-258869. National Institute for Occupational Safety and Health, Cincinnati, OH 1976 pp83-89

91 Schneider T: Man-made mineral fibres and other fibres in the air and in settled dust. Environ Int 1986 (12):61-65

92 Rindel A, Bach E, Breum NO, Hugod C, Schneider T: Correlating health effects with indoor air quality in kindergartens. Int Arch Occup Environ Hlth 1987 (59):363-373

93 Berglund B, Johansson I, Lidvall TH: Volatile organic compounds from building materials in a simulated chamber study. In: Seifert B (ed) Indoor Air '87, Vol 1. Institute for Water, Soil and Air Hygiene, Berlin, 1987 pp16-21

94 Hollowell CD, Miksch RR: Sources and concentration of organic compounds in indoor air environments. Bull NY Acad Med 1981 (57):962-967

95 De Bortoli M, Knoeppel H, Peccio E, Peil A, Rogora L, Schauenburg H: Concentrations of selected organic pollutants in indoor air In Northern Italy. In: Berglund U, Lidvall T, Spengler J, Sundell J (eds) Indoor Air Quality: Papers of the 3rd Int Conf on Indoor Air Quality and Climate. Stockholm. Environ Int 1984 (12):343-350

96 Gammage RB, White DA, Gupta KC: Residential measurements of high volatility organics and their sources. In: Berglund B, Lidvall T, Sundell J (eds) Indoor Air. Proc of the 3rd Int Conf on Indoor Air Quality and Climate. Vol 4. Chemical Characterization and Personal Exposure. Swedish Council for Building Research, Stockholm 1984 pp157-162 (NTIS, Report PB85-104214, Springfield, Va)

97 Molhave L, Moller J: The atmospheric environment in modern Danish dwellings - Measurements in 39 flats. In: Fanger PO, Valbjorn O (eds) Indoor Climate: Effects of Human Comfort, Performance and Health In Residential, Commercial and Light-Industry Buildings. Proceedings of the 1st Indoor Climate Symposium. Danish Building Research Institute, Copenhagen 1978 pp171-186

98 Seifert B, Abraham HJ: Indoor air concentrations of benzene and some other aromatic hydrocarbons. Ecotoxicol Saf 1982 (6):190-192

99 Wallace LA: The Total Exposure Methodology (TEAM) Study: Summary and Analysis. Vol 1. EPA Rept. No 600/6-87-002. U.S. Environmental Protection Agency, Washington, DC 1987

100 Pellizzari ED, Perrit K, Hartwell TD, Michael LC, Whitmore R, Handy RW: The Total Exposure Assessment Methodology (TEAM) Study: Selected Communities in Northern and Southern California. Vol III. EPA Rept. No 600/6-87-00C. U.S. Environmental Protection Agency, Washington, DC 1987

101 Krause C, Mailahn W, Nagel R, Schulz C, Seifert B, Ullrich D: Occurrence of volatile organic compounds in the air of 500 homes In the Federal Republic of Germany. In: Seifert B, Esdorn H,

Fischer M, Rueden H, Wegner J (eds) Indoor '87. Proceedings of the 4th Int Conf on Indoor Air Quality and Climate. Vol 1. Volatile Organic Compounds, Combustion Gases, Particles and Fibres and Microbiological Agents. Institute for Water, Soil and Air Hygiene, Berlin 1987 pp102-106

102. Sterling DA: Volatile organic compounds in indoor air: An overview of sources, concentrations and health effects. In: Gammage RB, Kaye SB, Jacobs VA (eds) Indoor Air and Human Health. Lewis Publ, Chelsea, MI 1985 pp387-402

103. Pleil JD: Volatile organic compounds in indoor air: A survey of various structures. In: Walkinshaw DS (ed) Indoor Air Quality in Cold Climates. Hazards and Abatement Measures. Air Pollut Control Assoc, Pittsburg, Pa 1986 pp237-249

104. Saarela K, Kaustia K, Kiviranta A: Emissions from materials: The role of additives in PVC. In: Bieva CJ, Courtois Y, Govaerts M (eds) Present and Future of Indoor Air Quality. Elsevier Science BV, Amsterdam 1989 pp329-336

105. Jungers RH, Sheldon LS: Characterization of volatile organic chemicals in public access buildings. Indoor Air '87. Vol 1. Institute of Water, Soil and Air Hygiene, Berlin 1987 pp144-148

106. Liu, KS, Huang FY, Hayward SB, Weslowski J, Sexton K: Irritant Effects of Formaldehyde Exposure in Mobile Homes. Environ Sci Technol 1991 (94):91-94

107. Sexton K, Petreas MX, Liu K: Formaldehyde exposures inside mobile homes. Environ Sci Technol 1990 (23):985-988

108. Hanrahan LP, Dally KA, Anderson HA, Kanerek MS, Rankin J: Formaldehyde vapor in mobile homes: A cross-section survey of concentrations and irritant effects. Am J Publ Hlth 1984 (74):1026-1027

109. Gupta KC, Ulsamer AG, Preuss PW: Formaldehyde in indoor air: Sources and toxicity. Environ Int 1982 (8):348-358

110. National Research Council: Formaldehyde and Other Aldehydes. National Academy Press, Washington, DC 1991 pp7-1-7-46

111. U.S.Environmental Protection Agency: Assessment of Health Risks to Garment Workers and Certain Home Residents from Exposure to Formaldehyde. Washington, DC 1987

112. Versar Inc: Maximum Levels of Formaldehyde Exposure in Residential Settings. U.S. EPA Contract No 68-02-3968. Springfield, Va 1986

113. Ritchie LM, Lehnen RG: An analysis of formaldehyde concentrations in mobile and conventional homes. J Environ Hlth 1985 (47):300-305

114. Godish T: Residential formaldehyde. J Environ Hlth 1990 (53):34-37

115. Hemminki K: Environmental carcinogens. In: Cooper CS, Glover PL (eds) Handbook of Experimental Pharmacology. Springer-Verlag, Heidelberg 1989 pp31-61

116. Waldman JM, Lioy PJ, Greenberg A, Butler JP: Analysis of human exposure to benzo(a)pyrene via inhalation and food ingestion in the total human environmental exposure study (THEES). J Expos Anal Environ Epidemiol 1991 (1):193-225

117. Menzie CA, Potocki BB, Santodonato J: Exposure to carcinogenic PAHs in the environment. Environ Sci Technol 1992 (26):1278-1284

118. Lewtas J, Goto S, Williams K, Chuang JC, Petersen BA, Wilson NK: The mutagenicity of indoor air particles in a residential pilot field study: Application and evaluation of new methodologies. Atmos Environ 1987 (21):443-449

119. IARC: IARC Monographs on the Evaluation of the Carcinogenic Risk of Chemicals to Humans. Vol 32. Polynuclear Aromatic Compounds. Part 1. Chemical, Environmental and Experimental Data. International Agency for Research on Cancer, Lyon 1983

120. Mumford JI, Williams RW, Walsh DB, Burton RM, Svendsgaard DJ, Chuang JC, Houk VS, Lewtas J: Indoor air pollutants from unvented kerosene heaters. Emissions in mobile homes: Studies on particles, semi-volatile organics, CO and mutagenicity. Environ Sci Technol 1991 (25):1732-1736

121. Wilson NK, Chuang JC: Indoor air levels of polynuclear aromatic hydrocarbons and related compounds in an eight-home pilot study. In: Proceedings of the 11th Int Symp on Polynuclear Aromatic Hydrocarbons. Gaithersburg, Md, Gordon and Breech, New York 1987

122. Smith KR, Apte M, Menon P, Shrestha M: Carbon monoxide and particulates from cooking stoves: Results from a simulated village kitchen. In: Berglund B, Lindvall T, Sundell J (eds) Indoor Air: Proceedings of the 3rd Int Conf on Indoor Air Quality and Climate. Vol 4. Chemical Characterization and Personal Exposure. Swedish Council for Building Research, Stockholm 1984 pp389-395

123. Dockery DW, Spengler JD: Indoor-outdoor relationships of respirable sulfates and particles. Atmos Environ 1981 (15):335-343

124. Sexton K, Webber LM, Hatward SB, Sextro RG: Characterization of particle composition, organic vapor constituents and mutagenicity of indoor air pollutant emissions. Environ Int 1986 (12):351-362

125. Repace JL: Indoor Concentrations of Environmental Tobacco Smoke: Field Surveys. In: O'Neill IK, Brunnemann KD, Dodet B, Hoffmann D (eds). Environmental Carcinogens- Methods of Analysis and Exposure Measurement. Vol.9. Passive Smoking. IARC Sci. Publ No.81. International Agency for Research on Cancer, Lyon 1987 pp141-162

126. Highsmith VR, Rodes CE, Hardy RJ: Indoor Particle Concentrations Associated With Use of Tap Water In Portable Humidifiers. Environ Sci Technol 1983 (17):369-371

127. Geoghlou PE, Blagden P, Snow DA, Winsor L, Williams DT: Mutagenicity of indoor air containing environmental tobacco smoke: Evaluation of a portable PM-10 impactor sampler. Environ Sci Technol 1991 (25):1496-1500

128. Highsmith VR, Hardy RJ, Costa DL, Germani MS: Physical and chemical characteristics of indoor aerosols resulting from the use of tap water in portable home humidifiers. Environ Sci Technol 1992 (26):673-680

129 Traynor GW, Allen JR, Apte MG: Pollutant emissions fom portable kerosene-fired space heaters. Environ Sci Technol 1983 (17):369-371

130 Barnes J, Holland P, Mihlmester P: Characterization of Populations and Usage of Unvented Kerosene Space Heaters. EPA Rept. No 600/7-90-004. U.S. Environmental Protection Agency, Washington, DC 1990 pp1-37

131 WHO: HEAL (Human Exposure Assessment Location) Project: Indoor Air Pollution Study, Maragua Area, Kenya. United Nations Environment Programme, World Health Organization, Geneva 1987 pp18-19

132 Lewis RG, Bond AE, Johnson DE, Hsu JP: Measurement of atmospheric concentrations of common household pesticides; A pilot study. Environ Monit Assess 1988 (10):59-73

133 Lewis RG, MacLeod KE: Portable sampler for pesticides and semi-volatile industrial organic chemicals in air. Anal Chem 1986 (54):310-315

134 Lewis RG, Bond AE, Fitzsimons TR, Johnson DE, Hsu JP: Monitoring for non-occupational exposure to pesticides in indoor air and personal respiratory air. Presented at 79th Annual Meeting of the Air Pollution Control Association, Minneapolis, MN June 17, 1986 Paper No 86-37.4

135 Anderson DJ, Hites RA: Chlorinated pesticides in indoor air. Environ Sci Technol 1988 (22):717-720

136 Wright CG, Leidy RB: Chlordane and heptachlor in the ambient air of houses treated for termites. Bull Environ Contam Toxicol 1981 (27):406-411

137 Livingston JM, Jones CR: Living area contamination by chlordane used for termite treatment. Bull Environ Contam Toxicol 1981 (27):406-411

138 Laxen DPH, Raab GM, Fulton M: Children's blood lead and exposure to lead in household dust and water - A basis for an environmental standard for lead in dust. Sci Total Environ 1987 (66):235-244

139 Hunt A, Johnson DL, Watt JM, Thornton I: Characterizing the sources of particulate lead in house dust by automated scanning electron microscopy. Environ Sci Technol 1992 (26):1513-1526

140 Ripley PJ, Murdock BS: Environmental issues in primary care. Minnesota Dept of Health, Minneapolis, MN 1991

141 Nagao M, Honda M, Seino Y, Yahagi T, Sugimura T: Mutagenicities of some smoke condensates and the charred surface of fish and meat. Cancer Lett 1989 (2):221-226

142 Rappaport SM, McCartney MC, Wei ET: Volatilization of Mutagens From Beef During Cooking. Cancer Lett 1979 (8):139-145

143 IARC: IARC Monographs on the Evaluation of the Carcinogenic Risk of Chemicals to Humans. Vol 40 Some Naturally Occurring and Synthetic Food Components, Furocoumarins and Ultraviolet Radiation. International Agency for Research on Cancer, Lyon 1986

144 Ahlbom A, Gerhardson M, Hogstedt C, Lundberg I, Plato N, Stelbeck G, Tornling G: Yrke och Cancer, Arbeten utsatta for sarkilda halsorisker, bilagadel D. Stockholm 1989

145 Felton JS, Healy S, Stuermer D, Berry C, Timoutian H, Hatch F, Morris M, Bjeldanes L: Mutagens from the cooking of foods. I. Improved extractions and characterization of mutagenic fractions from cooked ground beef. Mutat Res 1981 (88):33-44

146 Sugimura T: Food as a source of complex mixtures of mutagens and carcinogens. In: Vainio H, Sorsa M, McMichael A (eds) Complex Mixtures and Cancer Risk. IARC Sci Publ No 104. International Agency for Research on Cancer, Lyon 1990 pp399-407

147 Vainiotalo S, Hameila M, Matveinen K, Nylund L, Tornaeus J, Hesso A: Karyista aiheutuvat haitat eralla elintarviketeollisuuden ja ravintola-alan tyopaikoilla. Tyoterveyslaitos Tyosuojelurahasto 1991

Environmental Carcinogens: Assessment of Exposure and Effect

Kari Hemminki[1], Herman Autrup[2] and Aage Haugen[3]

1   Centre for Nutrition and Toxicology, Karolinska Institute, Novum, 141 57 Huddinge, Sweden
2   Steno Institute of Public Health, University of Aarhus, 8000 Aarhus, Denmark
3   National Institute of Occupational Health, P.O. Box 8149 Dep, 0033 Oslo, Norway

In the previous monograph the chapter on exposure monitoring covered air and biological sampling [1]. An analysis was given of parent compounds and, in the case of biological monitoring, of their metabolites in the body. In the present chapter we discuss a new form of biological monitoring: measurement of covalent reaction products (adducts) of the carcinogen with DNA and protein. In addition, we discuss the consequences of the adducts, i.e., mutations. The examples are taken from environmental exposures.

Mechanisms of Environmental Carcinogenesis

Cancer, induced by chemical or physical agents, is believed to be a multistage process in which damage to DNA in important growth-controlling genes or loci leads to aberrant cellular growth [2]. Many carcinogenic chemicals cause DNA damage through adduct formation in target and non-target tissue. Adducts are also formed in RNA and proteins and they can be used as surrogate indicators of DNA binding [3,4]. DNA and RNA adducts are released spontaneously by DNA repair or RNA turnover, and are excreted in urine. Urinary adducts can also be used as a measure of exposure.
DNA adducts can lead to mutations by causing misreading during DNA replication or errors in DNA repair [5]. Most of the mutations (or DNA sequence alterations) are likely to affect sequences or genes that are not critical to the control of cell growth. However, mutations in oncogenes, tumour suppressor genes and other important genes and loci may lead to malignant transformation and appearance of clinically manifest tumours [2,6]. Mutations lead to expression of mutant proteins, which is used as a selection mechanism in many mutation assays, as will be discussed later.

DNA Adducts - Postlabelling

The ^{32}P-postlabelling assay, described in the early 1980s [7-9], is a sensitive technique which is now extensively used in human biomonitoring. The sensitivity of the technique depends on the use of highly specific-activity ^{32}P-ATP in the kinase reaction, where a radioactive phosphate group is transferred to 3'-nucleotides (Fig. 1) [10]. The method has improved in specificity and cost effectiveness since nuclease P1, butanol and high-performance liquid chromatographic techniques (HPLC) have been used to prepurify adducts before the kinase reaction [11].
In a recent review Beach and Gupta [11] list examples of the application of the ^{32}P-postlabelling technique to human tissues and cells (Table 1). Most of the studies have focused on tobacco smoking, occupational exposures and cancer chemotherapy patients. Following exposure to complex mixtures, multiple radioactive spots (called diagonal radioactive zone, DRZ) have been detected (Table 1). The quantitation covers many types of adducts and may be imprecise. Few studies have reported specific adducts in humans (e.g., O^6- and N-7-methylguanine, 4-aminobiphenyl-C8-guanine adduct).

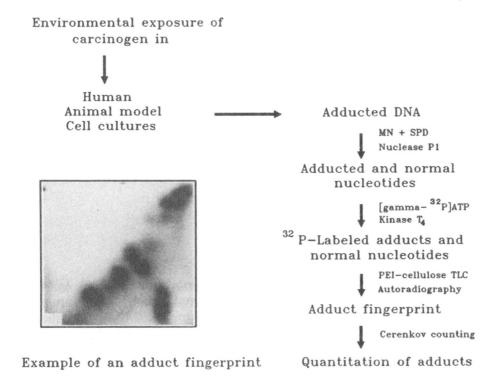

Fig. 1. A scheme of the postlabelling protocol used for aromatic DNA adducts [10]

In environmental studies on a Silesian population living in a highly industrial area, the aromatic adduct levels in total white cell DNA exceeded 2 to 3 times those measured in a control population in eastern Poland [12,13]. Recently, it has been shown that the adduct levels are higher in winter than in summer, coinciding with the level of air pollution [14,15]. In the same individuals differences were also seen in chromosomal aberrations and sister chromatid exchanges [14].

The postlabelling assay is sensitive enough to show adducts in apparently unexposed individuals. This applies to aromatic adducts as well as to specific adducts such as N-7-methylguanine [16]. The origin of these adducts is unknown; in the case of aromatic adducts (if they really are such) the origin is likely to be environmental and/or dietary; food contains aromatic compounds as contaminants and as products of cooking [17,18].

DNA Adducts - Immunoassays and Fluorescence

Antibodies might be useful in studies of structural modifications in DNA. Over the last decade highly specific polyclonal and monoclonal antibodies have been developed for detection of carcinogen-modified DNA, for example DNA adducts produced by polycyclic aromatic hydrocarbons, aromatic amines, mycotoxins, alkylating agents and ultraviolet light [19]. Immunological techniques that are currently available for such studies vary in sensitivity and specificity. The development of highly sensitive enzyme immunoassays, for example the radioimmunoassay (RIA), the enzyme-linked immunosorbent assay (ELISA) and the ultrasensitive enzyme radioimmunoassay (USERIA), represents an important advance for the specific detection of DNA modification by carcinogens at low levels. Assay sensitivity depends on the antibody used (i.e., affinity constant) and on the assay. The assays are generally sensitive enough to detect one adduct in 10^8 nucleotides in 50 µg DNA [20]. Assay specificity depends upon the cross-reactivity of the antibody with other DNA adducts. For instance, antibodies raised against BP-DNA adducts cross-react with other aromatic hydrocarbons such as chrysene and benz(a)anthracene due to their similar chemical structure and therefore detect a broad spectrum of PAH-DNA adducts [21]. This may be an advantage in environmental monitoring. A major limitation of this

Table 1. DNA adduct data compiled from ^{32}P-postlabelling analysis of various human tissues and cells [11]

Exposure/tissue	Enhancement procedure	No./nature of adducts[a]	Adduct levels[b] adducts/10^9 nucleotides
Cigarette smokers			
Lung	P$_1$	DRZ[c]	6-340
Lung/heart	P$_1$	DRZ	10-250
Lung	HPLC	O^6-methyl-dG	100-5200
Lung	HPLC	O^6-ethyl-dG	200-3600
Lung	HPLC	N^7-methyl-dG	1400-7200
Lung	HPLC	dG-C8-ABP	10-850
Lung	P$_1$	DRZ/dG-N^2-B[a]P[d]	19-340[d]
Lung	P$_1$	DRZ	14-134
Lung/heart	P$_1$/butanol	2-6	≤100
Lung	ATP-deficient	4-7	170-290
Bronchoalveolar lavagate	P$_1$/butanol	2-4	≤200
Placenta	ATP-deficient	1-4	5-12
Placenta	P$_1$/butanol	dG-N^2-B[a]P	≤200[e]
Bladder	P$_1$/butanol	6-9	≤50
Bladder	P$_1$/butanol	up to 5	13-270
Urothelial cells	P$_1$/butanol	2-6	1-25
Urinary mutagens	P$_1$/butanol	up to 7[f]	not applicable[g]
PBL	P$_1$	1-6	≤10
WBC	P$_1$	DRZ	20-25
WBC	P$_1$	4	very low[h]
PBL	P$_1$	10	100-600
PBL	butanol	2-5	≤30
Monocytes	P$_1$	2	not reported
Tobacco chewers/cigarette smokers			
Oral mucosa	ATP-deficient	up to 5	1-100
Oral mucosa	butanol	up to 16	5-200
Oral mucosa	butanol	DRZ	up to 1600
Occupationally exposed			
WBC (foundry)	P$_1$	up to 15	2-200
WBC (foundry)	P$_1$	DRZ	90-260
WBC (coke oven)	P$_1$	DRZ	27-530
WBC (roofers)	P$_1$	2-3	2-130
WBC (styrene)	none	2	2200
Clinically exposed			
Skin (coal/juniper tar)	P$_1$	DRZ	2-150
Liver (mitomycin C)	P$_1$	up to 4	6-30
WBC (mitomycin C)	P$_1$	up to 4	≤10
WBC (procarbazine/darbazine)	HPLC	N^7-methyl-dG	250-5700
Undefined exposure			
Bone marrow	ATP-deficient	5	10-90
Gastric/duodenal	P$_1$	DRZ	1-40/1-109
Colon	P$_1$	1-2	10
Mammary	P$_1$	1-2	4-30

[a] Except when indicated, the only class of compounds analysed were aromatic/lipophilic adducts
[b] Levels where reported in femto or attomol/μg DNA were converted to adducts/10^9 nucleotides, considering 1 μg DNA = 3x10^9 amol
[c] DRZ = diagonal radioactive zone of unresolved radioactive compounds
[d] Part (2-42 adducts/10^9 nucleotides) of the adduct radioactivity was attributed to the presence of dG-N^2-B[a]P
[e] Estimated from data of known standards
[f] PhIP identified as the major metabolite
[g] It seems difficult to correlate levels of DNA-reactive metabolites (DRM) to tissue DNA adducts
[h] Actual levels not reported, probably in the range of 10-30 adducts/10^9 nucleotides

approach is the need to develop antibodies for each adduct of interest. At present the list of antibodies is relatively short. An additional problem in using immunological detection for the quantification of carcinogen adducts in humans has been the use of highly modified DNA as a competitor in ELISA and USERIA. The antibody affinity might depend on the level of DNA modification. Recent studies have shown that the use of highly modified DNA in an immunoassay leads to erroneous results when analysing DNA from biological samples [22]. Therefore, one should be cautious when comparing adduct levels between different studies because of the use of different antibodies and assay methods. An advantage of the immunoassay is that a large number of samples can be analysed.

Occupational Exposure

Polycyclic aromatic hydrocarbons (PAHs) are among of the most widespread environmental pollutants known today, and comprise a group of compounds which are suspected to induce cancer in man [23]. The highest PAH concentrations are found in occupational settings, e.g. coke oven plants, aluminium industry, foundries, and during handling of tar, pitch and asphalt. The most important emission sources are coal tar and pitch. Immunoassays for DNA adduct measurement have been applied in several studies on occupational hazards connected with PAH exposure (Table 2).
White blood cell (WBC) DNA has often been used as a surrogate in these studies since

Table 2. Detection of PAH-DNA adducts in DNA by immunoassay

Population	DNA source	Assay	No. detected/ assayed	Adduct level (10^8 nucleotides)	Reference
Occupational Exposure					
Coke oven workers					
USA	PBL	USERIA	18/27 (67%)	12-1029[a]	Harris et al. [25]
Norway	PBL	USERIA	13/38 (34%)	3-411[a]	Haugen et al. [26]
- after vacation	PBL	USERIA		3.3-5[a]	ibid.
Poland	WBC	ELISA	31	15.3[b]	Hemminki et al. [12]
the Netherlands	WBC	ELISA	24/51 (47%)	5.1±5.1[c]	van Schooten et al. [27]
Norway	WBC	USERIA	36/97 (37%)	6-23.8[a]	Øvrebø et al. [29]
- high exposure	WBC	USERIA	11/31 (35%)	9.2-23.8[a]	ibid.
- medium exposure	WBC	USERIA	12/44 (27%)	7.3-20.5[a]	ibid.
- low exposure	WBC	USERIA	13/40 (32%)	6-18.8[a]	ibid.
- controls	WBC	USERIA	8/13 (61%)	6-16.5[a]	ibid.
Foundry workers					
USA	PBL	ELISA	7/20 (35%)		Shamsuddin et al. [24]
Finland					
- high exposure	WBC	ELISA	4/4 (100%)	24-84[a]	Perera et al. [28]
- medium exposure	WBC	ELISA	13/13 (100%)	3-60[a]	ibid.
- low exposure	WBC	ELISA	13/18 (72%)	0.9-25.8[a]	ibid.
- controls	WBC	ELISA	2/10 (20%)	0.9-9[a]	ibid.
Finland					
- at work	WBC	ELISA	9	30.8±6.9	Hemminki et al. [30]
- after vacation	WBC	ELISA	9	3.9-1.6	ibid.
Fire fighters					
USA	WBC	ELISA	15/43 (35%)	56.1±48.6[d]	Liou et al. [31]
- controls	WBC	ELISA	13/38 (34%)	34.5±13.8[d]	ibid.
Roofers					
USA	PBL	ELISA	7/28 (25%)	1.2-72[a]	Shamsuddin et al. [24]
Environmental Exposure					
Poland					
- urban	WBC	ELISA	15	13[b]	Hemminki et al. [12]
- rural	WBC	ELISA	13	2.3[b]	ibid.

[a] range; [b] arithmetic mean; [c] mean ± SD; [d] mean ± SE

WBC can be obtained easily. The studies cleary showed PAH-DNA adducts in some individuals and the mean levels of PAH-DNA adducts were generally higher in groups at high exposure to PAH. For instance coke-oven workers, foundry workers and roofers are occupationally exposed to high levels of PAHs and have an increased risk of developing lung cancer. DNA adducts were found more frequently in the high-risk individuals when the ELISA/USERIA methods were used. In an early study Shamsuddin et al. detected PAH-DNA adducts in 7 of 28 samples from roofers and 7 of 20 samles from foundry workers [24]. Using USERIA Harris et al. and Haugen et al. analysed WBC DNA from coke oven workers and 18 of 27 and 13 of 38 had detectable levels of PAH-DNA adducts [25,26]. In a recent study by van Schooten, 24 of 51 subjects were found to have detectable levels of PAH-DNA adducts [27]. In a Polish study by Hemminki et al., 31 workers had detectable levels of PAH-DNA adducts [12]. Perera et al. and Øvrebø et al. demonstrated a dose-response relationship between adduct levels in WBC DNA from foundry and coke oven workers and exposure [28,29]. Studies have shown that the mean levels of PAH-DNA adduct levels in WBC decreased after 3 weeks' vacation [26,30]. Recently, WBC DNA from fire fighters was studied by ELISA. PAH-DNA adducts were detected in 15 of 43 subjects. After adjustment for charcoal-broiled food consumption, fire fighters had a significanlty higher level of PAH-DNA adducts than controls [31].

Environmental Exposure and Smoking

Immunoassays have also been employed to monitor DNA adducts in humans exposed to PAHs in outdoor air (Table 2). PAHs are present in emissions from various industries and in engine exhaust, smoke associated with fuel burning and tobacco smoke. More than 500 PAHs have been detected in outdoor air [23]. In a Polish study by Hemminki et al. individuals living in a highly polluted area close to a coke oven plant had levels of PAH-DNA adducts in lymphocyte DNA similar to coke oven workers [12]. Seasonal variations in PAH-DNA adduct levels in WBC have been described by Perera et al. and Øvrebø et al. [28,29].

The influence of smoking on adduct levels has been determined with immunoassay techniques (Table 3). Increased PAH-DNA adduct levels were found in lung tissue and bronchial epithelium from smokers [33,34]. In some of the human lung studies PAH-DNA adduct levels correlated with the number of cigarettes smoked. On the other hand, in a recent study by Weston and Bowman where a fluorescence detection method was used, no association was found between the benzo-(a)pyrene-7,8-diol-9,10-epoxide (BPDE)-DNA adduct level and cigarette smoking [35]. However, adduct levels are determined by many different factors, e.g. exposure, age and metabolic phenotype. Using an immunofluorescence technique, Baan et al. detected BPDE-DNA adducts in human bronchial cells from smokers [36]. PAH-DNA adducts have

Table 3. Detection of PAH-DNA adducts in human tissue by immunoassay

	Subjects	Assay	No. detected/ assayed	Adduct level (10^8 nucleotides)	Reference
Lung	Lung cancer patients	ELISA	5/27 (19%)	4.2-5.4[a]	Perera et al. [43]
Lung	Lung cancer patients	ELISA	16/29 (55%)	6.3-2.7[a]	Perera et al. [32]
Lung	Controls	ELISA	4/8 (50%)	6.9-4.5[b]	ibid.
Lung	Smokers	USERIA	4/10 (40%)	>10	Wilson et al. [42]
Lung	Non-smokers	USERIA	5/7 (71%)	>10	ibid.
Lung	Lung cancer patients	ELISA	6/21 (29%)	2-134[a]	Van Schooten et al. [44]
Fetal lung	Spontaneous abortions	ELISA	5/12 (42%)	3-7.9[a]	Hatch et al. [38]
Fetal liver	Spontaneous abortions	ELISA	4/15 (27%)	6.3-25.1[a]	ibid.
Placenta	Spontaneous abortions	ELISA	6/14 (43%)	11.9-17.8[a]	ibid.

[a] range; [b] mean ± SE

also been detected in placental and foetal tissues by immunoasssay [37,38]. In a recent study by Manchester et al. the PAH-DNA adducts in human placenta were determined by means of immunoaffinity chromatography columns and high pressure liquid chromatography-synchronous fluorescence spectroscopy (HPLC-SFS). Benzo(a)pyrene (BP) tetrols were detected in 5 of 7 smokers and 3 of 9 non-smokers [39]. Several studies have been conducted that were designed to determine the influence of smoking on PAH adduct levels in WBC DNA. The data show no clear relationship between cigarette smoking and adduct level in WBC [29,40,41].

Adducts Excreted in Urine

One of the disadvantages of using carcinogen-DNA adducts as the measure of exposure to genotoxic compounds is their instability due to 1) existence of DNA-repair enzymes, which remove the damage, and 2) spontaneous depurination of some adducts. The excretion of the released products in urine may serve as an alternative method to detect carcinogen exposure. The possibility of detecting DNA damage by measurement of adducts in the urine has the advantage of being completely non-invasive as compared to tests requiring blood sampling.

The major carcinogen-DNA adduct formed by the carcinogenic mycotoxin aflatoxin B1 (AFB) has been identified as aflatoxin-N7-guanine. This adduct is quite unstable, with a half-life of less than 12 hours in rats, and has been detected in urine. A positive association has been observed between the exposure level, DNA adduct levels in the target tissue and the level of AFB-guanine detected in urine. Using HPLC with UV detection a weak association between exposure to aflatoxin, measured by the detection of AFB-guanine in urine, and the incidence of liver cancer was established in a cross-sectional study in Kenya [45]. A positive correlation between the dietary intake of AFB and the level of urinary AFB-guanine has been established in both a West African and a Chinese population using immunoaffinity chromatography in combination with HPLC to isolate and quantitate AFB-guanine [46,47].

Oxidative damage to cellular DNA is considered one of the major contributors to cancer and cellular ageing processes. The major adducts are thymine glycol, 5-hydroxymethyluracil and 8-hydroxyguanosine. These damaged DNA bases are released by excision repair and are excreted into the urine. A specific method using HPLC with radiochemical detection has been developed to detect 8-hydroxyguanine in urine [48]. Using this method, Poulsen et al. (unpublished result) have shown that smokers have a 50% increased oxidative DNA damage.

Methylating agents react with a number of different sites in DNA, the N-7 position of guanine being the predominant reaction site. This N-7 adduct together with another methylpurine, 3-methyladenine (3-MeAde), is excreted in the urine. A sensitive analytical technique using immunoaffinity purification in combination with GC-MS has been used to detect 3-MeAde. The level of this adduct showed great daily variation. It was suggested that this was caused by preformed adduct in the diet and that the level of 3-MeAde can be reduced to a low, stable level by a controlled diet [49]. This approach is being developed with the objective to detect human exposure to alkylating nitrosamines.

The major BP-DNA adduct is formed with the exocyclic amino group in guanine but an adduct formed with the N-7 position has been identified by a number of groups. This adduct is unstable just like most alkylated N-7 guanine adducts, and has been detected in the urine of rats treated with BP and in the urine of a heavy smoker [50]; however, this approach to detect exposure to PAH has not been pursued.

A major disadvantage of using carcinogen-DNA base adducts in urine as a measure of genotoxic exposure is that the measured level will only be representative for the exposure within the last days, due to the fact that the adducts in DNA are quite unstable. Furthermore, RNA adducts are also excreted and, unless thymine adducts are measured, are indistinguishable from DNA adducts. A contribution of dietary sources of adducts may be an interfering factor.

Protein Adducts

A number of studies have demonstrated that most, if not all, chemical carcinogens bind to proteins. Although DNA binding is considered to be the critical initiation step in chemical carcinogenesis, binding of carcinogens to protein has been suggested as an alternative technique to monitor human exposure to environmental carcinogens. A selected number of human studies is represented in Table 4. Aromatic amines react more efficiently with haemoglobin than with albumin, and no hydrolyzable albumin adducts could be detected after treatment with most aromatic amines [67,68]. The serum albumin adduct of 4-aminobiphenyl (ABP) differs from the adduct to haemoglobin, as albumin adduct formation requires N-acetylation prior to nucleophilic substitution by the amino-acid side chain at the ortho-position to the amino group [69]. In contrast, aflatoxin B1 (AFB) binding has been detected only to albumin and not haemoglobin. A list of desirable properties of a protein adduct dosimetry has been suggested by Skipper and Tannenbaum [70] and includes: 1) chemical stability under biological conditions; 2) adduct formation should not influence the stability of the protein; 3) easy accessibility; 4) relationship between protein dose and DNA dose; 5) a record of exposure should be provided over a significant fraction of the lifetime of the protein.

Haemoglobin Adducts

Haemoglobin dosimetry as a tool for monitoring exposure to alkylating agents was first introduced by Lars Ehrenberg and associates [71]. Human erythrocytes have a lifespan of approx. 120 days. Since there is no evidence for preferential clearance of carcinogen-modified haemoglobin, the steady-state level of carcinogen-haemoglobin adducts represents a measure of the accumulated dose of 120 days, i.e., the haemoglobin dosimetry reflects a record of 4 months' average exposure.

Table 4. Human exposure to carcinogens detected by carcinogen-protein adducts

Carcinogen	Protein	Method	Exposure	Reference
Aflatoxin B1	Albumin	IAC/ELISA ELISA/HPLC	Occupation General	Autrup et al. [52] Wild et al. [53]
4-Aminobiphenyl	Haemoglobin	GC/MS	Smokers Transplacental	Bartsch et al. [54] Bryant et al. [55] Coghlin et al. [56]
Aromatic amines	Haemoglobin	GC/MS	Smokers Occupation	Hecht et al. [57] Lewalter et al. [58]
Benzopyrene	Albumin Haemoglobin	ELISA GC/MS	Occupation General Smokers	Sherson et al. [60] Lee et al. [61] Autrup et al. [51] Weston et al. [62]
Chrysene	Haemoglobin	IAC/HPLC	Smokers	Day et al. [63]
Ethylene oxide	Haemoglobin	GC/MS RIA	Smokers Occupation Occupation	Bailey et al. [64] Törnqvist [65] Wraith et al. [66]
NNK/NNN	Haemoglobin	GC/MS	Smokers	Hecht et al. [57]
Trp-P1	Haemoglobin	GC/MS	General	Umemoto et al. [59]

ELISA, enzyme-linked immunosorbent assay; GC/MS, gas chromatography/mass spectrophotometry; HPLC, high pressure liquid chromatography; IAC, immunoaffinity chromatography; RIA, radioimmunoassay

Table 5. Preferential sites of reaction between carcinogens and amino acids in serum proteins

Carcinogen	Protein	Amino acid(s)
Acrylamide	Haemoglobin	Valine/cysteine
Aflatoxin B1	Albumin	Lysine
Aromatic amines	Haemoglobin	Cysteine
Benzene	Haemoglobin	Cysteine
Benzopyrene	Haemoglobin	Carboxylic group of aspartic acid and glutamic acid or C-terminal carboxylic group
Methylating agents	Haemoglobin	Cysteine
Ethylene oxide	Haemoglobin	Valine, histidine

Most of the studies using carcinogen-haemoglobin adducts in biomonitoring have been conducted on simple alkylating agents and aromatic amines, whereas there is little information on polycyclic aromatic hydrocarbons (PAHs). Higher binding to haemoglobin was seen for direct acting carcinogens compared to carcinogens that have to be metabolically activated to their biologically active form. However, the level of binding, the haemoglobin binding index, can not directly be used as an indicator of carcinogenic potency. The target amino acid in haemoglobin will depend on the biologically active form of the carcinogen (Table 5).

Highly specific and sensitive analytical procedures have been developed to detect haemoglobin adducts. Most of these methods are based on chromatographic separation followed by mass-spectrometry (MS) detection and quantification. The development of new detection modes and tandem MS-MS has made this approach very powerful. Immunological techniques have only been used for ethylene oxide and benzo(a)pyrene diolepoxide (BPDE)-haemoglobin adducts.

Ethylene Oxide

The N-terminal amino acid, valine, in haemoglobin is a major reaction site for epoxides and other alkylating agents. The resulting adducts can be degraded by the N-alkyl Edman degradation procedure, and the products analysed with high sensitivity and specificity by gas chromatography/mass spectrometry (GC/MS) [65]. N-(2-hydroxyethyl)valine is the major adduct formed after exposure to ethylene oxide or ethylene that can be detected by the N-alkyl Edman procedure. Adducts formed at other nucleophilic sites, e.g. histidine, have also been identified. The level of N-(2-hydroxyethyl)valine was significantly higher in smokers than in non-smokers, and a good correlation between adduct level and number of cigarettes smoked has been established [64]. The adduct was also detected in non-smokers. This could be due to either endogenously formed ethylene, e.g. by degradation of unsaturated lipids by intestinal bacteria, or to the presence of ethylene as a general pollutant in urban air. Inhaled ethylene requires metabolic activation to ethylene oxide prior to reaction with haemoglobin. In rats and hamsters exposed to diesel exhaust, approximately 5-10% of inhaled ethylene was metabolised to ethylene oxide. Using N-(2-hydroxyethyl)valine as the indicator, it has been estimated that the Swedish population (8 million) has an average exposure to ethylene in the range of 10-20 ppb. Using the rad-equivalence concept it was estimated that the exposure to 10 ppb ethylene is associated with approx. 80 cancer deaths per year in Sweden [73]. Using antibodies raised against an ethylene heptapeptide released form ethylene oxide modified haemoglobin in a radioimmunoassay, exposure to ethylene oxide was detected in occupationally exposed individuals [66].

Aromatic Amines

Aromatic amines, when activated by N-hydroxylation, bind to sulphydryl groups of cysteine to yield sulphinamides. Haemoglobin binds aromatic amines particularly well because the erythrocytes accelerate the rate of nitroso arene formation from hydroxylamine. The binding occurs at the ß-93 cysteine residue in human haemoglobin. Since the oxidation of N-hydroxy-arylamine to nitroso arenes occurs in erythrocytes, the active metabolite reacting with DNA is not the same as that reacting with haemoglobin, so that the correlation between binding to haemoglobin and DNA is poor. However, an association exists between haemoglobin binding and the biologically active dose of the aromatic amine [74].

Quantitative analysis of aromatic amine haemoglobin adducts is based upon release of the aromatic amine by mild acid hydrolysis and GC-MS following derivatisation with, for example, 3,5,-bis(trifluoromethyl)benzyl bromide. The level of binding to haemoglobin is higher than the binding to albumin due to the formation of nitroso arene within the erythrocytes in the course of methaemoglobin production.

A number of aromatic amine haemoglobin adducts, e.g. 4-ABP and 3-ABP, have been detected in erythrocytes from both smokers and non-smokers. The level of adducts depends on the number of cigarettes smoked and the type of tobacco used. High levels of 4-ABP adducts have also been detected in non-smokers, which could be due to exposure to environmental tobacco smoke or to a general environmental pollutant such as 4-nitrobiphenyl [55]. The level of 3-ABP is lower than that of 4-ABP, but it is a more specific indicator of the exposure to aromatic amines in cigarette smoke as the background level is very low. Transplacental exposure to 4-ABP in smoking mothers has been assessed by quantification of 4-ABP-haemoglobin in umbilical cord blood, the level in maternal blood being 2-fold higher [56]. N-oxidation and N-acetylation are important metabolic processes in the bioactivation of aromatic amines. The level of 4-ABP-haemoglobin adducts was dependent on the metabolic phenotype, and a higher 4-ABP adduct level was seen in the slow acetylator phenotype, but the highest level of 4-ABP-haemoglobin adduct was seen in the slow acetylator/fast oxidizer phenotype [57]. The slow acetylators had a higher level of aniline-haemoglobin adducts following accidental exposure to aniline, and were more subject to intoxication [58]. However, there was no association between the level of 4-ABP-haemoglobin adducts and the debrisoquine metabolic phenotype [75].

3-Amino-1,4-dimethyl-5H-pyrido[4,3-b]indole (Trp-P1), a dietary carcinogen which is also present in extracts from urban air particulates, binds to both haemoglobin and serum albumin in experimental animals. Using HPLC with fluorescence detection following acid hydrolysis of haemoglobin, exposure to Trp-P1 was detected in human volunteers at the level of 0.23-4.33 pmol/g haemoglobin; however, the source of Trp-P1 was not identified [58]. The level of Trp-P1 haemoglobin was 10-fold lower than the level of 4-ABP-haemoglobin in non-smokers.

Polycyclic Aromatic Hydrocarbons (PAHs)

This group of compounds is formed by incomplete combustion of fossil fuels and is found in emissions from mobile and stationary sources. PAHs are ubiquitous carcinogens, which are also present in cigarette smoke. Fluoranthene (FA) is always found at higher levels than benzo(a)pyrene (BP) as an environmental pollutant. Therefore, adducts formed between FA and macromolecules might be a better marker for exposure to PAHs than BP.

FA binding to target cell DNA and haemoglobin has only been studied in experimental animals. The active form of FA binds to cysteine-125 in haemoglobin in rats treated with FA. Only 0.12% of the administered dose bound to haemoglobin, and the half-life of this adduct was identical to that of rat erythrocytes [76]. In contrast to FA, no reaction between the cysteine residue and the anti-diol epoxide of benzo(a)pyrene, the ultimate carcinogenic form, has been detected. The major adducts (80% of the total) were formed by the reaction of BPDE with the free carboxylic acid groups, e.g. side chains of the glutamic or aspartic residues or the C-terminal carboxylic group [77]. Minor adducts were formed by the reaction with amino groups and heterocyclic nitrogen atoms. Two different approaches have been adopted to quantitate the BP-haemoglobin adduct level. Both methods are based upon the release of BP-tetrols from the haemoglobin either by proteolytic digestion or acid hydrolysis. The former appears to be the most efficient. The released metabolites can be detected by HPLC in combination with fluorescence spectroscopy. An immunological method has been developed to quantitate

BP-tetrols using the 8E11 antibody [78]. Significant cross-reactivity of the antibody was found with other BP metabolites as well as with other PAH tetrols. For application to human samples it was recommended that an immunoaffinity purification step should be included, as the sensitivity might otherwise be too low [79]. Using GC-MS analysis with positive chemical ionisation, adduct levels of 1 to 5 pmol/g haemoglobin have been found in smokers [62].

In a survey of human blood samples to assess reactions with other PAHs and haemoglobin, an adduct formed between chrysene diol epoxide and haemoglobin was identified by GC-MS following HPLC purification of protease-digested globin [63].

Immunological techniques have been used to monitor exposure to BP in the occupational environment. Different sample preparations were employed in the investigations, and this may explain the difference found in adduct levels when the same monoclonal antibody was used. BP tetrols were either released by proteolysis [61] or acid hydrolysis [60]. The level was higher in foundry workers than in a reference group. A higher level of adducts was observed in workers who were concomitantly exposed to mineral dust that might have served as a carrier of BP [60]. A high level of PAH-albumin adducts was also found among non-smokers and individuals who were not occupationally exposed to PAH. The high level of adducts could be related to factors of life style: for example, two individuals who cycled to work over highly trafficked roads in Copenhagen, had an adduct level corresponding to the level seen in regular smokers [51].

Tobacco Smoke-Specific Carcinogens

Tobacco-specific nitrosamines are formed from nicotine and other tobacco alkaloids. 4-(methyl-nitrosamino)-1-(3-pyridyl)-1-butanone (NNK) and N'nitrosonornicotine (NNN) are strong carcinogens in this group. Both compounds form haemoglobin adducts after biological activation. Keto-alcohols are released by mild basic hydrolysis of the isolated globin, and these metabolites can be detected by GC-MS following derivatisation and HPLC purification. In rats only 0.02% of the dose of NNK was released as the keto-alcohol. In humans, the level of haemoglobin adducts was significantly higher in snuff-dippers than in smokers and non-smokers [57]. Other haemoglobin adducts detected in erythrocytes of smokers include adducts with aromatic amines, ethylene oxide and methylating agents.

Benzene

Humans are exposed to benzene in both occupational and environmental settings, and specific and sensitive methods to assess human exposure to this carcinogen are important. Two major benzene-haemoglobin adducts that cochromatographed with chemically synthesised standards have been identified as phenylcysteine and S-(2,5-dihydroxyphenyl)cysteine [80]. In rodents the benzene-haemoglobin adduct accumulated linearly with the administered dose. However, better method development is required before binding of benzene to haemoglobin can be used as a biological monitoring assay. S-phenylcysteine could not be detected in haemoglobin isolated from workers who were exposed to 28 ppm benzene for 8 h/day, 5 days/week. Acid hydrolysis of serum albumin from the same workers showed the formation of S-phenylcysteine [80].

Albumin Adducts

One of the advantages of using serum albumin as the surrogate target compared to erythrocytes is that the protein is synthesised in the hepatocytes with a high level of enzymes involved in the bioactivation of indirectly acting carcinogens. Consequently, the active form of the carcinogen does not have to pass the cell membrane prior to the reaction with the nucleophilic site. The half-life of human albumin is 20-25 days, compared to 120 days for haemoglobin, which makes albumin a short-term dose monitor in comparison with haemoglobin.

In conclusion, recent methodological development has extended the scope of human biomonitoring to DNA and protein adducts. Urinary excretion products of nucleic acid adducts can also be assayed. Mutation assays have been extended beyond the traditional cytogenetic assays to molecular analysis of point mutations and larger DNA lesions.

REFERENCES

1. Hemminki K: Measurement and monitoring of individial exposures. In: Tomatis L (ed) Air Pollution and Human Cancer. European School of Oncology Monograph Series. Springer-Verlag, Berlin 1990 pp 33-47
2. Harris CC: Chemical and physical carcinogenesis: advances and perspectives for the 1990s. Cancer Res 1991 (51):5023s-5044s
3. Ehrenberg L, Moustacchi E, Osterman-Golkar S: Dosimetry of genotoxic agents and dose-response relationships in their effects. Mutat Res 1983 (123):121-182
4. Neumann H-G: Analysis of hemoglobin as a dose monitor for alkylating and arylating agents. Arch Toxicol 1984 (56):1-6
5. Hutchinson F: Use of data from bacteria to interpret data on DNA damage processing in mammalian cells. Mutat Res 1989 (220):269-278
6. Vogelstein B, Fearon ER, Kern SE, Hamilton SR, Preisinger AC, Nakamura Y, White R: Allelotype of colorectal carcinomas. Science (Washington DC) 1989 (244):207-211
7. Randerath K, Reddy MV, Gupta RC: 32 P-postlabeling test for DNA damage. Proc Natl Acad Sci 1981 (78):6126-6129
8. Gupta RC, Reddy MV, Randerath K: 32 P-postlabeling analysis of non-radioactive aromatic carcinogen-DNA adducts. Carcinogenesis 1982 (3):1081-1092
9. Reddy MV, Randerath K: Nuclease P 1-mediated enhancement of sensitivity of 32 P-postlabeling test for structurally diverse DNA adducts. Carcinogenesis 1986 (7):1543-1551
10. Savela K: Characterization and Human Monitoring of DNA Adducts Formed by Aromatic Carcinogens. Institute of Occupational Health, Helsinki 1991
11. Beach AC, Gupta RC: Human biomonitoring and the 32 P-postlabeling assay. Carcinogenesis 1992 (13):1053-1074
12. Hemminki K, Grzybowska E, Chorazy M, Twardowska-Saucha K, Sroczynski JW, Putman KL, Randerath K, Phillips DH, Hewer A, Santella RM, Young T-L, Perera FP: DNA adducts in humans environmentally exposed to aromatic compounds in an industrial area of Poland. Carcinogenesis 1990 (11):1229-1231
13. Hemminki K, Reunanen A, Kahn H: Use of DNA adducts in the assessment of occupational and environmental exposure to carcinogens. Eur J Cancer 1991 (27):289-291
14. Perera FP, Hemminki K, Grzybowska E, Motykiewicz G, Michalska J, Santella RM, Young T-L, Dickey C, Brandt-Rauf P, De Vivo I, Blaner W, Tsai W-Y, Chorazy M: Molecular damage from environmental pollution in Poland (submitted)
15. Grzybowska E, Hemminki K, Chorazy M: Seasonal variations in levels of DNA adducts and x-spots in the human populations living in different parts of Poland. Environ Health Perspect (in press)
16. Mustonen R, Försti A, Hietanen P, Hemminki K: Measurement by 32 P-postlabeling of 7-methylguanine levels of white blood cell DNA of healthy individuals and cancer patients treated with dacarbazine and procarbazine. Human data and method development for 7-alkylguanines. Carcinogenesis 1991 (12):1423-1431
17. Hemminki K, Mustonen R, Reunanen A, Kahn H: Application of DNA adduct measurements for dietary studies. In: Kok FJ, van 't Veer P (eds) Biomarkers of Dietary Exposure. Smith-Gordon, London 1991 pp 59-66
18. Sugimura T: Past, present and future of mutagens in cooked foods. Environ Health Perspect 1986 (67):5-10
19. Phillips D: Modern methods of DNA adduct determination. In: Cooper ES, Grover PL (eds) Chemical Carcinogenesis and Mutagenesis I. Springer-Verlag, Berlin-Heidelberg 1990 pp 503-546
20. Santella RM: Application of new techniques for the detection of carcinogen adducts to human population monitoring. Mutat Res 1988 (205):271-282
21. Weston A, Rowe M, Poirier M, Trivers G, Vähäkangas K, Newman M, Haugen A, Manchester D, Mann D, Harris CC: The application of immunoassays and fluorometry to the detection of polycyclic hydrocarbon-macromolecular adducts and anti-adduct antibodies in humans. Int Arch Occup Environ Health 1988 (60):157-162
22. Van Schooten FJ, Kriek E, Steenwinkel M-JST, Noteborn HPJM, Hillbrand MJX, Van Leeuwen FE: The binding efficiency of polyclonal and monoclonal antibodies to DNA modified with benzo(a)pyrene diol epoxide is dependent on the level of modification. Implications for quantitation of benzo(a)pyrene-DNA adducts in vivo. Carcinogenesis 1987 (8):1263-1269
23. International Agency for Research on Cancer: Monographs on the Evaluation of the Carcinogenic Risk to Humans. Vol 32. IARC, Lyon 1983 pp 95-451
24. Shamsuddin AK, Sinopoli NT, Hemminki K, Boesch RR, Harris CC: Detection of benzo(a)pyrene - DNA adducts in human white blood cells. Cancer Res 1985 (45):66-68
25. Harris CC, Vähäkangas K, Newman NJ, Trivers GE, Shamsuddin A, Sinopoli N, Mann DL, Wright W: Detection of benzo(a)pyrene diol epoxide-DNA adducts in peripheral lymphocytes and antibodies to the adducts in serum from coke oven workers. Proc Natl Acad Sci USA 1985 (82):6662-6676
26. Haugen A, Becher G, Benestad C, Vähäkangas K, Trivers GE, Newman MJ, Harris CC: Determination of polycyclic aromatic hydrocarbons in the urine, benzo(a)pyrene diol epoxide-DNA adducts in lymphocyte DNA, and antibodies to the adducts in sera from coke-oven workers exposed to measured amounts of polycyclic aromatic hydrocarbons in the work atmosphere. Cancer Res 1986 (46):4178-4183

27. Van Schooten FJ, Leeuwen FE, Hillbrand MJX, de Rijke ME, Hart AAM, van Veen HG, Oosterick S, Kriek E: Determination of benzo(a)pyrene diol epoxide-DNA adducts in white blood cell DNA from coke-oven workers: the impact of smoking. JNCI 1990 (82):77-83
28. Perera FP, Hemminki K, Young T-L, Brenner D, Kelly G, Santella RM: Detection of polycyclic aromatic hydrocarbon - DNA adducts in white blood cells of foundry workers. Cancer Res 1988 (48):2288-2291
29. Øvrebø S, Haugen A, Phillips DH, Hewer A: Detection of polycyclic aromatic hydrocarbon-DNA adducts in white blood cells from coke oven workers: correlation with job categories. Cancer Res 1992 (52):1510-1514
30. Hemminki K, Randerath K, Reddy MV, Putman KL, Santella RM, Perera FP, Young T-L, Phillips DH, Hewer A, Santella K: Postlabeling of immunoassay of polycyclic aromatic hydrocarbons-adducts of deoxyribonucleic acid in white blood cells of foundry workers. Scand J Work Environ Health 1990 (16):158-162
31. Liou S-H, Jacobsen-Kram D, Poirier MC, Nguyen D, Strickland PT, Tockman MS: Biological monitoring of fire fighters: sister chromatide exchange and polycyclic aromatic hydrocarbon-DNA adducts in peripheral blood cells. Cancer Res 1989 (49):4929-4935
32. Perera FB, Mayer J, Jaretzki A, Hearne S, Brenner D, Young T-L, Fischman HK, Grimes M, Grantham S, Tang MX, Tsai W-Y, Santella RM: Comparison of DNA adducts and sister chromatid exchanges in lung cancer cases and controls. Cancer Res 1989 (49):4446-4451
33. Everson RB, Randerath E, Santella RM, Cefalo RC, Aritts TA, Randerath K: Detection of smoking-related covalent DNA adducts in human placenta. Science 1986 (231):54-57
34. Phillips DH, Hewer A, Martin CN, Garner RC, King MM: Correlation of DNA adduct levels in human lung with cigarette smoking. Nature 1988 (336):790-792
35. Weston A, Bowman ED: Fluorescence detection of benzo(a)pyrene - DNA adducts in human lung. Carcinogenesis 1981 (12):1445-1449
36. Baan RA, Van der Berg PTM, Steenwinkell M-JST, van der Wulp CJM: Detection of benzo(a)pyrene DNA adducts in cultured cells treated with benzo(a)pyrene diol epoxide by quantitative immunfluorescence microscopy and ^{32}P-postlabelling; immunofluorescence analysis of benzo(a)pyrene - DNA adducts in bronchial cells from smoking individuals. In: Bartsch H, Hemminki K, O'Neill IK (eds) Methods for Detecting DNA Damaging Agents in Humans: Applications in Cancer Epidemiology and Prevention. IARC Scientific Publications, Lyon 1988 (89) pp 146-154
37. Manchester DK, Bowman ED, Parker NB, Caporaso NE, Weston A: Determination of polycyclic aromatic hydrocarbon - DNA adducts in human placenta. Cancer Res 1992 (52):1499-1503
38. Hatch MC, Warburton D, Santella RM: Polycyclic aromatic hydrocarbon-DNA adducts in spontaneously aborted fetal tissue. Carcinogenesis 1990 (11):1673-1675
39. Savela K, Hemminki K: DNA adducts in lymphocytes and granulocytes of smokers and non-smokers deteected by the 32P-postlabelling assay. Carcinogenesis 1991 (12):503-508
40. Phillips DH, Schoket B, Hewer A, Bailey E, Kostic S, Vincze I: Influence of cigarette smoking on the levels of DNA adducts in human bronchial epithelium and white blood cells. Int J Cancer 1990 (46):569-575
41. Vincze I: Influence of cigarette smoking on the levels of DNA adducts in human bronchial epithelium and white blood cells. Int J Cancer 1990 (46):569-575
42. Wilson VL, Weston A, Manchester DK, Trivers GE, Roberts DW, Kadlubar FF, Wild CP, Montesano R, Willey JL, Mann DL, Harris CC: Alkyl and aryl carcinogen DNA adducts detected in human peripheral lung. Carcinogenesis 1989 (10):2149-2153
43. Perera FP, Poirier MC, Yuspa SH, Nakayama J, Jaretski A, Curnen MM, Knowles DM, Weinstein IB: A pilot project in molecular cancer epidemiology: determination of benzo(a)pyrene-DNA adducts in animal and human tissues by immunoassays. Carcinogenesis 1982 (3):1405-1410
44. van Schooten FJ, Hillebrand MJX, van Leeuwen FE, van Zandwijk N, Jansen HM, den Engelse L, Kriek E: Polycyclic hydrocarbon-DNA adducts in white blood cells from lung cancer patients: no correlation with adduct levels in lung. Carcinogenesis 1992 (13):987-993
45. Autrup H, Seremet T, Wakhisi J, Wasunna A: Aflatoxin exposure measured by urinary excretion of aflatoxin B1-guanine adducts and hepatitis B virus infection in areas with different liver cancer incidence in Kenya. Cancer Res 1987 (47): 3430-3433
46. Groopman JD, Hall AJ, Whittle H, Hudson GJ, Wogan GN, Montesano R, Wild CP: Molecular dosimetry of aflatoxin-N7-guanine in human urine obtained in Gambia, West Africa. Cancer Epid Biomarkers Prev 1992 (1):221-227
47. Groopman JD, Zhu J, Donahue PR, Pikul A, Zhang L, Chen J-S, Wogan GN: Molecular dosimetry of urinary aflatoxin DNA adducts in people living in Guangxi autonomous region, People's Republic of China. Cancer Res 1992 (52):45-52
48. Ames BN: Measuring oxidative damage in humans: relation to cancer and ageing. IARC Scientific Publications 1988 (89):407-416
49. Shuker DEG: Urinanalysis: review of methods. In: Garner RC, Farmer FB, Steel GT, Wright AS (eds) Human Carcinogen Exposure - Biomonitoring and Risk Assessment. IRL Press, Oxford 1991 pp 47-59
50. Autrup H, Seremet T: Excretion of benzo(a)pyrene-gua adduct in urine of benzo(a)pyrene treated rats. Chem-Biol Interactions 1986 (60):217-226
51. Autrup H, Seremet T, Sherson D: Quantitation of polycyclic aromatic hydrocarbon-serum protein and lymphocyte DNA adducts in Danish foundry workers using immunoassays. In: Garner RC, Farmer FB, Steel GT, Wright AS (eds) Human Carcinogen Exposure - Biomonitoring and Risk Assessment. IRL Press, Oxford 1991 pp 207-213

52 Autrup JL, Schmidt J, Seremet T, Autrup H: Determination of exposure to aflatoxins among Danish workers in animal-feed production through analysis of aflatoxin B1 adducts to serum albumin. Scand J Work Environ Health 1991 (17):436-440

53 Wild CP, Jiang Y-Z, Sabbioni G, Chapot B, Montesano R: Evaluation of methods for quantification of aflatoxin-albumin adducts and their application to human exposure assessment. Cancer Res 1990 (50):245-251

54 Bartsch H, Caporaso N, Coda M, Kadlubar F, Malaveille C, Skipper PL, Talaska G, Tannenbaum SR, Vineis P: Carcinogen hemoglobin adducts, urinary mutagenicity, and metabolic phenotype in active and passive cigarette smokers. JNCI 1990 (82):1826-1831

55 Bryant SM, Vineis P, Skipper PL, Tannenbaum SR: Haemoglobin adducts of aromatic amines in people exposed to cigarette smoke. IARC Scientific Publications 1988 (89):133-136

56 Coghlin J, Gann PH, Hammond SK, Skipper PL, Taghizadeh K, Paul M, Tannenbaum SR: 4-aminobiphenyl hemoglobin adducts in fetuses exposed to tobacco smoke carcinogen in utero. JNCI 1991 (83):274-280

57 Hecht SS, Kagan M, Kagan SS, Carmella SG: Quantitation of tobacco-specific nitrosamine-globin adducts in humans. In: Garner RC, Farmer FB, Steel GT, Wright AS (eds) Carcinogen Exposure - Biomonitoring and Risk Assessment. IRL Press, Oxford 1991 pp 267-274

58 Lewalter J, Korallus U: Blood protein conjugates and acetylation of aromatic amines: new findings on biological monitoring. Int Arch Occup Environ Health 1985 (56):179-196.

59 Umemoto A, Monden Y, Grivas S, Yamashita K, Sugimura T: Determination of human exposure to the dietary carcinogen 3-amino-1,4-dimethyl-5H-pyrido[4,3-b]indole from by hemoglobin adduct: the relationship to DNA adducts. Carcinogenesis 1992 (13): 1025-1030

60 Sherson D, Sabro P, Sigsgaard T, Autrup H: Biological monitoring of foundry workers exposed to polycyclic aromatic hydrocarbons. Br J Ind Med 1990 (47):448-453

61 Lee BM, Baoyun Y, Herbert R, Hemminki K, Perera FP, Santella RM: Immunological measurement of polycyclic aromatic hydrocarbon-albumin adducts in foundry workers and roofers. Scand J Work Environ Health 1991 (17):190-194

62 Weston A, Rowe ML, Manchester DK, Farmer PB, Mann DL, Harris CC: Fluorescence and mass spectral evidence for the formation of benzo(a)pyrene anti-diol-epoxide-DNA and haemoglobin adducts in humans. Carcinogenesis 1989 (10):251-257

63 Day BW, Skipper PL, Wishnok JS, Coghlin J, Hammond SK, Gann P, Tannenbaum SR: Identification of an in vivo chrysene diol epoxide adduct in human hemoglobin. Chem Res Toxicol 1990 (3):340-343

64 Bailey E, Brooks AGF, Dollery CT, Farmer PB, Passingham BJ, Sleightholm MA, Yates DW: Hydroxyethylvaline adduct formation in haemoglobin as a biological monitor of cigarette smoke intake. Arch Toxicol 1988 (62):247-253

65 Törnqvist M: The N-alkyl Edman method for haemoglobin adduct measurement: updating and applications to humans. In: Garner RC, Farmer FB, Steel GT, Wright AS (eds) Carcinogen Exposure - Biomonitoring and Risk Assessment. IRL Press, Oxford 1991 pp 411-419

66 Wraith MJ, Watson WP, Eadsforth CV, van Sittert NJ, Törnqvist M, Wright AS: An immunoassay for monitoring human exposure to ethylene oxide. IARC Scientific Publications 1988 (89):271-274

67 DeBord GD, Swearengin TF, Cheever KL, Booth-Jones AD, Wissinger LA: Binding characteristics of ortho-toluidine to rat hemoglobin and albumin. Arch Toxicol 1992 (66): 231-236

68 Sabbioni G, Neumann H-G: Quantification of haemoglobin binding of 4,4'-methylenebis(2-chloroaniline (MOCA) in rats. Arch Toxicol 1990 (64): 451-458

69 Skipper PL, Naylor S: Mass spectrometric analysis of protein-carcinogen adducts. In: Garner RC, Farmer FB, Steel GT, Wright AS (eds) Human Carcinogen Exposure - Biomonitoring and Risk Assessment. IRL Press, Oxford 1991 pp 61-68

70 Skipper PL, Tannenbaum SR: Protein adducts in the molecular dosimetry of chemical carcinogens. Carcinogenesis 1990 (11):507-518

71 Ehrenberg L, Hiesche KD, Osterman-Golkar S, Wennberg I: Evaluation of the genetic risks of alkylating agents: tissue doses in the mouse from air contaminated with ethylene oxide. Mutat Res 1974 (24):83-103

72 Törnqvist M, Ehrenberg L: On cancer risk estimation of urban air pollution. Environ Health Perspectives 1993 (in press)

73 Neumann H-G, Birner G, Sabbioni G: Hemoglobin adducts of aromatic amines as a dosimeter for exposure control and risk assessment. In: Garner RC, Farmer FB, Steel GT, Wright AS (eds) Human Carcinogen Exposure - Biomonitoring and Risk Assessment. IRL Press, Oxford 1991 pp 337-344

74 Weston A, Caporaso NE, Taghizadeh K, Hoover RN, Tannenbaum SR, Skipper PL, Resau JH, Trump BF, Harris CC: Measurement of 4-aminobiphenyl-hemoglobin adducts in lung cancer cases and controls. Cancer Res 1991 (51): 5219-5223

75 Hutchins DA, Skipper PL, Naylor S, Tannenbaum SR: Isolation and characterization of the major fluoranthene-hemoglobin adducts formed in vivo in the rat. Cancer Res 1988 (48):4756-4761

76 Naylor S, Gan L-S, Day BW, Pastorelli R, Skipper PL, Tannenbaum SR: Benzo(a)pyrene diol epoxide adduct formation in mouse and human hemoglobin: Physicochemical basis for dosimetry. Chem Res Toxicol 1990 (3):111-117

77 Santella RM, Lin CD, Dharmaraja N: Monoclonal antibodies to a benzo(a)pyrene diolepoxide modified protein. Carcinogenesis 1986 (7): 441-444

78 Lee BM, Santella RM: Quantitation of protein adducts as a marker of genotoxic exposure: immunological detection of benzo(a)pyrene-globin adducts in mice. Carcinogenesis 1988 (9):1773-1777

79 Melikian AA, Prahalad AK, Coleman S: Isolation and characterization of two benzene-derived hemoglobin adducts in vivo in rats. Cancer Epidemiol Biomarker Prevention 1992 (1): 307-313

80 Bechtold WE, Willis JK, Sun JD, Griffith WC, Reddy TV: Biological markers of exposure to benzene: S-phenylcysteine in albumin. Carcinogenesis 1992 (13): 1217-1220

Experimental Evidence for the Carcinogenicity of Indoor and Outdoor Air Pollutants

Joellen Lewtas

Health Effects Research Laboratory, U.S. Environmental Protection Agency, MD 68A, Research Triangle Park, N.C. 27711, U.S.A.

The role of air pollution in human lung cancer has been difficult to assess or quantitate due to the many confounding exposures and factors that influence human cancer (see the chapters by Pershagen and Simonato in this volume). This is especially true for cancers of the respiratory tract where the vast majority of cancers have been related to cigarette smoking. Much of our understanding of the potential human risk from air pollution is derived from experimental cancer studies on both individual chemicals and mixtures of air pollutants [1]. This chapter discusses the experimental evidence for the carcinogenicity of air pollutants in long-term animal cancer studies and from short-term bioassays. The evidence is organised and discussed in three categories of exposures: a) individual chemicals found as air pollutants (e.g., formaldehyde), b) mixtures emitted from air pollution sources (e.g., automotive emissions, tobacco smoke, and industrial sources), and c) mixtures of air pollution taken from ambient indoor air or outdoor air (e.g., urban air particulate matter).

Although definitive evidence of carcinogenicity in humans can be provided only by human epidemiological and clinical studies, experimental studies in animals and short-term bioassays provide evidence that is considered relevant to the classification and prediction of potential human cancer risk [2]. This chapter will consider the following two types of experimental evidence for carcinogenicity of air pollutants: animal cancer bioassays that are generally considered to be long-term tests and short-term bioassays for genetic and related effects.

Animal Cancer Bioassays

A large proportion of the chemicals or mixtures that are known from epidemiological studies to be carcinogenic to humans and that are suitable for a long-term animal cancer bioassay, have been shown to induce cancer in animals in at least one species through experimental methods [3,4]. The fraction of animal carcinogens that are also human carcinogens is unknown. The International Agency for Research on Cancer (IARC) [2] has stated in its Monographs on the Evaluation of Carcinogenic Risks to Humans, the view that is also held by many other international and national health organisations, namely that "...in the absence of adequate data on humans, it is biologically plausible and prudent to regard agents and mixtures for which there is sufficient evidence of carcinogenicity in experimental animals as if they presented a carcinogenic risk to humans..." [2].

The evidence relevant to carcinogenicity in experimental animals is classified by IARC into one these following categories: sufficient evidence[1], limited evidence[2], inadequate

---

[1] Generally this evidence is provided by positive carcinogenicity studies in 2 or more species of animals or in 2 or more independent studies in one species but at different times and under different laboratory conditions. In exceptional cases, a single study in one species may provide sufficient evidence of carcinogenicity when the cancer occurs to an unusual degree with regard to incidence, site, type of tumour or age of onset.

[2] Generally this evidence is provided by either positive carcinogenicity in a single experiment or unresolved questions regarding the adequacy of positive studies, or

evidence[3], and evidence suggesting lack of carcinogenicity[4]. Similar classification schemes for carcinogens have been used by other organisations [5].

As scientific research has advanced our understanding of the mechanisms by which chemical and physical agents may induce cancer [6], this information should be incorporated into both qualitative classification of human cancer risk and quantitative cancer risk assessment.

Short-Term Bioassay for Genetic and Related Effects: the Mechanism of Cancer Induction

Evidence has been growing since the 1960s to support the theory that electrophilic chemicals react covalently with the nucleophilic centres in DNA and subsequently induce genetic changes (e.g., mutations). When such reactive electrophilic chemical mutagens react with DNA, this event may become the initiating event in a multistage process leading to cancer [6-8]. The mutational theory of cancer is supported by evidence that many electrophilic mutagens also induce cancer in animals [8] and that carcinogens induce mutations in specific genes involved in the carcinogenic process: oncogenes and tumour suppressor genes [10,11]. Oncogenes introduced into normal cells can transform these cells into cancer cells. The oncogenes that have been identified so far (over 50) result from mutational changes in normal genes (proto-oncogenes) that lead to changes in the regulation of cell division and eventually cancer. Mutational changes may also adversely modify normal tumour suppressor genes that are involved with controlling cell division. Loss of the control of cell division through mutations in tumour suppressor genes is also thought to play a role in uncontrolled cell growth and cancer. This theory that the event that initiates cancer is caused by a genetic change in DNA, and the evidence supporting it has become the basis for using short-term genetic bioassays to detect carcinogens. There are, however, many aspects of the carcinogenic process that are unknown or only partly understood.

There is growing evidence suggesting that chemical and physical agents may act at different stages in the carcinogenic process and by different mechanisms, including, in some cases, "non-genotoxic" mechanisms [6,12,13] that may influence the promotion or progression stages of cancer rather than the initiation stage. This recognition has encouraged the scientific development of short-term bioassays for the detection of carcinogens that act at other stages in the cancer process. There are a number of short-term bioassays which detect changes in cells that are not necessarily the result of genetic changes but are thought to have specific relevance to the process of carcinogenesis. These bioassays include tests for tumour-promoting activity, cellular proliferation, intercellular communication, and neoplastic cell transformation [8,12,13].

Short-term bioassays are often classified by the following phylogenetic groups: prokaryotes, fungi, plants, insects, mammalian cells (*in vitro*), mammalian cells (*in vivo*) and human (tissues/body fluids) [2,8,16]. Short-term bioassay data are evaluated and interpreted based on the biological endpoints detected, which include the following: DNA damage, gene mutation, sister chromatid exchange, micronuclei, chromosomal aberrations, aneuploidy and cell transformation [16]. Some of these endpoints are more directly related to a genotoxic event (e.g., gene mutations and chromosomal aberrations), while others are less clearly genetic but may be related to changes in DNA (e.g., unscheduled DNA synthesis, formation of DNA adducts) or cellular changes related to both tumour initiation and progression or promotion (e.g. oncogenic cell transformation).

Predicting which chemicals and mixtures will be carcinogenic to humans based on the use of short-term bioassays is certainly compli-

---

the agents or mixtures increase the incidence of only benign neoplasms or lesions of uncertain neoplastic potential (e.g., certain neoplasms may occur spontaneously in high incidence in certain strains of animals).

[3] If studies cannot be interpreted as showing either the presence or absence of a carcinogenic effect, then the evidence for carcinogenicity is considered inadequate.

[4] Generally this evidence is provided by adequate studies involving at least 2 species that show a lack of carcinogenicity. This evidence is limited to the species, tumour sites and levels of exposures studied.

cated by the complex multistage process of cancer [17]. Genetic bioassays are designed to detect chemicals that initiate cancer through one or more of types of genetic damage detected by different endpoints measured in short-term tests. The two main classes of genetic damage that are now readily evaluated by these tests are gene mutations and chromosomal alterations [18]. Based on several analyses of the chemicals classified by IARC as human carcinogens, it has been concluded that the Salmonella typhimurium mutagenicity assay [19] and an *in vivo* cytogenetic assay will detect all of the 31 organic human carcinogens, except benzene [20]. The most common variation on this initial 2-test approach is the use of either an *in vitro* mammalian cell cytogenetic assay or an *in vivo* cytogenetic assay together with the Salmonella mutation assay [21].

Identifying a Cancer Hazard Using Short-Term Bioassays

Many studies have evaluated the correlation between mutagenicity in short-term tests and carcinogenicity in animals. Studies of hundreds of chemicals in the 1970s demonstrated that bacterial mutagenicity assays detected over 90% of the animal carcinogens that had been identified up to that time [19,22,23]. Several changes occurred in the 1980s in rodent cancer bioassay protocols (e.g., testing up to the maximum tolerable dose) and the types of chemicals being tested [24]. The method of chemical selection was changed from selecting chemicals with electrophilic structures to high-volume industrial chemicals because these chemicals may have greater potential for human exposure. A recent report on 73 such chemicals showed that short-term genetic bioassays only predicted about 60% of these animal carcinogens [25]. This study has raised many critical issues related to predicting cancer risk in humans based on experimental data in both animals and short-term bioassays [24,26-28]. These issues include: 1) concordance between carcinogenicity results in rats and mice and the concordance between these rodents and short-term genetic bioassays [26,28]; 2) influence of chemical class on the sensitivity and specificity of genetic bioassays [29]; and 3) genotoxic versus non-genotoxic carcinogens [30]. It is clear that animal carcinogens that are also mutagenic are more likely to be carcinogenic across species and target organs and are carcinogenic at much lower doses [31]. Bioassays that detect, by definition, genotoxic agents would not be expected to detect agents that may induce cancer by a mechanism that does not involve interaction with DNA; mutation induction or other genetic effects. The tumours induced by non-mutagenic chemicals tend to be limited to one species and organ site [24], although the data base for supporting this conclusion is not large. The human cancer risk of these non-genotoxic rodent carcinogens may be questionable, particularly if the agent induces tumours in only one species and only at the maximum tolerable dose [26,28]. Although the list of recognised human carcinogens [2] is much smaller than the list of animal carcinogens, most of these human carcinogenic agents are positive in short-term bioassays [4,27,32]. The chemicals that are rodent carcinogens across several species and organ sites (trans-species carcinogens) are generally also mutagenic in short-term bioassays [24,31].

Although most of the chemicals classified by IARC as human carcinogens can be detected as genotoxic by using the Salmonella typhimurium mutagenicity assay [19] and either an *in vivo* or *in vitro* cytogenetic assay [20,21], there are still several important human carcinogens that are missed, notably benzene and the inorganic carcinogens (e.g. chromium). Modifications to a wider variety of short-term genetic bioassays will result in detection of several of these carcinogens that are not readily detected in the standardised short-term bioassays.

Quantitative Assessment of Cancer Risk

The classification of carcinogens according to their mechanisms of action [6,7] could facilitate both the qualitative and quantitative assessment of cancer risk, but until recently sufficient data on the mechanism of cancer induction by various agents was not known. Most international and national health and environmental agencies do not classify or regulate carcinogens according to their mechanisms of action [33,34]. This may change in the future when a better understanding of carcinogenesis mechanisms is achieved. The organisations that conduct quantitative carcinogen risk assessments have only made some attempts to classify carcinogens by their mechanism of action (e.g., genotoxic versus non-genotoxic carcinogens) for the purpose of extrapolation modelling at low doses. For quantitative cancer risk assessment to be scientifically defensible in the future, an understanding of the mechanism of an agent's action in inducing cancer may be required [7].

Quantitative cancer risk assessments using linear or other non-threshold low-dose extrapolations are based on the assumptions that involve the genetic mechanism of cancer induction [6,7]. If it can be shown that a carcinogen acts by a non-genotoxic mechanism that results in a threshold dose below which no excess cancers would be observed, then linear non-threshold low-dose extrapolations may be inappropriate models [33,34]. Quantitative cancer risk assessment as developed and applied by the U.S. Environmental Protection Agency (EPA) in the 1980s [35] was based on a methodology developed by Crump [36] to estimate cancer risk from chronic animal experiments. This approach is referred to as the linearised multistage model and is widely used to establish upper bounds on suspected cancer risk. One of the important deficiencies of this model is that it is not derived from an underlying biological theory of carcinogenesis and does not take into account agent-induced stimulation of cell proliferation.

A 2-stage model of carcinogenesis proposed by Armitage and Doll [37] was based on the biological evidence that stem cells are transformed into premalignant cells. They proposed that these premalignant cells divide at a constant rate, producing an exponential growth of preneoplastic clones. A preneoplastic cell is then transformed into a cancer cell, that may ultimately develop into a tumour. More recently, Moolgavkar and Knudson [38] have proposed a mathematical model that is based on the biological evidence linking mutation induction and tumour formation. This model assumes that the first critical event in a series of steps that can lead to cancer is the induction of a mutation in the DNA of a normal stem cell resulting in a preneoplastic cell. The second critical step is the transformation of a preneoplastic cell into a malignant cancer cell. Biologically motivated cancer risk models such as the 2-stage model have many advantages over purely mathematical approaches to risk assessment [7,39]. Importantly, the parameters in the model are interpretable in biological terms and may potentially be estimated from experimental cellular data including mutation and cell transformation data. These new biologically based dose-response models will take into account new knowledge on the molecular genetics and origins of cancer [10,11]. Cell proliferation and cellular toxicity (death) data may also be incorporated into this model [12-14].

Comparative methods for quantitative cancer risk assessment all rely on comparing the relative potency of one carcinogen either to a standard agent (e.g., radiation or a well studied chemical) or to other carcinogenic agents. The underlying assumption in all comparative methods is that the relative potency in humans is either equivalent or that it may be predicted from the relative potency in a laboratory bioassay.

The use of ionising radiation as a standard in the evaluation of risk from exposure to environmental chemicals was the first comparative risk method proposed in the 1970s [40]. Tornqvist and Ehrenberg [41] have used the radiation equivalent risk model most extensively to estimate the cancer risk in Sweden from a series of urban air pollutants, particularly gaseous alkenes (e.g., ethene).

The comparative potency method developed for complex mixtures of air pollutants from combustion sources [42] is based on the hypothesis that there is a constant relative potency across different bioassay systems (e.g., human and rodent), where relative potency is determined by the ratio of the slopes of the dose responses from the same bioassay, as shown below:

$$\text{relative potency} = \frac{\text{bioassay potency of carcinogen}_1}{\text{bioassay potency of carcinogen}_2}$$

This method was initially conceived for the purpose of comparing the mutagenic and carcinogenic activity of diesel vehicle emissions to 3 similar emissions for which human cancer risk data were available (coke ovens, roofing coal tar and cigarette smoke) [42]. The first application of this method was the cancer risk assessment of diesel emissions [43]. The constant relative potency assumptions is invoked in this method, the general expression for this assumption is the following:

$$\frac{\text{relative human potency}}{\text{relative bioassay potency}} = (k)$$

The constant relative potency assumption is implicit in any comparative method which utilises the relative genotoxic effect of two substances in animals to estimate their relative genotoxic risk in humans. The potency in this method directly employs the slope which may be expressed in response per unit exposure or per unit dose. This method has been most widely used in estimating the genotoxic and carcinogenic risk of complex mixtures of air pollutants containing polycyclic organic matter including ambient air particulate matter itself [44]. Figure 1 illustrates the application of the comparative potency method using mouse skin tumour initiation potency to predict the human lung cancer unit risk estimate of ambient particulate matter.

Individual Air Pollutant Chemicals

More than 2,800 different individual chemicals have been identified as atmospheric compounds [45]. These compounds represent almost every known chemical class. The number of chemicals identified in each class does not necessarily represent the distribution of chemicals by class in the air, since the chemicals that have been identified are highly dependent on our current chemical analytical detection methods. Graedel et al. [45] suggested that alcohols, carboxylic acids and nitrogen-containing organic compounds are underrepresented with respect to their actual occurrence in the ambient air. Table 1 shows the number of chemicals in each category that have been detected in atmospheres including ambient air, indoor air and air emission sources. Unfortunately, only about 10% of these chemicals have been evaluated in any bioassays. Table 1 shows the number of chemicals in each category for which either short-term bacterial genetic bioassay data or animal cancer data have been reported.

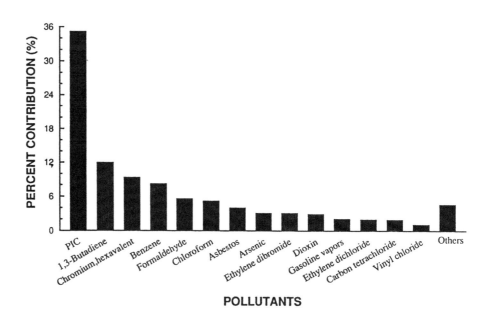

Fig. 1. Relative contribution to total estimated cancer cases per year by pollutant in the U.S. Adapted from US EPA, 1990. The values in this figure are not absolute predictions of cancer occurrence and are intended to be used for comparative purposes. The dose-response relationships and exposure assumptions have a conservative bias, but due to the omission of uncharacterised pollutants (either emitted directly or formed from atmospheric reactions) and emission sources, the long-range transport of pollutants and the lack of knowledge of total risk from multi-pollutant exposures may offset this bias to an unknown extent.

Table 1. Occurrence and bioassay results for airborne chemicals

Category	Number of compounds identified	Number bioassayed	Positive compounds Type of Bioassay	
			Animal	STT*
Inorganics	260	30	4	5
Hydrocarbons	729	51	19	12
Ethers	44	3	0	1
Alcohols	233	28	0	1
Ketones	227	11	0	0
Aldehydes	108	6	1	4
Carboxylic acid derivatives	219	6	2	0
Carboxylic acids	174	5	0	0
Heterocyclic oxygen compounds	93	16	7	4
Nitrogen-containing organics	384	59	12	22
Sulphur-containing organics	99	4	1	1
Halogen-containing organics	216	71	21	16
Organometallic compounds	41	13	0	6
GRAND TOTALS	2827	303	67	72

* STT=short-term tests as described in the text   Adapted from Graedel et al. [45]

Three categories (hydrocarbons, nitrogen-containing organics and halogenated organics) account for nearly 60% of the compounds that have been bioassayed. This table shows that the percentage of ketones, carboxylic acids and their derivatives that have been identified in the air is much greater than the percentage of those compounds with any bioassay data. Therefore, the contribution of these categories of chemicals to the potential airborne carcinogens cannot be estimated.

This computerised data base on the occurrence of atmospheric compounds has been merged with the largest evaluated bioassay data base. The bioassay data base was developed by the U.S. Environmental Protection Agency Gene-Tox Programme [16] with the assistance of many international experts who reviewed and evaluated the bioassay data. This entire bioassay data base contains bioassay results for 2346 compounds, only 303 of which are overlapping with the 2827 compounds that have been identified as air pollutants. As shown in Table 1, the three chemical categories that have the most bioassay data also have the highest number of positive bioassay results in both animal cancer tests and short-term bioassay tests. This data is very useful in summarising what is known and what is not known about the potential genotoxic and carcinogenic activity of compounds found in air pollution. Unfortunately, the distribution of both chemicals and positive bioassay results reflects the degree of attention paid by atmospheric chemists and toxicologists to specific classes of chemicals rather than the degree of potential hazard of these classes of chemicals compared to those classes that have not been investigated. This data base does not include the relative exposure concentrations of these chemicals, a critical factor in understanding the potential risk (see the chapter by Fishbein and Hemminki).

When the source of each atmospheric compound is included in the analysis of the occurrence of biologically active compounds, several conclusions become apparent [45]. Firstly, the sources that emit the highest number of bioassay-positive chemicals are sources involving combustion (e.g., tobacco smoke, automobile exhaust and coal combustion). Non-combustion sources including chemical manufacturing and pesticides are also significant but in this analysis rank below the combustion sources. Vegetation appears on the list because of the low molecular weight aldehydes frequently emitted by plants.

Nearly 300 different compounds from Table 1 [45] were identified in indoor air. Recent indoor air studies have identified many more indoor air pollutants and their sources (see the chapter by Fishbein).

Weight of Evidence for Human Cancer Risk of Individual Chemicals

The list of chemicals identified in air has been combined with the weight of evidence for those chemicals evaluated for carcinogenic risk to humans by the IARC evaluation [46] as shown in Table 2. Of those chemicals with sufficient evidence for human carcinogenicity, benzene is the one chemical with the highest and best characterised human exposure. Of those chemicals with limited evidence for human carcinogenicity but sufficient evidence for animal carcinogenicity (Group 2A), formaldehyde has the highest and best characterised human exposure. Of the other chemicals in the Group 2A and 2B category (sufficient evidence for animal carcinogenicity) identified in air with human exposure assessment data, the following have been identified as potentially important contributors to human cancer risk: 1,3-butadiene, ethylene dibromide, and carbon tetrachloride [47].

There are many uncertainties in evaluating the weight of evidence for human cancer risk of the chemicals found in air pollution. One of the most important of these is that other chemicals either not yet identified in air or not studied in animal cancer or short-term bioassays may eventually be shown to be more significant air pollutants in the future. There is recent evidence from studies of complex mixtures of urban air particles and gases that the major contributors to the genotoxic activity of urban air are mutagens that have not yet been identified and may be produced upon atmospheric transformation of organics emitted by many sources [48,49]. New bioassay-directed chemical identification techniques have identified polar organic species (e.g., hydroxylated and nitrated aromatic hydrocarbons) in urban air [48].

Quantitative Estimates of the Contribution of Individual Chemicals to Human Cancer Risk

Quantitation of cancer risk from individual chemicals in air has many uncertainties associated with both the exposure assessment and cancer potency assessment that are combined to produce an estimate of excess cancer cases. In spite of these large uncertainties, this procedure is being widely used in the U.S. to rank the importance of chemicals and sources associated with air pollution [36]. The total annual number of cancer cases for the U.S. estimated to be derived from outdoor air is approximately 2,000 per year, which is similar in magnitude to the estimated number of cancer cases from passive smoking and much less than the number of cancer deaths in the U.S. attributed to cigarette smoking. This analysis has many uncertainties and does not include in the analysis all possible sources or all chemicals that have been identified in the air as discussed above. Figure 2 illustrates the relative contribution of a number of individual chemicals and several mixtures to the total estimated U.S. cancer cases per year from outdoor air pollutants using this method [36]. The most dramatic observation from this analysis is the estimated importance of products of incomplete combustion (PIC), which is a very complex mixture of gases and particles. The other major contributing chemicals in this analysis include several that are either evaluated by IARC as having sufficient evidence (Group 1) to be carcinogenic to humans or are probably (2A) or possibly (2B) carcinogenic to humans including: 1,3 butadiene, benzene, formaldehyde, chloroform, asbestos, ethylene dibromide, and carbon tetrachloride. Of the remaining chemicals that this analysis estimates may be important, there are several where the weight of evidence for human cancer risk is lacking principally through a lack of an appropriate animal bioassay model that will detect inorganic carcinogens such as hexavalent chromium and arsenic.

Table 2. Summary of the weight of evidence for human cancer risk of individual airborne chemicals

CHEMICAL	Evidence for Carcinogenicity			OVERALL[c] EVALUATION
	HUMAN[a]	ANIMAL[a]	STT[b]	
ARSENIC and ARSENIC COMPOUNDS	S	S	+	1
BENZENE	S	S	+	1
BIS(CHLOROMETHYL)ETHER	S	S	+	1
CHLOROMETHYL METHYL ETHER	S	S	+	1
CHROMIUM (VI) COMPOUNDS	S	S	+	1
NICKEL and NICKEL COMPOUNDS	S	S	+	1
VINYL CHLORIDE	S	S	+	1
SULPHURIC ACID MISTS	S	-	-	1
ACRYLONITRILE	L	S	+	2A
BERYLLIUM (OXIDE) CPDS	L	S	+	2A
Cd (II) OXIDE	L	S	(+)	2A
EPOXYETHANE	L	S	+	2A
FORMALDEHYDE	L	S	+	2A
BUTADIENE, 1,3-	L	S	+	2A
DIMETHYL SULFATE	I	S	+	2A
DIBROMOETHYLENE	I	S	+	2A
EPOXYPROPANE, 1,2-	I	S	+	2A
EPICHLOROHYDRIN	I	S	+	2A
BENZO (A) PYRENE	ND	S	+	2A
DIBENZ (A,H) ANTHRACENE	ND	S	+	2A
N-NITROSODIMETHYLAMINE	ND	S	+	2A
ACETALDEHYDE	I	S	+	2B
CARBON TETRACHLORIDE	I	S	(+)	2B
CHLOROFORM	I	S	(-)	2B
DICHLOROPROPANE, 1,3-	I	S	+	2B
DIOXANE, 1,4-	I	S	(-)	2B
HYDRAZINE	I	S	+	2B
LEAD (INORGANIC)	I	S	(-)	2B
STYRENE	I	L	+	2B
VINYLIDENE CHLORIDE	I	L	+	3
BENZO (J) FLUORANTHENE	ND	S	(+)	2B
DIBENZO (A,E) PYRENE	ND	S	(+)	2B
DIBENZO (A,L) PYRENE	ND	S	ND	2B
DIBENZO (C,G) CARBAZOLE	ND	S	ND	2B
DIBENZ (A,H) ACRIDINE	ND	S	(+)	2B
DIBENZ (A,J) ACRIDINE	ND	S	+	2B
DICHLOROETHANE, 1,2-	ND	S	+	2B
DIMETHYLHYDRAZINE	ND	S	+	2B
DINITROPYRENE, 1,6-	ND	S	+	2B
DINITROPYRENE, 1,8-	ND	S	+	2B
INDENO (1,2,3-CD) PYRENE	ND	S	(+)	2B

Table 2. (continued)

CHEMICAL	Evidence for Carcinogenicity			
	HUMAN [a]	ANIMAL [a]	STT [b]	OVERALL [c] EVALUATION
NITROCHRYSENE, 6-	ND	S	+	2B
NITROFLUORENE, 2-	ND	S	+	2B
NITROPROPANE, 2-	ND	S	+	2B
NITROPYRENE, 1-	ND	S	+	2B
NITROPYRENE, 4-	ND	S	+	2B
N-NITROSODIETHANOLAMINE	ND	S	+	2B
N-NITROSOMORPHOLINE	ND	S	+	2B

a Degree of Evidence as evaluated by IARC (1987-1989) in the following catagories:
S = Sufficient evidence of carcinogenicity as evaluated by IARC
L = Limited evidence of carcinogenicity as evaluated by IARC
I = Inadequate evidence of carcinogenicity as evaluated by IARC
ND = No adequate data

b STT = Short term tests for genotoxicity, mutagenicity or cell transformation. This evidence has been summarised into + to indicate positive results, - to indicate negative results or () to indicate an inconclusive evaluation with either both + and - studies reported or an insufficient number of adequate STT to evaluate.

c Overall Evaluation category by Groups as evaluated by IARC (1987-1989):
Group 1 = carcinogenic to humans
Group 2A = probably carcinogenic to humans
Group 2B = possily carcinogenic to humans
Group 3 = not classifiable as to carcinogenicity to humans
Group 4 = probably NOT carcinogenic to humans (none listed)

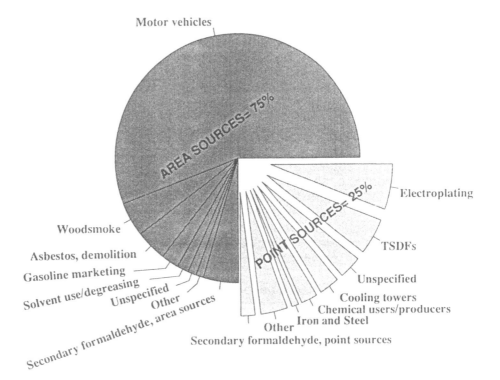

Fig. 2. Relative contribution of area and point sources to the total estimated cancer cases per year in the U.S. Adapted from US EPA, 1990. The data in this figure have the same limitations as described in Figure 1.

Mixtures of Air Pollutants

The first recognised chemical carcinogens were the coal tars and soots from chimneys that were found to induce not only scrotal cancer in humans but tumours in animals [50]. It is now recognised that combustion, pyrolysis and other types of thermal treatment of organic matter results in the formation of polycyclic aromatic compounds (PACs) such as the polycyclic aromatic hydrocarbon (PAH), benzo(a)pyrene. Many individual PACs are carcinogenic in animals (see Table 2) and genotoxic in short-term tests [51]. Humans, however, are not generally exposed to individual PACs, but to complex mixtures containing these compounds. These and other mixtures of air pollutants will be discussed as a) mixtures from sources emitted into the air, and b) mixtures of air pollution as they occur in urban, industrial, rural and indoor air.

Outdoor Sources

Many of the mixtures found in air that are listed in Table 3 as having an overall evaluation as carcinogenic to humans (Category 1), had sufficient evidence for excess cancer risk in humans exposed through occupational exposures (e.g. coke production, iron and steel founding). The industrial mixtures listed in Table 3 may not all have significant emissions to the outdoor air (e.g., boot and shoe manufacturing and repair). Several of these industrial sources are either not widely found or are not currently practiced throughout the world (e.g., shale oils and coal gasification). Other industrial source emissions can be significant sources of air pollution in industrial areas where they are present (e.g., coke production, iron and steel founding, aluminum production, lumber and paper industries). Two of these Category 1 carcinogens are primarily indoor air pollutants: asbestos and tobacco smoke.

The most widely distributed outdoor air pollutant is soot. Soot is a mixture of sub-micron carbonaceous particles that contain a relatively high percentage of condensed organic matter (tar). Although the first soot to be recognised as a human carcinogen was the soot from coal combustion [52], there is increasing evidence that soots from the combustion of other fuels (e.g., petroleum, wood) are similar in their composition, genetic activity and induction of tumours in animals [53,54]. A recent IARC evaluation of diesel and gasoline engine exhausts relied heavily on the animal evidence of carcinogenicity to evaluate these mixtures as probably and possibly carcinogenic to humans [55] (see Table 3). Vehicular emissions from automobiles, buses, trucks and other mobile sources are ubiquitous air pollutants in urban areas. Quantitative estimates of the possible contribution to human cancer risk in the United States suggest approximately half of the estimated cancer risk from outdoor air pollution may result from exposure to motor vehicle emissions and another one-fourth of the risk from other area sources [47].

Indoor Sources

The most important indoor air pollutant sources generally fall into one of the following categories: indoor combustion, building materials, household products, biologicals, and outdoor sources. The indoor air pollutants recognised as human carcinogens include tobacco smoke, asbestos, radon, and coal tars and soots. In addition to the human epidemiological evidence that these sources are carcinogenic, experimental evidence in animal cancer bioassays and/or short-term genetic bioassays has provided additional evidence that these sources are genotoxic and/or carcinogenic. There are many other indoor air pollutants where the only evidence for carcinogenicity is from experimental studies in animals and/or short-term tests on selected components in the emissions. These pollutant sources include: 1) mixtures of volatile organics emitted from building materials, furniture, glues, and fabrics, and 2) mixtures of household products such as cleaners, pesticides, and cosmetics.

Animal cancer studies support the large epidemiological data base showing that radon produces lung cancer [56]. The animal studies have the advantage of controlling such variables as the fraction, of radon not at-

Table 3. Summary of the weight of evidence for human cancer risk of airborne pollutant mixtures

MIXTURES	Evidence for Carcinogenicity			OVERALL [c] EVALUATION
	HUMAN [a]	ANIMAL [a]	STT [b]	
ASBESTOS	S	S	(+)	1
COAL-TAR PITCHES	S	S	+	1
COAL-TARS	S	S	+	1
SHALE OILS	S	S	+	1
TOBACCO SMOKE	S	S	+	1
RUBBER INDUSTRY	S	I	+	1
SOOTS	S	I	+	1
FURNITURE and CABINET MAKING	S	I	ND	1
ALUMINUM PRODUCTION	S		+	1
BOOT and SHOE MANUFACTURE and REPAIR	S		ND	1
COAL GASIFICATION	S		+	1
COKE PRODUCTION	S		+	1
IRON and STEEL FOUNDING	S		+	1
DIESEL				
WHOLE DIESEL ENGINE EXHAUST	L	S	+	2A
GAS-PHASE DIESEL ENGINE EXHAUST (PARTICLES REMOVED)		I	(+)	
EXTRACTS OF PARTICLES		S	+	
PETROL				
WHOLE PETROL ENGINE EXHAUST	I	I	+	2B
CONDENSATES/EXTRACTS OF PETROL ENGINE EXHAUST		S	+	
ENGINE EXHAUSTS (UNSPECIFIED)	L		+	
LUMBER & SAWMILL INDUSTRIES (INCLUDING LOGGING)	I		ND	3
PULP and PAPER MANUFACTURING	I		+	3

a   Degree of Evidence as evaluatuated by IARC (1987-1989) in the following catagories:
S = Sufficient evidence of carcinogenicity as evaluated by IARC
L = limited evidence of carcinogenicity as evaluated by IARC
I = inadequate evidence of carcinogenicity as evaluated by IARC
ND = no adequate data

b   STT = Short term tests for genotoxicity, mutagenicity or cell transformation. This evidence has been summarised into + to indicate positive results, - to indicate negative results or () to indicate an inconclusive evaluation with either both + and - studies reported or an insufficient number of adequate STT to evaluate.

c   Overall Evaluation category by Groups as evaluated by IARC (1987-1989):
Group 1 = carcinogenic to humans
Group 2A = probably carcinogenic to humans
Group 2B = possily carcinogenic to humans
Group 3 = not classifiable as to carcinogenicity to humans
Group 4 = probably NOT carcinogenic to humans (none listed)

tached to particles, particle size, and radon progeny concentration. Animal studies conducted in several species at various exposure levels are also useful for quantitative dose-response extrapolations from animals to humans.

Environmental tobacco smoke (ETS) from sidestream cigarette smoke is the largest source of elevated human exposures to particles and gases in indoor environments. In addition to the evidence that tobacco smoke as a mixture is carcinogenic in humans [57], ETS contains relatively high concentrations of chemicals for which there is sufficient evidence of carcinogenicity in animals including polynuclear aromatic hydrocarbons, N-nitrosamines, benzene, formaldehyde, and 1,3 butadiene. Carcinogenicity testing of tobacco smoke in animals has primarily been conducted with animals exposed to whole tobacco smoke [58]. The only study comparing the carcinogenicity of sidestream smoke to mainstream smoke was conduced on mouse skin [59]. This study showed that the smoke condensate from sidestream smoke was more tumorigenic on mouse skin than the mainstream smoke.

Combustion sources other than tobacco represent the other major sources of mutagenic activity detected indoors. These sources include unvented kerosene, coal and gas heaters and stoves used indoors. Cooking, even with an electric source of heat, can under certain circumstances result in airborne emissions of mutagenic activity [60]. The other combustion sources studied indoors that emit mutagenicity include incense smoke and insecticidal coils [60].

Ambient Indoor and Outdoor Air Mixtures

Particulate matter collected from the ambient air contains condensed organic matter similar to that described above for soot. A number of studies have shown that this organic extractable matter from air particles is carcinogenic in animals [61-63] and mutagenic in short-term bioassays [48,64-66]. Short-term mutagenicity bioassays have been used in ambient air monitoring studies and chemical characterisation studies in order to identify the major sources and compounds that contribute to the mutagenic activity of air particulate extracts [48,67]. Small area combustion sources that include vehicles and home heating sources have been shown to account for most of the mutagenic activity associated with air particulate matter in many urban areas [68], whereas in highly industrialised areas there is evidence of a significant contribution by coke ovens and other sources known to emit significant quantities of mutagenic polycyclic organic matter [69].

The first short-term bioassay study of indoor air mixtures was conducted in a large office building in Stockholm [60]. This study, and a number of other studies in restaurants, bars, apartments and houses, have concluded that the presence of ETS from smokers accounts for most of the mutagenic activity detected in particulate matter from indoor air [60]. In the presence of smokers, indoor air concentrations of particles and mutagenic activity can, in the worst case, reach exceptionally high concentrations (10-100 times the concentrations in the absence of smoking). In the absence of tobacco smoking, other sources of mutagenic particulate matter have been identified as outdoor air, cooking, kerosene heaters, and fireplaces.

Gaseous mixtures of air pollutants studied in short-term mutagenesis bioassays in plants and bacteria are mutagenic particularly after atmospheric transformations [70-72]. These studies suggest that highly reactive nitrogen-containing gases, such as peroxyacetyl nitrate (PAN), formed from ozone and nitrogen oxides reacting with simple non-mutagenic hydrocarbons, may produce genotoxic gases present in the urban air. Atmospheric transformations by ozone and nitrogen oxides have also been shown to increase the mutagenic activity of particulate matter and alter the nature of the mutagens to form more polar mutagens including nitroarenes [73].

Summary

Experimental evidence in animal studies and short-term bioassays provides much of the evidence that certain indoor and outdoor air pollutants are carcinogenic. Of the nearly 3,000 chemicals identified so far as air pollutants, only 10% have been studied in experimental bioassays. Many of the chemicals or mixtures that are carcinogenic to humans also induce tumours in animals and are genotoxic in short-term bioassays. There are many more air pollutants that have been shown to be carcinogenic in animals for which no adequate human data are available. In some cases human data for the individual chemicals may never be obtained since humans are only exposed to mixtures of these chemicals (e.g., PAH). In the absence of such human data, it is advisable to regard these air pollutants as presenting a carcinogenic risk to humans. There are many more air pollutants that have only been evaluated in short-term bioassays. The prediction of cancer risk based on only positive short term-tests is less certain, however, in the absence of other data, it would be advisable to avoid excessive and prolonged exposure to such agents.

Of all the air pollutants studied in humans and experimental systems, the greatest human exposure and risk appears to be associated with mixtures of polycyclic aromatic compounds, particularly those derived from incomplete combustion. The sources of greatest concern in indoor air are tobacco smoke, radon, certain building materials containing asbestos and formaldehyde, and unvented space heaters or cooking stoves. The sources of greatest concern in urban areas are usually the area sources such as motor vehicles and residential heating due to the high human exposure resulting from their proximity to population centres. In certain industrial areas, however, coke ovens, aluminium smelters, iron and steel foundries, chemical plants, power plants and other industrial sources have been shown to emit significant quantities of carcinogenic agents into the air.

Acknowledgements

The author acknowledges the assistance of Katherine Williams in the preparation of Tables 2 and 3. The research described in this paper has been reviewed by the Health Effects Research Laboratory, U.S. Environmental Protection Agency and approved for publication. Approval does not signify that the contents necessarily reflect the views and policies of the agency.

REFERENCES

1. Higginson, J, Jensen, OM: Epidemiological review of lung cancer in man. In: Mohr U, Schmahl D, Tomatis L (eds) Air Pollution and Cancer in Man. IARC Scientific Publications No 16. International Agency for Research on Cancer, Lyon 1977 pp 169-189
2. IARC: IARC Monographs on the Evaluation of Carcinogenic Risks to Humans, Suppl 7. Overall Evaluations of Carcinogenicity: An Updating of IARC Monographs Volumes 1-42. International Agency for Research on Cancer, Lyon 1987 pp 17-34
3. Wilbourn J, Haroun L, Heseltine E, Kaldor J, Partensky C, Vainio H: Response of experimental animals to human carcinogens: An analysis based upon the IARC Monographs Programme. Carcinogenesis 1986 (7):1853-1863
4. Tomatis L, Aitio, A, Wilbourn, J, and Shuker L: Human carcinogens so far identified. Jpn J Cancer Res 1989 (80):795-807
5. Huff JE, McConnell EE, Haseman, JK, Boorman, GA, Eustis SL, Schwartz BA, Rao GN, Jameson CK, Hart LG, and Rall D: Carcinogenesis studies: results of 398 experiments on 104 chemicals from the US National Toxicology Program. Ann NY Acad Sci 1988 (534):1-30
6. IARC: Approaches to Classifying Chemical Carcinogens According to Mechanism of Action. IARC Internal Technical Report No 83/001, Lyon 1983
7. IARC: Mechanisms of Carcinogenesis in Risk Identification. IARC Internal Technical Report No 91/002, Lyon 1991
8. Montesano, R, Bartsch, H, Vainio, H, Wilbourn, J, Yamasaki, H (eds) Long-Term and Short-Term Assays for Carcinogenesis - A Critical Appraisal. IARC Scientific Publications No 83. International Agency for Research on Cancer, Lyon 1986
9. Miller EC, Miller JA: The mutagenicity of chemical carcinogens: Correlations, problems, and interpretations. In: Hollaender A (ed) Chemical Mutagens: Principles and Methods for Their Detection, Vol 1. Plenum Press, New York 1971 pp 83-94
10. Bishop JM: The molecular genetics of cancer. Science 1987 (235): 305-311
11. Weinberg R (ed) Oncogenes and the Molecular Origins of Cancer. Monograph 18, Cold Spring Harbor Laboratory Press, NY 1990
12. Butterworth, BE: Consideration of both genotoxic and nongenotoxic mechanisms in predicting carcinogenic potential. Mutat Res 1990 (239):117-132
13. Weinstein BI: Mitogenesis is only one factor in carcinogenesis. Science 1991 (251): 387-388
14. Butterworth B, Slaga T, Farland W, McClain W (eds): Chemically Induced Cell Proliferation: Implications for Risk Assessment. Wiley-Liss Inc, New York 1989
15. Trosko JE and Chang CC: Non-genotoxic mechanisms in carcinogenesis: role of inhibited intercellular communication. In: Hart RW and Hoerger FD (eds) Carcinogen Risk Assessment, Banbury Report 31. Cold Spring Harbor Laboratory, Cold Spring Harbor, New York 1988 pp139-174
16. Waters MD, Auletta A: The GENE-TOX program: genetic activity evaluation. J Chem Inf Comput Sci 1981(21): 35-38
17. Yamasaki H: Multistage carcinogenesis: implications for risk estimation. Cancer Metastasis Rev 1988 (7): 5-18
18. Ashby J: The prospect for a simplified internationally harmonized approach to the detection of possible human carcinogens and mutagens. Mutagenesis 1986 (1): 3-16
19. McCann J, Choi E, Yamasaki E and Ames BN: Detection of carcinogens as mutagens in the salmonella/microsome test: Assay of 300 chemicals. Proc Natl Acad Sci USA 1975 (72):5135-5139
20. Shelby MD and Zeiger E: Activity of human carcinogens in the salmonella and rodent bone-marrow cytogenetics tests. Mutation Res 1990 (234): 257-261
21. Ashby J and Morrod, RS: Detection of human carcinogens. Nature 1991 (352):185-186
22. Bartsch H: Predictive value of mutagenicity tests in chemical carcinogenesis. Mutat Res 1976 (38):177-190
23. Sugimura TS, Sato M, Nagao T, Yahagi T, Matsushima Y, Seino M, Takeuchi and Kawachi T: Overlapping of carcinogens and mutagens. In: Magee PN, Takayama S, Sugimura T and Matsushima T (eds) Fundamentals of Cancer Prevention. University Park Press, Baltimore, MD 1976 pp191-213
24. Ashby J and Tennant RW: Chemical structure, Salmonella mutagenicity and extent of carcinogenicity as indicators of genotoxic carcinogenesis among 222 chemicals tested in rodents of the U.S. NCI/NTP. Mutat Res 1988 (204):17-115
25. Tennant RW, Margolin BH, Shelby MD, Zeiger E, Haseman JK, Spalding, J, Caspary W, Resnick M, Stasiewicz S, Anderson B, Minor R: Prediction of chemical carcinogenicity in rodents from in vitro genetic toxicity assays. Science 1987 (236): 933-941
26. Brockman HE and DeMarini DM: Utility of short-term tests for genetic toxicity in the aftermath of the NTP's analysis of 73 chemicals. Environ Mol Mutagen 1988 (11):421-435
27. Bartsch H and Malaveille C: Prevalence of genotoxic chemicals among animal and human carcinogens evaluated in the IARC Monograph Series. Cell Biol Toxicol 1989 (5):115-127
28. Lave LB, Ennever FK, Rosenkranz HS and Omenn GS: Information value of the rodent bioassay. Nature 1988 (336):431-433
29. Claxton LD, Stead AG and Walsh D: An analysis by chemical class of Salmonella mutagenicity tests as predictors of animal carcinogenicity. Mutat Res 1988 (205):197-225
30. Ashby J: The separate identities of genotoxic and non-genotoxic carcinogens. Mutagenesis 1988 (3):365-366

31 Gold LS, Slone TH, Backman GM, Eisenberg S, DaCosta M, Wong M, Manley, NB, Rohrbach L, and Ames BN: Third chronological supplement to the carcinogenic potency database: Standardized results of animal bioassays published through December 1986 and by the National Toxicology Program through June 1987. Environ Health Perspect 1990 (84):215-286

32 Garrett, NE, Stack, HF, Gross, MR, Waters, MD: An analysis of the spectra of genetic activity produced by known or suspected human carcinogens. Mutat Res 1984 (134):89-111

33 Ames BM, Magaw R and Gold LS: Ranking possible carcinogenic hazards. Science 1987 (236):271

34 Ames BN, Magaw R and Gold LS: Response to letter: Risk assessment. Science 1987 (237):235

35 Anderson EL and the Cancer Assessment Group of the US Environmental Protection Agency: Quantitative approaches in use to assess cancer risk. Risk Anal 1983 (3):277-295

36 Crump KS: An improved procedure for low-dose carcinogenic risk assessment from animal data. J Environ Pathol Toxicol 1981 (5):675-684

37 Armitage P and Doll R: A two-stage theory of carcinogenesis in relation to the age distribution of human cancer. Br J Cancer 1957 (11):161-169

38 Moolgavkar SH and Knudson AG: Mutation and cancer: A model for human carcinogenesis. JNCI 1981 (66):1037-1052

39 Thorslund TW, Brown CC, and Charnley G: Biologically motivated cancer risk models. Risk Anal 1987 (7):109-119

40 Committee 17: Environmental mutagenic hazards. Science 1975 (187):503-514

41 Tornqvist M and Ehernberg L: Risk estimation of urban air pollution: Information sources and methods. Environ Int 1985 (11):401-406

42 Lewtas J: Development of a comparative potency method for cancer risk assessment of complex mixtures using short-term in vivo and in vitro bioassays. Toxicology and Industrial Health 1985 (4):193-203

43 Albert R, Lewtas, J, Nesnow, S, Thorslund, T and Anderson, E: Comparative potency method for cancer risk assessment: Application to diesel particulate emissions. Risk Analysis 1983 (3):101-117

44 Lewtas J: Complex mixtures of air pollutants: Characterizing the cancer risk of polycyclic organic matter (POM). Environ Health Perspect 1992 (100) in press

45 Graedel TE, Hawkins DT, Claxton LD: Atmospheric Chemical Compounds: Sources, Occurrence, and Bioassay. Academic Press Inc, Orlando, FL 1986 p 732

46 IARC: IARC Monographs on the Evaluation of Carcinogenic Risks to Humans, Volumes 1-46. International Agency for Research on Cancer, Lyon

47 US Environmental Protection Agency: Cancer Risk from Outdoor Exposure to Air Toxics. Office of Air Quality Planning and Standards, Research Triangle Park, NC 27711. EPA-450/2-89

48 Lewtas J: Genotoxicity of complex mixtures: Strategies for the identification and comparative assessment of airborne mutagens and carcinogens from combustion sources. Fundam Appl Toxicol 1988 (10):571-589

49 Claxton LD: Assessment of bacterial bioassay methods for volatile and semivolatile compounds and mixtures. Environ Int 1985 (11):375-382

50 Searle CE (ed) Chemical Carcinogens. ACS Monograph No 173. American Chemical Society, Washington DC 1976

51 IARC: IARC Monographs on the Evaluation of Carcinogenic Risks to Humans. Polynuclear Aromatic Compounds, Part 1: Chemical, Environmental and Experimental Data, Vol 32. International Agency for Research on Cancer, Lyon 1982-1987 pp 17-34

52 IARC: IARC Monographs on the Evaluation of Carcinogenic Risks to Humans. Polynuclear Aromatic Compounds, Part 4: Bitumens, Coal-tar and Derived Products, Shale Oils and Soots, Vol 35. International Agency for Research on Cancer, Lyon 1985

53 Hoffman D, Wynder EL: Environmental respiratory carcinogenesis. In: Searle CE (ed) Chemical Carcinogens. ACS Monograph 173. American Chemical Society, Washington, DC 1976 pp 324-365

54 Lewtas J: Combustion emissions: Characterization and comparision of their mutagenic and carcinogenic activity. In: Stich HF (ed) Carcinogens and Mutagens in the Environment. Volume V: The Workplace. CRC Press, Boca Raton, F 1985 pp 59-74

55 IARC: IARC Monographs on the Evaluation of Carcinogenic Risks to Humans. Diesel and Gasoline Engine Exhausts and Nitroarenes, Vol 46. International Agency for Research on Cancer, Lyon 1989

56 Guilmette RA, Johnson NF, Newton GJ, Thomassen DG, and Yeh HC: Risks from radon progeny exposure: What we know, and what we need to know. Ann Rev Pharmacol Toxicol 1991 (31):69-601

57 US Environmental Protection Agency: Respiratory Health Effects of Passive Smoking: Lung Cancer and Other Disorders. Office of Research and Development, Washington, DC 20460. May 1992, SAB Draft, EPA/600/6-90/006B

58 US Department of Health and Human Services: The Health Consequences of Involuntary Smoking: A Report of the Surgeon General. Office on Smoking and Health, Rockville, MD 20857, 1986

59 Wynder EL and Hoffman D: Tobacco and Tobacco Smoke: Studies in Experimental Carcinogenesis. Academic Press, New York 1967

60 Lewtas, J, Claxton, L, Mumfortd, J and Lofroth G: Bioassay of Complex Mixtures of Indoor Air Pollutants. IARC Monograph on Indoor Air Methods. IARC, Lyon 1992 pp 65-75

61 Leiter J, Shimkin MB, Shear MJ: Production of subcutaneous sarcomas in mice with tars extracted from atmospheric dusts. JNCI 1942 (3):155-165

62 Kotin P, Falk HL, Mader P, Thomas M: Aromatic hydrocarbons. 1. Presence in the Los Angeles atmosphere and the carcinogenicity of atmospheric extracts. Arch Indust Hyg 1954 (9):153-163

63 Hueper WC, Kotin P, Tabor EC, Payne W, Falk HL, Sawiciki E: Carcinogenic bioassays on air pollutants. Arch Pathol 1962 (74):89-116
64 Alfheim I, Lofroth G, Moller M: Bioassay of extracts of ambient particulate matter. Environ Health Persp 1983 (47):227-238
65 Matsushita H, Goto S, Takagi Y: Human exposure to airborne mutagens indoors and outdoors using mutagenesis and chemical analysis methods. In: Waters MD, Daniel FB, Lewtas J, Moore MM, Nesnow S (eds) Short-Term Bioassays in the Analysis of Complex Environmental Mixtures VI. Plenum Press, New York 1990 pp 33-56
66 Barale R, Migliore L, Cellini B, Francioni L, Giogelli F, Barai I, Loprieno N: Genetic toxicology of airborne particulate matter using cytogenetic assays and microbial mutagenicity assays. In: Waters MD, Daniel FB, Lewtas J, Moore MM, Nesnow S (eds) Short-Term Bioassays in the Analysis of Complex Environmental Mixtures VI. Plenum Press, New York 1990 pp 57-71
67 Schuetzle D, Lewtas J: Bioassay-directed chemical analysis in environmental research. Anal Chem 1986 (58):1060A-1075A
68 Lewis CW, Baumgardner RE, Claxton LD, Lewtas J, Stevens RK: The contribution of woodsmoke and motor vehicle emissions to ambient aerosol mutagenicity. Environ Sci Technol 1988 (22):968-971
69 Tokiwa H, Morita K, Takeyoshi H, Takahashi K, Ohnishi Y: Detection of mutagenic activity in particulate air pollutants. Mutat Res 1977 (48):237-248
70 Tice RR, Costa DL, Schaich KM: Genotoxic Effects of Airborne Agents, Vol 25, Environmental Science Research. Plenum Press, New York 1980
71 Claxton LD, Kleindienst TE, Perry E and Cupitt LT: Assessment of the mutagenicity of organic air pollutants before and after atmospheric transformation. In: Waters MD, Daniel FB, Lewtas J, Moore MM, Nesnow S (eds) Short-Term Bioassays in the Analysis of Complex Environmental Mixtures VI. Plenum Press, New York 1990 pp 103-111
72 Kleindienst TE, Shepson PB, Edney EO, Claxton LD, Cupitt LT: Wood smoke: measurement of the mutagenic activities of its gas-and particulate-phase photooxidation products. Environ Sci Technol 1986 (20): 493-501
73 Kamens RM, Rives GD, Perry JM, Bell DA, Paylor RF, Goodman RG, Claxton LD: Mutagenic changes in dilute wood smoke as it ages and reacts with ozone and nitrogen dioxide: An outdoor chamber study. 1984 Environ Sci Technol 1984 (18,7):523-530

Epidemiological Evidence on Indoor Air Pollution and Cancer

Lorenzo Simonato [1] and Göran Pershagen [2]

1 Cancer Registry of the Veneto Region, Via Giustiniani 7, 35128 Padova, Italy
2 Department of Epidemiology, Institute of Environmental Medicine, Karolinska Institute, Box 60208, 104 01 Stockholm, Sweden

Epidemiological evidence is accumulating on cancer risks related to non-occupational exposures with primary sources indoors, such as environmental tobacco smoke, radon, cooking fumes and mineral fibres. Most of the data is focused on lung cancer risks and on women because they are believed to receive the heaviest residential exposures. For clarity the different exposure factors will be treated separately, although it is realised that they often occur together, and that interactions may be of importance.

Environmental Tobacco Smoke (ETS)

While the carcinogenic risk from direct inhalation of tobacco smoke was demonstrated some 40 years ago, the hypothesis that involuntary exposure to tobacco smoke from active smokers might increase the risk of lung cancer has been tested by epidemiological research only during the last decade. In very few years, however, several analytical studies were carried out on this subject and the epidemiological evidence available in 1986 led the Surgeon General to conclude in its report that ETS should be regarded as a cause of lung cancer [1]. Similar conclusions were reached by an expert group assembled at the International Agency for Research on Cancer [2].
It is now widely acknowledged that ETS, which is present in different types of environment (i.e., home, workplace, offices, public spaces), is a major component of indoor air pollution.

The purpose of this chapter is to provide the main information on the numerous epidemiological studies that have investigated the association between lung cancer and exposure to ETS. An effort has been made to select and summarise the results, with particular attention to the available evidence on the effects of different types of exposure in the 3 main geographical areas where the studies were conducted.
In 1981, 2 studies carried out more or less simultaneously in Greece and in Japan [3,4] reported an increased lung cancer risk among non-smoking women who were exposed to tobacco smoke from their husbands. Trichopoulos and colleagues carried out and subsequently updated [3,5] a case-control investigation on women admitted to the main hospitals in Athens with a diagnosis of lung cancer. After excluding adenocarcinomas, 77 cases were left in the study. The control group comprised 225 patients hospitalised in the Athens Hospital for Orthopaedic Disorders. All study subjects were interviewed by the same physician using a standard questionnaire.
The overall risk due to tobacco exposure from husbands was 2.1 (95% confidence interval: 1.2-3.8), indicating also a statistically significant increasing trend of the risk with exposure. The Relative Risk (RR) was 1.9 when husbands were ex-smokers, 2.4 when husbands smoked up to 20 cigarettes per day, and 3.4 when they smoked more than 20 cigarettes per day.
Similar results were obtained by an independent study conducted in Japan [4]. This was part of a large population-based perspective study including 265,118 persons aged at

least 40 years which was carried out in 29 health districts from 1966 to 1979.

The mortality from lung cancer of 91,540 non-smoking wives was analysed separately, using the available information of the smoking habits of the husbands. Non-smoking wives of ex-smokers or daily smokers of 1-19 cigarettes had a RR of 1.61, while non-smoking wives of men who smoked 20 or more cigarettes per day had a RR of 2.08 for lung cancer as compared to non-smoking wives of non-smokers.

A subsequent updating of the study [6] confirmed the results among females with a RR of 1.63 (95% CI: 1.25-2.11) and further supported the hypothesis of a link between lung cancer excess and exposure to ETS, showing an increased risk also among non-smoking males married to smoking wives (RR=2.25; 95% CI: 1.04-4.86).

Following the same approach, Garfinkel [7] analysed the data from the American Cancer Society perspective study which observed non-smoking women in relation to the smoking habits of their husbands. The results showed a slightly increased risk of lung cancer (RR=1.18; 95% CI: 0.90-1.54), with an inverse relationship between the number of cigarettes smoked daily by the husband and lung cancer mortality.

This first report from the U.S. was somewhat conflicting with the 2 previous studies and raised the hypothesis that exposure to ETS might vary from country to country and that exposure to a smoking spouse is not necessarily the most relevant type of exposure.

A large case-control study of lung cancer was subsequently conducted in the U.S. by Correa et al. [8], with a study population of 1338 lung cancer patients and 1393 hospital controls in Louisiana. Non-smoking subjects were interviewed about potential exposure to smoke from spouses and from parents during their childhood. The results, although based on only 30 cases, indicated a 2-fold increased risk in relation to the spouse's smoking habits, showing an increasing trend with amount of smoke.

The risk of lung cancer was also increased when the mother smoked, with an Odd Ratio (OR) of 1.36 ($p < 0.05$) after adjusting for direct tobacco smoking; exposure to a smoking father was not linked with an increased risk.

A similar hospital-based case-control study was carried out in the U.S. by Kabat and Wynder [9]. The matched analysis of 53 cases and controls did not indicate any difference between exposure and non-exposure to ETS for any of the 3 (i.e., home, workplace, spouse's smoke) types of exposure that were investigated.

The negative results from this study are consistent with a previously published case-control study [10] carried out in Hong Kong, which failed to demonstrate any association between lung cancer risk and smoking habits of husbands. The study population consisted of 84 non-smoking, female lung cancer patients and 139 hospital controls. The relative risk for lung cancer in relation to husbands' smoke was 0.75 (95% CI: 0.45-1.31).

A population-based perspective study was carried out in 2 urban communities in the West of Scotland using the data from a screening survey and the record linkage with the Registrar General for Scotland [10]. A 3-fold excess of lung cancer among non-smoking males exposed to ETS was reported (RR=3.25; 95% CI: 0.60-17.65), while no excess was apparent among the same category of females. ETS exposure was defined as marriage to a smoking spouse. This study was subsequently updated by Hole et al. [12]. Within the data from a multi-site case-control study investigating the relationship between childhood exposure and cancer risk in adulthood, Sandler and colleagues [13,14] analysed the relationship between exposure to ETS and lung cancer risk. The results indicated an effect of exposure to ETS in relation to the number of smokers in the household increasing from a RR of 1.5 with 1 smoker to 2.8 with 3 smokers (x^2 for trend statistically significant, $p < 0.01$). Separate analysis for exposure during childhood and adulthood indicated a RR of 1.48 (95% CI: 1.33-1.63) and 1.58 (95% CI: 1.33-1.88), and a RR of 2.71 (95% CI: 2.34-3.14) when both are present. Most of the other cancer sites, however, also showed an effect from cumulative exposure to ETS and in this study it was not possible to interview 30% of the cases and 40% of the controls.

Garfinkel et al. [15] conducted a hospital-based case-control study of 134 lung cancer cases and 402 colon-rectum controls among women. The ORs among non-smoking women exposed to husband's smoke were 1.23 (95% CI: 0.81-1.86) and 2.11 (95% CI: 1.13-3.95) if the husbands smoked more than 20 cigarettes per day at home, while the number of hours of exposure did not show any association with the risk. Exposure to smoke of others did not show any consistent effect on lung cancer at home or at work, while exposure to ETS during the last 25 years in other areas was associated with an increased OR of 1.42 (95% CI: 0.89-2.26).

Within a population-based case-control study on lung cancer among white women in Los Angeles County, Wu and colleagues [16] analysed non-smokers individually in order to investigate the risk associated with exposure to ETS. Only 45% of the eligible cases were alive at the time of the study and agreed to an interview. For each case one control was selected, matched for date of birth and neighbourhood. All interviews were conducted by telephone. Due to the small number, squamous cell carcinomas could not be analysed. Only a limited increase in the risk (RR=1.2; 95% CI: 0.5-3.3) was found for exposure to spouse's smoke, and for exposure to ETS at work (RR=1.3; 95% CI: 0.5-3.3), while no excess was associated with exposure to ETS from either parent (RR=0.6; 95% CI: 0.2-1.7). A statistically non-significant, increasing trend of the risk with the number of years of exposure was associated with exposure to ETS from spouse and at work.

In an extension of a hospital-based case-control study of the relation between tobacco smoke and lung cancer, chronic bronchitis, ischaemic heart disease and stroke, Lee and colleagues [17] interviewed the spouses of 56 non-smoking lung cancer patients and 112 matched non-smoking controls. In this way it was possible to compare the information on ETS from the index subject with that from the spouse of the index subject. The results showed important discrepancies, with an OR of 1.5 for males and 0.8 for females when the former was used, and 1.01 for males (95% CI: 0.44-5.78) and 1.60 for females (95% CI: 0.23-4.41) when the latter was used. The use of both sources of information resulted in an OR of 1.3 (95% CI: 0.37-4.54) among males and 1.03 (95% CI: 0.41-2.58) among females. This study pointed to the importance of the potential bias due to misclassification of smokers as non-smokers in ETS studies. An increasing trend in ORs was found among males in relation to exposure to ETS during leisure. For none of the other categories of exposure to ETS a consistent excess was present. The analysis was sometimes limited by the small numbers involved.

A case-control study of lung cancer within the cohort of the Hiroshima and Nagasaki survivors was conducted with the aim of investigating possible effects of exposure to husband's smoke [18]. Most of the interviews were taken from relatives of dead cases and matched controls. Ninety-four female cases and 270 controls were included in the analysis.

The overall OR was 1.5 (90% CI: 1.0-2.5) and an increasing trend was observed with the daily number of cigarettes smoked by the husband but not with smoking duration, nor with the number of cigarettes smoked in the course of a marriage. The analysis also indicated an excess risk related to the last 10 years of exposure to husband's smoke.

Data on non-smoking subjects from 3 large hospital-based case-control studies of lung cancer conducted in Louisiana, Texas and New Jersey were pooled together for a common analysis [19], including the data already reviewed here of Correa et al. [8]. The 2 studies are, therefore, not fully independent. The information on smoking was collected either from the index subject or from a surrogate respondent. A total of 99 non-smoking lung cancer cases and 736 non-smoking controls were included in the analysis. The results indicated an adjusted OR of 1.47 (95% CI: 0.76-2.83) for non-smokers married to a smoking spouse.

The OR was higher (2.71; 95% CI: 0.84-8.52) when the spouse smoked 280 cigarettes per week but no increasing trend was apparent in relation to duration of smoking, while a cumulative dose in pack years of exposure was positively correlated with the risk.

As part of a population-based case-control study of lung cancer in New Mexico, Humble and colleagues investigated the relationship between lung cancer and ETS [20]. Cases were obtained from the New Mexico Tumour Registry between 1980 and 1984. Sex, race and age-matched controls were randomly selected from the general population census. In 19 out of 28 cases the information on the smoking habits of the spouses of the non-smoking patients had to be collected from surrogate respondents. The 8 male cases were subsequently excluded from the analysis due to the small number. The results revealed a relative risk of 1.7 (90% CI: 0.6-4.3) for females married to a smoking husband. The OR was more elevated among females with more than 26 years of exposure to ETS, while an inverse relationship with the mean daily consumption of cigarettes was suggested.

Lung cancer risk in relation to ETS among Chinese women in Hong Kong was investigated by Lam and colleagues [21]. Exposure to ETS was defined as marriage to a smoking husband. A total of 199 non-smoking cases and 335 non-smoking population controls were included in this study.

An overall RR of 1.65 (95% CI: 1.16-2.35) was found, which was higher when the analysis was restricted to adenocarcinomas but did not show any relation with daily amount of tobacco smoked by the husband.

Using the data from a cross-sectional survey of smoking habits among women conducted in Sweden in the early 1960s and data from the Swedish twin register from the same period, Pershagen and colleagues [22] conducted a case-control study of non-smoking, female lung cancer patients through a linkage with the Swedish Cancer Registry and the National Registry of the Causes of Death. A total of 92 cases of cancer of the respiratory tract were thus identified. Two control groups were selected from the same cohort: the first matched for year of birth, and the second for year of birth and vital status, amounting to a total of 368 controls. The information on smoking was updated by means of a questionnaire mailed to the index subject or, if deceased, to her next of kin. A slight elevation (RR=1.2; 95% CI: 0.6-2.2) was present for exposure to smoking husbands. The RR rose to 3.2 (95% CI: 1.0-9.5) in the category with high exposure to tobacco smoke from the husband (i.e., more than 15 cigarettes per day during 30 years or more of marriage). A relative risk close to 2 was present for women with at least one smoking parent, but only for squamous or small cell carcinoma.

Exposure to ETS was investigated among 88 female lung cancer cases who never smoked and 137 female controls who never smoked within a larger case-control study of lung cancer conducted in Hong Kong by Koo and colleagues [23]. The relative risk due to exposure to husband's smoke was 1.64 (95% CI: 0.87-3.09) and was not associated with increasing daily cigarette consumption.

Exposure to ETS in the household was associated with a 2-fold increase in the RR (2.07; 95% CI: 0.51-5.15) during childhood, and up to 1.65 (95% CI: 0.62-5.45) during adulthood, but the increase tended to disappear when both exposures were considered together. Some of these analyses were, however, based on small numbers. Different types of dose estimates did not show any consistent association with lung cancer risk when all histological types were combined, while an increasing trend of the RR was detectable when the analysis was limited to squamous or small cell carcinoma.

Gao and colleagues [24] conducted a large case-control study on female lung cancer patients in China, which was focused on several risk factors including active and passive smoking. Overall exposure to ETS during childhood or adulthood was not associated with an increased risk of lung cancer among non-smokers. When the data were analysed in relation to husband's smoking habits, a slightly elevated RR was discernible (OR = 1.19; 95% CI: 1.16-1.22), which tended to increase with the number of years of marriage to a smoking husband. The RR in the group with 40 or more years of exposure (OR = 1.7; 95% CI: 1.0-2.9) was even higher when the analysis was restricted to squamous or small cell carcinomas (OR = 2.9; 95% CI: 1.0-8.9).

A case-control study carried out by Inoue and Hirayama [25] in the Kanagawa prefecture, Japan, focused on lung cancer risk among females. Thirty-seven cases of lung cancer were compared to 74 cerebrovascular deaths matched by age, year of death and district of residence. The number of non-smokers among cases and controls was 28 and 62, respectively. For about one-fourth of cases and controls, the husband's smoking habits were unknown. The relative risk for non-smoking wives with smoking husbands was 2.55 (95% CI: 0.91-7.10), showing an increasing trend with the number of cigarettes.

Another case-control investigation of lung cancer in non-smoking women was conducted in Nagoya (Japan) by Shimizu and colleagues [26]. A total number of 90 cases was included in the study together with 163 non-lung cancer controls matched by age, hospital, and date of admission. The Relative Risk was high for passive exposure to mother's smoke (RR=4.0; 95% CI: 1.6-12.2) and to husband's father's smoke (RR=3.2; 95% CI: 1.9-8.0), while it was close to 1 for all other familial exposures.

Geng and colleagues [27] carried out a case-control study on 157 incident lung cancer cases among females resident in the Tianjin province of China. An equal number of population controls were matched by age, race and marital status. There were 54 non-smokers among the cases and 93 among the controls, the OR from passive exposure to a smoking husband was 2.16 (95% CI = 1.03-4.53) and was reported to increase both with the amount of tobacco smoked by the husband and with years of smoking.

The prospective cohort study carried out by Gillis et al. [11] was updated by Hole and colleagues [12]. This study included all residents in the age range 45-64, in 2 towns of West Scotland between 1972 and 1976. A self-administered questionnaire including smoking behaviour was completed by 15,399 residents (80% of the eligible cohort) and 7997 attended for multiphasic screening with a cohabitee. The cohort was followed till the end of 1985. The Relative Risk for passive smoking computed comparing non-smokers with a smoking cohabitee, was, for lung cancer, 2.41 (95% CI = 0.45-12.83).

A population-based case-control study of female lung cancer cases in relation to various risk factors was conducted in Sweden by Svensson and colleagues [28]. A total of 210 incident cases and 209 age-matched population controls were included in the study. Forty-two percent of the controls were interviewed by telephone. Only 38 cases were non-smokers, thus affecting the statistical power of the analysis. Exposure to ETS during childhood (0-9 years) from parents showed an increased risk when the mother smoked (RR=3.3; 95% CI: 0.5-18.8); the risk was not increased with a smoking father. Exposure to ETS during adulthood was associated with a more elevated RR (RR=2.1; 95% CI: 0.6-0.81) when exposure occurred both at home and at work. Similarly, lifetime exposure to ETS both as child and adult appeared to increase the risk (RR=1.9; 95% CI: 0.2-3.7) more than exposure either during childhood or adulthood (RR=1.4; 95% CI: 0.2-2.5).

A hospital-based case-control study was conducted in 7 hospitals of the Greater Athens region between 1987 and 1989, investigating risk and protective factors for lung cancer among non-smoking women [29]. A multiple logistic regression analysis indicated a statistically significant increase in the RR (RR=2.1; 95% CI: 1.1-4.1) for women married to a smoker. An increased risk was also present in relation to household exposure to ETS from others and in the workplace, neither of them being statistically significant.

Janerich and colleagues [30] conducted a population-based case-control study of incident cases occurring in New York State from 1982 to 1985. One hundred and ninety-one lung cancer cases that did not smoke more than 100 cigarettes were enrolled in the study, with the same number of individually matched controls. Matching criteria were age, sex, county of residence, and type of interview (direct or surrogate). The study did not reveal an increased risk for lung cancer in relation to ETS exposure during childhood (RR=0.9; 95% CI: 0.5-1.4), although a tendency to increase with the amount of exposure was present; however, a RR of 1.3 (95% CI: 0.8-2.1) was associated with exposure during childhood and adolescence. A cumulative dose of smoker-years of exposure was calculated and analysed in relation to the lung cancer risk. The results indicated a 2-fold increase in the lung cancer risk for the subjects in the highest category of exposure during childhood and adolescence. No similar effect was found in relation to exposure during adulthood. No effect of exposure to ETS in the workplace or in social settings was detected.

A large hospital-based case-control study of lung cancer conducted in Osaka, Japan, by Sobue [31] offered the opportunity to investigate the lung cancer risk among non-smoking women in relation to ETS exposure. The analysis included 156 non-smoking cases and 786 hospital controls affected by diseases other than lung cancer. A moderately increased risk of lung cancer (RR=1.33; 95% CI: 0.74-2.37) was associated with childhood ETS exposure from the mother but not from the father. The RR in adulthood in relation to exposure from the husband was close to 1, while a statistically significant increased risk (RR=1.57; 95% CI: 1.07-2.31) was associated with exposure from other household members. A large case-control study of female lung cancer conducted in 2 provinces of north-east China included 965 cases and 959 population controls [32]. No elevation of the RR for lung cancer was reported in relation to passive exposure to cigarette smoke nor was there any association with the intensity and duration of the exposure.

A large, multicentre case-control study on lung cancer risk among non-smoking women was conducted in 5 major metropolitan areas of the United States by Fontham and colleagues [33]. Two control groups were selected: the first was a random sample from the Health Care Financing Administration, the second was composed of colon cancer cases. All controls were age, residence, and language matched to the eligible cases. Information on exposure was collected through the medical records, from family physicians and, when neither information was available, through direct interview by telephone. The completeness of the interviews ranged from 84% of the cases to 72% of the population controls.

Household exposure to ETS was associated with an OR of 1.21 (95% CI: 0.96-1.54) for a smoking spouse, and 1.23 (95% CI: 0.97-1.56) for other smoking members of the household. No clear increasing trend of the RR with years of exposure was present. Exposure to ETS in the workplace was associated with an OR of 1.34 (95% CI: 1.07-1.73), while the point estimate in relation to social exposure was 1.58 (95% CI: 1.22-2.04). In neither analysis could a dose-response relationship be observed. An increasing trend of lung cancer risk was discernible when analysed in relation to the amount (pack years) smoked by the spouse. The trend was more evident for adenocarcinomas. Childhood exposure to ETS did not increase the relative risk, independently of histological subtype or parent involved.

The lung cancer risk from environmental tobacco smoke has probably been the subject on which the largest number of epidemiological studies have been conducted in a very short period (approximately a decade), thus confirming the scientific and social importance of this issue. An important proportion of the studies, however, have not been specifically designed to test the hypothesis of the carcinogenic risk from ETS, but are a reanalysis or an updating of previous or ongoing studies on lung cancer whose data on non-smokers have been subsequently selected and analysed separately. This might have affected the quality of the information and might have resulted in a certain degree of misclassification.

The possibility of misclassification is indeed one of the major problems in the interpretation of the evidence from ETS. The potential impact of misclassification on the evaluation in causal terms of the association between lung cancer and ETS has been discussed on several occasions [34-36]. In principle, non-differential misclassification of exposure tends to dilute the association between exposure and effect. An attempt to estimate the magnitude of the effect for ETS [37,38] resulted in true point estimates between 1.5 and 1.6 as compared to an observed RR of 1.35.

However, the main problem with studies on ETS and lung cancer seems to be confounding by unreported active smokers. As smokers are more likely to marry smokers, misclassification of smokers as non-smokers leads to overestimation of the risk associated with passive exposure. The extent to which the relative risk is confounded depends obviously on the proportion of smokers, which has been estimated as up to 3% using validation by biological markers of nicotine [35,37,39,40]. Validation of the information on smoking has only been attempted in a very limited number of studies. It is, therefore, difficult to fully assess the effect of this bias on the point estimates published in the studies, although it is reasonable to believe that it should be within the range of 10-30% of the excess risk among females.

An overall evaluation of the epidemiological evidence is rather complex, considering the heterogeneity of the studies in relation to design, type of exposure investigated, and cultural habits of the country. The main results of the studies have been summarised and presented separately by geographic area in Tables 1 to 3, in relation to the different types of exposure investigated. Both the risk esti-

Table 1. Risk of lung cancer associated with different types of exposure to ETS in Europe

		TYPE OF EXPOSURE							
		Spouse		Household Childhood Adulthood				Workplace	Others
Study		RR	Dose response	RR	Dose response	RR	Dose response	RR Dose response	RR Dose response
Trichopoulos [3,5]	females	2.1*	YES*						
Gillis [11]	females	1.0	NO						
	males	3.3	YES						
Lee [17]	females	1.0		0.8#	____both____ NO			0.6 ____both____ NO	
Pershagen [22]	females	1.2	YES						
	males	3.3*°	YES*						
Hole [12]	both sexes	2.4							
Svensson [28]				0.9 (father) 3.3 (mother)					1.4 (child/adult) 1.9 (both)
Kalandidi [29]	females	2.1*	YES	1.8	|___both___| NO			1.4 NO	

* statistically significant at least at 0.05 level; ° squamous or small cell carcinoma; # crude estimate by the reviewer

Table 2. Risk of lung cancer associated with different types of exposure to ETS in Eastern Asia

		TYPE OF EXPOSURE							
		Spouse		Household Childhood Adulthood				Workplace	Others
Study		RR	Dose response	RR	Dose response	RR	Dose response	RR Dose response	RR Dose response
Japan									
Hirayama [4,6]	females	1.6*	YES*						
	males	2.3*	YES*						
Akiba [18]	females	1.5	YES						
Inoue [25]	females	2.6	YES						
Shimizu [26]	females	1.1		1.1 (father) 4.0 (mother) 3.2 (husband's father) 0.8 (husband's mother)		1.2			

Table 2. Risk of lung cancer associated with different types of exposure to ETS in Eastern Asia (contd.)

	TYPE OF EXPOSURE								
	Spouse		Household				Workplace		Others
			Childhood		Adulthood				
Study	RR	Dose response	RR	Dose response	RR	Dose response	RR	Dose response	RR Dose response
Sobue [30]	females 1.1		1.6* (any) 0.8 (father) 1.3 (mother) 1.2 (others)						
Hong Kong									
Chan [10]	females 0.8								
Lam [21]	females 1.7*	YES							
Koo [38]	females 1.6	NO	2.0				1.7		
China									
Gao [24]	females 1.2	YES	1.1				0.9		
Geng [27]	females 2.2	YES							
Wu [16]	females 0.7	NO	0.9 (mother) 1.1 (father)	NO NO					

* statistically significant at least at 0.05 level

mates and the dose-response effects, when reported, are shown.

In the European studies exposure from the spouse is associated with RRs ranging from 1.0 to 3.3. About half of the studies also collected further information on exposure in household and workplace. All studies where an increased risk was found show at least one positive association with dose, whatever the definition of exposure. Exposure during childhood is frequently associated with an increased risk, as is exposure at work and in social settings, when investigated.

Numerous studies have been conducted in Eastern Asia (Table 2), most of them focused on female exposure from husband's smoke. The RRs range from 0.7 to 2.6, with 10 out of 12 estimates in excess of 1, while the dose-responses are not consistently associated with the various parameters of exposure. Two of 3 studies show an effect from exposure during childhood while exposures in the workplace or in other environments are not considered. The United States contribute, as shown in Table 3, the largest part of the epidemiological evidence. The risk estimates range from 0.8 to 2.1, but are characterised by a larger variability both across studies and within studies in relation to the different types of exposure.

Most of these studies do not limit the investigation to ETS exposure from the spouse in view of the hypothesis that, particularly in the U.S., exposure to ETS in the workplace and in other social settings might be as important as that from the spouse. The inconsistencies across studies are difficult to interpret as they could be ascribed to the different study designs, to the different types and degrees of misclassification, and to the different social and cultural habits of the populations studied. The risk of lung cancer has been mainly in-

Table 3. Risk of lung cancer associated with different types of exposure to ETS in the United States

		TYPE OF EXPOSURE								
		Spouse		Household Childhood		Adulthood		Workplace		Others
Study		RR	Dose response	RR	Dose response	RR	Dose response	RR	Dose response	RR Dose response
Garfinkel [7]	females	1.2	NO							
Correa [8]	females males	2.1 2.0	YES YES	1.4* (mother) 0.8 (father) _____both_____						
Kabat [9]	females males	0.8 1.0	NO NO	0.9 1.2			NO NO	0.8 1.6*	NO YES*	
Sandler [13,14]	females males	1.5* 2.0*		1.8*			YES			
Garfinkel [15]	females	1.2	YES					0.9		
Wu [16]	females	1.2	YES	0.6				1.3	YES	
Dalager [19]	both sexes	1.5	YES							
Humble [20]	females	1.7	YES/NO							
Janerich [30]	females	0.9	YES	1.3#	YES	0.9	YES	0.9	NO	
Fontham [33]	females	1.3 1.5**	NO YES*			1.2	YES	1.3*	YES*	1.6* YES*

* statistically significant at least at 0.05 level; ** adenocarcinomas; # crude estimate by the reviewer

vestigated among women but it is noticeable how the few studies which have included males in the study population give the highest and the most consistent estimates of lung cancer risk.

The differences among geographical regions are not striking while the majority of the studies consistently indicate an elevation of the RR for lung cancer below 2.

Saracci and Riboli, in a recent metanalysis [41], computed an overall risk of 1.35. This estimate, although computed after pooling data from studies with different designs and methods, is quite consistent with estimates of the relative risk due to exposure to 0.5-1 cigarette equivalent in active smokers [42].

Pershagen [36] estimated the aetiologic fraction (EF) of lung cancer cases among non-smokers attributable to exposure to passive smoking. Assuming a relative risk of 1.23 and a proportion of women married to a smoker between 50% and 75%, the aetiologic fraction was 10% to 15%. For males, the EF ranged from 3% to 25% based on a RR of 1.82 and a proportion of men married to a smoker between 4% and 40%.

Other sites have been rarely investigated in relation to the carcinogenic risk from ETS, probably due to the difficulties in testing this hypothesis for sites at lower risk than the lung. The prospective study by Hirayama [6], however, suggested an increased risk for brain and for nasal cancer, the latter presenting a positive association with the number of cigarettes smoked by the husband which was statistically significant.

Residential Radon

A number of epidemiological investigations show that underground miners exposed to high levels of radon daughters have an increased risk of lung cancer [43]. Studies in experimental animals confirm that inhalation of radon daughters can induce lung cancer. The increased radon concentrations that are found in many homes of various countries suggest that residential radon exposure is an important risk factor for lung cancer in the general population. However, quantitative assessments of population risks based on the data in miners and experimental animals are uncertain. For example, aerosol size distribution, unattached fraction, breathing rate and route may differ in the various exposure situations [44]. Additional sources of uncertainty include age at exposure, sex, cigarette smoking and the effects of environmental contaminants other than radon.

The lung cancer risks related to residential radon exposure have been studied using ecological, cohort as well as case-control designs [45]. Ecological studies are unsuitable for the assessment of causal relationships and such investigations will not be further discussed. Earlier cohort and case-control studies based their estimation of exposure primarily on housing characteristics and/or geology [46-53]. Many of these studies showed an association between estimated radon exposure and lung cancer risk, however, limited study size and imprecision in the exposure estimates make it difficult to use the data for quantitative risk assessments.

Five recent case-control studies based the exposure estimation on radon measurements in the homes of the study subjects, covering about 10-30 years of residency [54-58]. These studies also contained detailed information on smoking and other potential confounding factors. Axelson et al. [54] included 125 male and 52 female deceased lung cancer cases diagnosed between 1960 and 1981 in 14 municipalities in the central part of southern Sweden, as well as 379 male and 294 female deceased non-cancer controls from the same area. Subjects had lived in the same house during at least 30 years. Radon daughter measurements using alpha-track detectors exposed during 2 months could be performed in the homes of 142 cases and 264 controls.

A weakly positive trend in lung cancer risk with increasing radon daughter concentration was suggested in the rural part of the population, with a relative risk of 1.4 (90% CI: 0.6-3.2) in the category >150 Bq/m^3 (corresponding to 300 Bq/m^3 as radon)[*] compared to the reference category with radon daughter levels below 50 Bq/m^3 (100 Bq/m^3 as radon). A weakly negative trend with measured radon daughter exposure was suggested in the urban population.

In a study from the heavily industrialised city of Shenyang, China, radon concentrations were measured during 1 year in the homes of 308 women with lung cancer diagnosed between 1985 and 1987 and of 356 controls [55]. The median time of residence in the homes was 24 years and the geometric mean radon level was 2.4 pCi/L (corresponding to 89 Bq/m^3). No association between radon and lung cancer was observed, except for non-significant positive trends among heavy smokers and for lung cancers of the small cell type. Relative risks (and 95% CIs) for all types of lung cancer adjusted for age, education, smoking status, and indoor air pollution were 1.0 (reference), 0.9 (0.6-1.3), 0.9 (0.5-1.4) and 0.7 (0.4-1.3) in the exposure categories below 1.9 pCi/L (70 Bq/m^3), 2.0-3.9 pCi/L (74-144 Bq/m^3), 4.0-7.9 pCi/L (148-292 Bq/m^3) and above 8.0 pCi/L (296 Bq/m^3).

An investigation from New Jersey, USA, included 403 women with lung cancer diagnosed during the period 1982-1983, and 402 controls for whom residential radon was

---

[*] Concentrations of radon gas are expressed as Bq/m^3 or pCi/L (1 pCi/L = 37 Bq/m^3). The major part of the radiation dose to the bronchial epithelium is delivered by the radon daughters, and the indoor radon daughter concentration is usually about half of the radon gas concentration.

measured with alpha-track detectors during 1 year in houses occupied for at least 10 years [56]. Relative risks (and 90% CIs) adjusted for age, smoking, occupation and respondent type were 1.0 (reference), 1.1 (0.8-1.7), 1.3 (0.6-2.9) and 4.2 (1.0-17.5) at exposure levels of <1.0 pCi/L (37 Bq/m^3), 1.0-1.9 pCi/L (37-70 Bq/m^3), 2.0-3.9 pCi/L (74-144 Bq/m^3) and 4.0-11.3 pCi/L (148-418 Bq/m^3), indicating a positive trend (p=0.04). The trend was strongest for light smokers and for undifferentiated carcinomas.

A total of 238 male lung cancer cases diagnosed in the period from 1980 to 1985 and 434 controls from southern Finland were included in a study by Ruosteenoja [57]. Radon measurements during 2 months could be performed in about half of the dwellings of the study subjects between 1950 and 1975, covering an average of about 15 years of residential time. The average radon concentrations for measured houses of cases and controls were 217 and 212 Bq/m^3, respectively. Relative risks (and 95% CIs) adjusted for smoking were 1.0 (reference), 0.8 (0.4-1.5), 1.7 (1.0-3.0), 1.8 (1.0-3.0) and 1.2 (0.7-2.1) in men exposed to radon levels of <109, 109-150, 151-196, 197-264 and ≥265 Bq/m^3, respectively. The trend was stronger in heavy smokers and for epidermoid carcinoma.

A study from Stockholm, Sweden, included 210 female lung cancer cases diagnosed between 1983 and 1986 and 400 controls [58]. Radon concentrations were measured in 72.6% of the dwellings lived in from 1945, covering an average of more than 25 years of residency. The geometric mean radon concentration was 96 Bq/m^3. Lung cancer risks tended to increase with estimated radon exposure, reaching an age, smoking and urban residence-adjusted relative risk of 1.7 (95% CI: 1.0-2.9) at an average radon level exceeding 150 Bq/m^3. Stronger associations were indicated in younger persons and for poorly differentiated tumours. Positive trends were suggested both for non-smokers and current smokers.

The risk estimates in the studies on residential radon exposure and lung cancer may be compared with those obtained from miners. Risk estimations based on the mining data often used relative risk models, either constant [59] or modified by age and time since exposure [43]. The risk estimates from the residential radon studies by Schoenberg et al. [56], Ruosteenoja [57] and Pershagen et al. [58] appear to lie within the same range as those projected from miners, while the study by Blot et al. [55] suggests lower risks. There are considerable uncertainties in the comparisons with the mining data. For example, age differences in risk or consequences of a non-multiplicative interaction between radon and smoking have not been considered.

Several attempts have been made to assess the aetiologic fraction for lung cancer in the general population related to residential radon exposure. Using risk estimates derived from underground miners, which appear to be consistent with some of the residential data, and results from radon measurements in quantitative samples of dwellings, it has been estimated that approximately 10-20% of all lung cancer cases may be attributed to residential radon in Finland, Norway and the United States [57,60,61]. If the interaction between radon exposure and smoking is multiplicative, the estimates of attributable risk are independent of the proportion of smokers in the population. These risk estimates suggest that residential radon exposure is the second most important cause of lung cancer in some countries. There is still a substantial uncertainty in the risk projections and a number of large epidemiological investigations are ongoing in several countries which will provide more precise risk estimates within the next years.

The type of interaction between radon exposure and smoking is of importance for the risk assessment. In miners a multiplicative or submultiplicative interaction was often found but the data are not fully consistent [43]. A major difficulty in the interpretation arises from the fact that the number of lung cancers is low among non-smokers, although the data clearly indicate that the risk is elevated also in this group among radon-exposed miners [62]. For residential exposure only limited evidence is available and no clear pattern of interaction between smoking and radon exposure has emerged.

Other cancer risks have also been investigated in relation to residential radon exposure. Two recent ecological studies reported a correlation between radon exposure in homes and acute myeloid leukaemia in the U.K. [63], and the international incidence of myeloid leukaemia, cancer of the kidney, melanoma and certain childhood cancers [64]. However, subsequent studies failed to show a consistent association between indoor radon levels and childhood cancer risks in the U.K. [65,66]. Swedish case-control studies have shown an increased risk of acute myeloid leukaemia related to background indoor gamma radiation from building materials, which also emit radon [67].

A correlation between residential radon and leukaemia may thus occur which does not represent a causal association. In any case, the ecological evidence is unsuitable for assessment of causal relationships and the doses delivered to other tissues following inhalation of radon daughters are much lower than for the bronchial epithelium.

Cooking Fumes

Several epidemiological studies have investigated the lung cancer risk in relation to exposure to combustion products in homes. The sources include fuels used for cooking and heating, such as coal and kerosene, as well as vegetable oils used for frying, etc. Most of the studies come from China, where indoor air pollution levels from such sources may be substantial [68]. In this context it is worth noting that increased lung cancer risks have been reported both among cooks and bakers [69,70], and among coke oven workers [71].

Vegetable Oils

Two case-control studies on female lung cancer from China suggest that cooking oil fumes may be of importance for lung cancer. One study involved 672 lung cancer cases diagnosed from 1984 to 1986 in Shanghai and 735 population controls [24]. Information on cooking practices and risk factors for lung cancer were obtained from interviews. There was a relative risk of 1.4 (95% CI: 1.1-1.8) for lung cancer associated with the use of rapeseed oil for cooking compared to soya bean oil. The lung cancer risk was also related to the degree of smokiness during cooking and the number of dishes prepared per week. On the other hand, no significant effects were seen in relation to the type of fuel used for cooking.

Another study was based in the industrial cities of Shenyang and Harbin and included 965 female lung cancer cases diagnosed from 1985 to 1987 and 959 controls [32]. The women were interviewed regarding cooking practices and risk factors for lung cancer. Increased risks of lung cancer were related to the number of meals prepared by deep frying and to eye irritation during cooking. For women reporting deep frying 3 times or more per month, the relative risk was 1.9 (95% CI: 1.4-2.7) compared to that for women who never used this type of cooking. Similar effects were seen in smokers and non-smokers.

Coal Burning

In parts of China, indoor burning of coal for domestic cooking and heating is common. Two types of coal used are "smoky coal", which smokes heavily on firing, and "smokeless coal", which produces little smoke. Lung cancer rates in Xuan Wei county among both men and women living in areas where "smoky" coal was the predominant fuel were substantially higher in the period from 1973 to 1979 than in areas where "smokeless" coal or wood was used [68].

A subsequent case-control study indicated that domestic coal use was a stronger risk factor for lung cancer in females than smoking and that the risk was related to the duration of exposure [72]. In the study from Shenyang and Harbin mentioned in the previous section, lung cancer risks in relation to heating practices were also analysed [32]. There was an elevated risk related to the number of years during which coal was used for domestic heating. More than 20 years' use of devices that burn the fuel directly under the bed was associated with a relative risk of 1.5 (95% CI: 1.1-2.0).

A case-control study including 224 male and 92 female lung cancer cases and a similar number of controls from Guangzhou, China, showed that several variables indicating poor kitchen and domestic ventilation were associated with an increased lung cancer risk [73]. Coal was the predominant fuel used in this area. The increased risk persisted after control for several potential confounding factors, including smoking.

An elevated relative risk associated with residential coal burning during childhood was observed in a U.S. study of 220 female lung cancer cases and a similar number of controls [16].

The majority of the tumours were adenocarcinomas, which showed a relative risk of 2.3 (95% CI: 1.0-5.5) after adjustment for smoking. No data were provided on current exposure to cooking fumes.

Other Sources

A case-control study including 200 female lung cancer cases and controls from Hong Kong [74] indicated an increased risk associated with kerosene use during more than 30 years (RR=1.6, $p = 0.02$). A positive interaction between smoking and kerosene use was suggested. No excess risk was observed for other types of fuels, such as wood/grass or liquid petroleum gas.

In a study from Osaka, Japan, including 120 female lung cancer cases and 519 controls, an increased lung cancer risk was related to the use of straw or wood as cooking fuel [75]. The relative risks for straw/wood use at ages 15 and 30 were 1.3 (0.9-2.0) and 1.9 (1.1-3.3), respectively. No elevated risk was associated with the use of other types of fuels.

Mineral Fibres

An excess rate of pleural mesothelioma, and to some extent also lung cancer, has been reported from some villages in the Cappadocian region of Turkey [76,77]. Environmental investigations revealed a high proportion of erionite fibres in dust swept from walls and floors of houses from these villages. This mineral belongs to the zeolite family and has a finely fibrous wool-like structure. Erionite fibres were identified in lung tissue samples in cases of pleural mesothelioma, supporting a causal relationship.

Non-occupational exposure to asbestos fibres near some industries has also resulted in an increased incidence of mesothelioma [78,79].

Conclusions

It may be concluded that the indoor environment can be of importance for cancer induction, primarily in the respiratory tract. In some situations, for example in parts of China where smoking is rare and indoor burning of coal is common, it seems to be the dominant cause of lung cancer. It is possible that fumes from vegetable oils used for cooking may also play a role, but these data need confirmation. According to current risk estimates based on data from miners, residential radon exposure seems to be in some countries the second most important cause of lung cancer after smoking. The aetiologic fraction in the U.S. and some Nordic countries has been estimated at 10-20%. Some support for this estimate is given by recent epidemiological studies on residential radon exposure and lung cancer, however, further data are needed to increase the precision of the risk estimation.

More than 25 epidemiological studies have been published on passive smoking and lung cancer. The most common approach in the analysis has been to base the exposure classification on smoking habits of spouses. Taking together the studies, a statistically significant increase (20-30%) has been observed in the lung cancer risk of non-smokers who are married to smokers. Higher risks in those married to heavy smokers were often observed, supporting a causal association. Part of the risk increase related to smoking spouses might be explained by confounding by smoking. On the other hand, non-differential misclassification of ETS exposure, resulting from crude exposure measures, will give rise to an underestimation of the true risks. The available empirical data suggest that bias cannot explain the observed association between ETS exposure and lung cancer. An overall assessment which takes into consideration the presence of carcinogens in ETS, exposure estimates in passive smokers, exposure-response relationships in smokers, and the epidemiological evidence on lung cancer in passive smokers, indicates that ETS is of carcinogenic importance.

Non-occupational exposure to mineral fibres (erionite and asbestos) has resulted in an increased incidence of mesothelioma. It is possible that mineral fibres may be of importance also for lung cancer induction in non-occupational exposure situations.

REFERENCES

1. U.S. Surgeon General: The Health Consequences of Involuntary Smoking. U.S. DHHS, Rockville, MD 1986
2. International Agency for Research on Cancer. Tobacco smoking. IARC Monographs on the evaluation of the carcinogenic risk of chemicals to humans. International Agency for Research on Cancer, Lyon 1986
3. Trichopoulos D, Kalandidi A, Sparros L and MacMahon B: Lung cancer and passive smoking. Int J Cancer 1981 (27): 1-4
4. Hirayama T: Non-smoking wives of heavy smokers have a higher risk of lung cancer: a study from Japan. Br Med J 1981 (282): 183-185
5. Trichopoulos D, Kalandidi A and Sparros L: Lung cancer and passive smoking: conclusion of Greek study. The Lancet 1983 (ii): 677-680
6. Hirayama T: Cancer mortality in nonsmoking women with smoking husbands based on a large-scale cohort study in Japan. Prev Med 1984 (13): 680-690
7. Garfinkel L: Time trends in lung cancer mortality among nonsmokers and a note on passive smoking. JNCI 1981 (66): 1061-1066
8. Correa P, Pickle LW, Fontham E, Lin Y and Haenszel W: Passive smoking and lung cancer. Lancet 1983 (ii): 595-597
9. Kabat GC and Wynder EL: Lung cancer in nonsmokers. Cancer 1984 (53): 1214-1221
10. Chan WC and Fung SC: Lung cancer in nonsmokers in Hong Kong. In: Grundmann E, Clemmesen J, Muir C (eds) Geographical Pathology in Cancer Epidemiology. Gustav Fischer Verlag, New York 1982 pp 199-202
11. Gillis CR, Hole DJ, Hawthorne VM and Boyle P: The effect of environmental tobacco smoke in two urban communities in the West of Scotland. Eur J Respir Dis 1984 (suppl 133): 121-126
12. Hole DJ, Gillis CR, Chopra C and Hawthorne VM: Passive smoking and cardiorespiratory health in a general population in the West of Scotland. Br Med J 1989 (299): 423-427
13. Sandler DP, Everson RB and Wilcox AJ: Passive smoking in adulthood and cancer risk. Am J Epid 1985 (121 No 1): 37-48
14. Sandler DP, Wilcox AJ and Everson RB: Cumulative effects of lifetime passive smoking on cancer risk. The Lancet 1985 (129 No 1): 312-315
15. Garfinkel L, Auerbach O and Joubert L: Involuntary smoking and lung cancer: a case-control study. JNCI 1985 (75): 463-469
16. Wu AA, Henderson BE, Pike MC and Yu MC: Smoking and other risk factors for lung cancer in women. JNCI 1985 (74):747-751
17. Lee PN, Chamberlain J and Alderson MR: Relationship of passive smoking to risk of lung cancer and other smoking-associated diseases. Br J Cancer 1986 (54): 97-105
18. Akiba S, Kato H and Blot WJ: Passive smoking and lung cancer among Japanese women. Cancer Res 1986 (46): 4804-4807
19. Dalager NA, Pickle LW, Mason TJ, Correa P, Fontham ETH, Stemhagen A, Buffler PA, Ziegler RG and Fraumeni JF: The relation of passive smoking to lung cancer. Cancer Res 1986 (46):4808-4811
20. Humble CG, Samet JM and Pathak DR: Marriage to a smoker and lung cancer risk. Am J Public Health 1987 (77 No 5): 598-602
21. Lam TH, Kung ITM, Wong CM, Lam WK, Kleevens JWL, Saw D, Hsu C, Seneviratne S, Lam SY, Lo KK and Chan WC: Smoking, passive smoking and histological types in lung cancer in Hong Kong Chinese women. Br J Cancer 1987 (56): 673-678
22. Pershagen G, Hrubec Z and Svensson C: Passive smoking and lung cancer in Swedish women. Am J Epidemiol 1987 (125 No 1): 17-24
23. Koo LC, Ho JHC Saw D and Ho CY: Measurements of passive smoking and estimates of lung cancer risk among non-smoking Chinese females. Int J Cancer 1987 (39): 162-169
24. Gao YT, Blot WJ, Zheng W, Ershow AG, Hsu CW, Levin LI, Zhang R and Fraumeni JF: Lung cancer among Chinese women. Int J Cancer 1987 (40): 604-609
25. Inoue R and Hirayama T: Passive smoking and lung cancer in women. In: Aoki M, Hisamichi S and Tominaga S (eds) Smoking and Health. Elsevier, Amsterdam 1988 pp 283-285
26. Shimizu HM, Morishita K, Mizuno K, Masuda T, Ogura Y, Santo M, Nishimura M, Kunishima K, Karasawa K, Nishiwaki K, Yamamoto M, Hisamichi S and Tominaga S: A case-control study of lung cancer in nonsmoking women. Tohoku: J Exp Med 1988 (154): 389-397
27. Geng GY, Liang ZH, Zhang AY and Wu GL: On the relationship between smoking and female lung cancer. In: Aoki M, Hisamichi S and Tominaga S (eds) Smoking and Health. Elsevier, Amsterdam 1988 pp 483-490
28. Svensson C, Pershagen G and Klominek J: Smoking and passive smoking in relation to lung cancer in women. Acta Oncologica 1989 (28 No 5): 623-629
29. Kalandidi A, Katsouyanni K, Voropoulou N, Bastas G, Saracci R and Trichopoulos D: Passive smoking and diet in the etiology of lung cancer among non-smokers. Cancer Causes and Control 1990 (1): 15-21
30. Janerich DT, Thompson WD, Varela LR, Greenwald P, Chorost S, Tucci C, Zaman MB, Melamed MR, Kiely M and McKneally MF: Lung cancer and exposure to tobacco smoke in the household. N Engl J Med 1990 (323): 632-636
31. Sobue T: Association of indoor air pollution and lifestyle with lung cancer in Osaka, Japan. Int J Epid 1990 (19 no 3): 562-566
32. Wu-Williams AH, Dai XD, Blot WJ, Xu ZY, Sun XW, Xiao HP, Stone BJ, Yu SF, Feng YP, Ershow AG, Sun J, Fraumeni JF and Henderson BE: Lung cancer among women in North-East China. Br J Cancer 1990 (62): 982-987

33 Fontham ETH, Correa P, Wu-Williams AH, Reynolds P, Greenberg RS, Buffler PA, Chen VW, Boyd P, Alterman T, Austin DF, Liff J and Greenberg D: Lung cancer in nonsmoking women: a multicenter case-control study. Cancer Epidemiology, Biomarkers & Prevention 1991 (1): 35-43
34 Lee PN: Misclassification of Smoking Habits and Passive Smoking. Springer Verlag, Berlin 1988
35 Riboli E, Preston-Martin S, Saracci R, Haley N, Trichopoulos D, Becker N, Burch JD, Fontham ETH, Gao YT, Jindal SK, Koo LC, Le Marchand L, Segnan N, Shimizu H, Stanta G, Wu-Williams AH and Zatonski W: Exposure to nonsmoking women to environmental tobacco smoke: a ten-country collaborative study. Cancer Causes Control 1990 (1): 243-252
36 Pershagen G: Passive smoking and lung cancer. In: Samet JM (ed) Epidemiology of Lung Cancer. Marcel Dekker Publ, New York (in press)
37 Wald NJ, Nanchahal K, Thompson SG and Cuckle HS: Does breathing others people's tobacco smoke cause lung cancer? Br Med J 1986 (293): 1217-1222
38 Gann P, Coghlin-Strom J and Hammond K: Measurement of bias due to misclassification in epidemiologic studies of passive smoking. Am J Epidemiol 1988 (128): 920
39 Lee PN: Passive smoking and lung cancer association: A result of bias? Hum Toxicol 1987 (6): 517-524
40 Thompson SG, Stone R, Nanchahal K and Wald NJ: Relation of urinary cotinine concentrations to cigarette smoking and to exposure to other people's smoke. Thorax 1990 (45): 356-361
41 Saracci R and Riboli E: Passive smoking and lung cancer: current evidence and ongoing studies at the International Agency for Research on Cancer. Mutation Research 1989 (222): 117-127
42 Darby SC and Pike MC: Lung cancer and passive smoking: Predicted effects from a mathematical model for cigarette smoking and lung cancer. Br J Cancer 1988 (58): 825-831
43 National Academy of Sciences. Radon and Other Internally Deposited Alpha-Emitters. BEIR IV. National Academy Press, Washington, DC 1988
44 National Academy of Sciences. Comparative Dosimetry of Radon in Miners and Homes. National Academy Press, Washington, DC 1991
45 Samet JM: Radon and lung cancer. JNCI 1989 (81): 745-757
46 Axelson O, Edling C and Kling H: Lung cancer and residency - A case-referent study on the possible impact of exposure to radon and its daughters in dwellings. Scand J Work Environ Health 1979 (5): 10-5
47 Simpson SG and Comstock GW: Lung cancer and housing characteristics. Arch Environ Health 1983 (38): 248-251
48 Edling C, Kling H and Axelson O: Radon in homes - A possible cause of lung cancer. Scand J Work Environ Health 1984 (10): 25- 34
49 Pershagen G, Damber L and Falk R: Exposure to radon in dwellings and lung cancer: A pilot study. In: Berglund B, Lindvall T, Sundell J (eds) Indoor Air. Vol 2. Swedish Council for Building Research, Stockholm 1984 pp 73-78

50 Lanctot EM: Radon in the domestic environment and its relationship to cancer: An epidemiological study. Doctoral thesis. State University of New York, Stony Brook 1985
51 Damber L and Larsson LG: Lung cancer in males and type of dwelling - An epidemiologic pilot study. Acta Oncol 1987 (26): 211-215
52 Lees RE, Steele RR and Roberts JH: A case-control study of lung cancer relative to domestic radon exposure. Int J Epidemiol 1987 (16): 7-12
53 Svensson C, Eklund G and Pershagen G: Indoor exposure to radon from the ground and bronchial cancer in women. Int Arch Occup Environ Health 1987 (59): 123-131
54 Axelson O, Andersson K, Desai G, Fagerlund I, Jansson B, Karlsson C and Wingren G: Indoor radon exposure and active and passive smoking in relation to the occurrence of lung cancer. Scand J Work Environ Health 1988 (14):286-292
55 Blot WJ, Xu ZY, Boice JD Jr, Zhao DZ, Stone BJ, Sun J, Jing LB and Fraumeni JF: Indoor radon and lung cancer in China. JNCI 1990 (82): 1025-30
56 Schoenberg JB, Klotz JB, Wilcox HB, Nicholls GP, Gil-del-Real MT, Stemhagen A and Mason TJ: Case-control study of residential radon and lung cancer among New Jersey women. Cancer Res 1990 (50): 6520-6524
57 Ruosteenoja E: Indoor radon and risk of lung cancer: An epidemiological study in Finland. Doctoral thesis. Finnish Centre for Radiation and Nuclear Safety, Helsinki 1991
58 Pershagen G, Liang ZH, Hrubec Z, Svensson C and Boice JD Jr: Residential radon exposure and lung cancer in women. Health Phys 1992 (63): 179-86
59 International Commission on Radiological Protection. Lung cancer risk from indoor exposures to radon daughters. Report No 50. Ann ICRP 1987 (17): 1-60
60 Lubin JH, Boice JD Jr: Estimating Rn-induced lung cancer in the United States. Health Phys 1989 (57): 417-427
61 Sanner T and Dybing E: Indoor radon exposure in Norway and lung cancer risk. In: International Symposium on Radon and Radon Reduction Technology. Atlanta, Georgia 1990
62 Roscoe RJ, Steenland K, Halperin WE, Beaumont JJ and Waxweiler RJ: Lung cancer mortality among nonsmoking uranium miners exposed to radon daughters. JAMA 1989 (262): 629-633
63 Lucie NP: Radon exposure and leukemia. Lancet 1989 (ii): 99-100
64 Henshaw DL, Eatough JP and Richardson RB: Radon as a causative factor in induction of myeloid leukaemia and other cancers. Lancet 1990 (i): 1008-12
65 Muirhead CR, Butland BK, Green BMR and Draper GJ: Childhood leukaemia and natural radiation. Lancet 1991 (i): 503-504
66 Wakefield M and Kohler JA: Indoor radon and childhood cancer. Lancet 1991 (ii): 1537-1538
67 Flodin U: Leukemia and multiple myeloma in relation to occupational and environmental exposures. Doctoral thesis. Linköping University Medical Dissertations No 308, 1990

68. Mumford JL, He XZ, Chapman RS, Cao SR, Harris DB, Li XM, Xian YL, Jiang WZ, Xu CW, Chuang JC, Wilson WE and Cooke M: Lung cancer and air pollution in Xuan Wei, China. Science 1987 (235):217-220
69. Coggon D, Pannett B, Osmond C and Acheson ED: A survey of cancer and occupation in young and middle aged men. I. Cancers of the respiratory tract. Br J Ind Med 1986 (43): 332-338
70. Tüchsen F and Nordholm L: Respiratory cancer in Danish bakers: A 10-year cohort study. Br J Ind Med 1986 (43): 516-521
71. Redmond CK: Epidemiological studies of cancer mortality in coke plant workers. In: Seventh Conference on Environmental T Toxicology 1976. Washington DC, US Environmental Protection Agency 1976
72. He XZ, Chen W, Liu Z and Chapman RS: An epidemiological study of lung cancer in Xuan Wei county, China: Current progress. Case-control study on lung cancer and cooking fuel. Environ Health Perspect 1991 (94): 9-13
73. Liu Q, Sasco AJ, Riboli E and Hu MX: Indoor air pollution and lung cancer in Guang Zhou, Peoples Republic of China. Am J Epidemiol 1992 (in press)
74. Koo LC, Lee N and Ho JHC: Do cooking fuels pose a risk for lung cancer? A case-control study of women in Hong Kong. Ecol Dis 1983 (2): 255-265
75. Sobue TR, Suzuki R, Nakayama N, Inubuse C, Matsuda M, Doi O, Mori T, Furuse K, Fukuoka M, Yasumitsu T, Kuwabara O, Ichigaya M, Kurata M, Kuwabara M, Nakahara K, Eudo S and Hattori S: Passive smoking among non smoking women and the relationship between indoor air pollution and lung cancer incidence. Results of a multicenter case-control study. Gan Rinsho 1990 (36): 329-333
76. Baris YI, Saracci R, Simonato L, Skidmore JW and Artvinli M: Malignant mesothelioma and radiological chest abnormalities in two villages in Central Turkey. Lancet 1981(ii):984-987
77. Baris YI, Simonato L, Artvinli M, Pooley FD, Saracci R, Skidmore JW and Wagner C: Epidemiological and environmental evidence of the health effects of exposure to erionite fibres: A four-year study in the Cappadocian region of Turkey. Int J Cancer 1987 (39): 10-17
78. Newhouse M and Thompson H: Mesothelioma of pleura and peritoneum following exposure to asbestos in the London area. Br J Ind Med 1966 (22): 261-269
79. Magnani C, Borgo G, Betta GP, Botta M, Ivaldo C, Mollo F, Scelzi M and Terracini B: Mesothelioma and non occupational environmental exposure to asbestos. Lancet 1991 (ii): 50

Epidemiological Evidence on Outdoor Air Pollution and Cancer

Göran Pershagen [1] and Lorenzo Simonato [2]

1 Department of Epidemiology, Institute of Environmental Medicine, Karolinska Institute, Box 60208, 104 01 Stockholm, Sweden
2 Cancer Registry of the Veneto Region, Via Giustiniani 7, 35128 Padova, Italy

Ambient air pollution may give rise to several types of health effects, ranging from annoyance reactions and acute irritation of eyes and airways to chronic inflammatory diseases, cancer and death [1]. Only malignant diseases will be discussed in this chapter, although it is realised that cancer may not represent the most important type of effect from a public health point of view.

Health effects of air pollution may be caused by direct exposure to pollutants or via indirect pathways. One example of indirect routes includes health effects related to increased exposure to heavy metals which are more easily mobilised as a result of acidification of soil and water. In some areas air pollution is a major contributor to acidification. Another example is skin cancer induced by ultraviolet radiation, which may increase due to the depletion of the ozone layer for which some air pollutants may be of importance. Such indirect effects of air pollution will not be treated here.

This chapter focuses on cancer risks related to exposure to ambient air pollution. Such exposure may take place both outdoors and indoors. The main emphasis is on air pollution in urban and industrialised areas. Exposures with primary sources indoors, such as radon and environmental tobacco smoke, are discussed in another chapter and will only be treated as possible confounders and/or effect modifiers in this chapter. Lung cancer risks have received the greatest attention and these data are evaluated most thoroughly.

Lung Cancer

Descriptive Studies

The relationship between lung cancer and air pollution has been investigated in different countries with different methodological approaches. A large number of descriptive studies are available from the literature, supplying an important body of knowledge on this issue. Descriptive studies are, however, limited by 3 main problems:
- The exposure either at population or at individual level is very difficult to assess. Air pollution is, in fact, a particularly complex mixture of chemicals and other substances which are rapidly modified by different atmospheric conditions and which, in addition, can interact with each other (see chapter 2).
- Descriptive and correlation studies examine the effects at group level (e.g., population resident in a town) and it is not possible to assess whether individuals affected by the disease investigated are those actually exposed or "more exposed".
- Particularly for lung cancer there are important confounding factors like tobacco smoke and occupational exposure which may contribute to an apparent association between air pollution and lung cancer risk. Information on confounding factors is generally not available in descriptive studies.

These limitations complicate the interpretation of descriptive studies due to the possibility of false-positive and false-negative results. The former situation is generally due to the lack of control of confounding factors, while the latter is related to the low sensitivity of the studies due to imprecise information on exposures at individual level.

An important section of the epidemiological evidence supporting the hypothesis of a carcinogenic risk related to exposure to air pollutants comes from descriptive studies investigating urban/rural differences of lung cancer rates. The major limitation to a definite evaluation of these studies probably resides in the overwhelming effect due to tobacco smoke and, to a lesser degree, occupational exposure to lung carcinogens. Tobacco smoke may increase the incidence of lung tumours up to 20 or 30 times in heavy smokers as compared to non-smokers. The increase is proportional to the average number of cigarettes smoked and is inversely related to the age of starting the habit. If we consider that the differences in lung cancer rates between urban and rural areas are, in general, around 100%, while even small variations in the amount smoked or in the age when smoking was started can result in 3- to 5-fold increases, we can estimate, at least in part, the urban-rural gradient as effected by historical differences in the diffusion of smoking habits. There is evidence that in many European countries smoking has increased more rapidly in urban than in rural populations. Still in the 1970s in England the average cigarette consumption per capita in urban areas was 12 and 6 cig/day in males and females, respectively, as compared to 5 and 3 in rural areas [2].

Several studies suggested an association between lung cancer and air pollution from the observation of an urban/rural gradient in lung cancer risk. In most of the countries from which mortality or incidence data for lung cancer were available in the 1950s and 1960s, the rates were 2- to 3-fold higher in urban areas compared to rural areas [3-7]. Stocks [3,8] observed that the mortality rate was higher in large towns than in small ones and that there was a correlation with the density of the population. The existence of an "urban factor" was subsequently supported by the results of many other descriptive studies [9,10]. Goldsmith [11] analysed U.S. mortality data during 1950-1960 in males, comparing urban and rural counties for a number of cancer sites. The results indicate a 2-fold ratio for lung cancer between urban and rural populations. Trichopoulos et al. [12] conducted an epidemiological study comparing the mortality from lung cancer in Athens during the period 1961-1980 with the pattern of mortality from the same tumour in towns of Greece which are known to be much less affected by air pollution. The results did not indicate any effect of air pollution either independent of or interactive with smoking on the population resident in Athens.

The urban/rural gradient has been progressively reduced in the last 20 years. However, the gradient still exists and is evident in the majority of the countries from which data are available. Some examples of lung cancer rates from rural and urban areas are reported in Table 1. The data reported appear somewhat conflicting as they compare similar patterns in areas with a different history of air pollution like the U.K. and Norway. Furthermore, the relative urban excess in females does not appear fully consistent across countries.

Additional evidence provided by descriptive epidemiological studies which might be of help in estimating the upper limit of the carcinogenic effect of air pollution on lung cancer comes from a comparison of the rates of this tumour in males and females. Until the 1970s, the lung cancer rates were 5 to 15 times higher in males than in females. Recent statistics show that lung cancer rates tend to level off among males while they are rapidly increasing among females. The phenomenon is somewhat conflicting with the pattern of air pollution exposures which have decreased, at least in England and the U.S., since the end of the 1950s. Thus, these two different trends of lung cancer rates in males and females appear to be unrelated to changes in exposure to air pollutants and are generally interpreted as the result of the different changes in smoking habits of the two sexes.

An attempt has been made to assess trends of lung cancer mortality in relation to reduction in air pollution, particularly in England and Wales in the 1920s and subsequently after the Clear Air Act of 1956. The major studies on this issue like those by the Royal

Table 1. Age-standardised rates per 100,000 population for mortality from carcinoma of the bronchus and trachea in urban and rural areas *

Registry	Males			Females		
	Urban	Rural	Ratio	Urban	Rural	Ratio
Japan, Miyagi	30.9	28.4	1.1	9.2	8.1	1.1
Czechoslovakia, Slovakia	68.2	70.5	1.0	9.4	6.5	1.4
FRG, Saarland	77.7	63.0	1.2	7.7	6.0	1.3
France, Calvados	46.1	39.6	1.2	3.4	2.9	1.2
France, Doubs	56.9	40.1	1.4	3.3	2.0	1.7
Hungary, Szabolcs	61.8	50.9	1.2	10.3	6.2	1.7
Norway	39.4	24.5	1.6	9.6	5.2	1.9
Romania, Cluj County	35.2	35.3	1.0	6.7	4.7	1.4
Switzerland, Vaud	63.8	56.6	1.1	8.7	5.6	1.6
UK, England and Wales	74.8	56.2	1.3	19.7	15.1	1.3
Australia, New South Wales	55.5	46.8	1.2	12.2	8.3	1.5

* from IARC [13]

College of Physicians [14] and by Lawther and Waller [15] indicate a beneficial effect on lung cancer risk due to the improved control of air pollution. The data do not take into account, however, changes in cigarette usage and in tar content that occurred during the same period.

Epidemiological investigations have been performed on migrants from areas characterised by high levels of air pollution. Most of these studies were carried out in the 1950s and 1960s within countries of the British Commonwealth, i.e., British citizens migrating to Australia, New Zealand or South Africa. The results tend to show that British citizens migrating to countries with lower levels of air pollution had lung cancer rates higher than the local white population [16-18]. Some of these studies collected information on smoking habits of lung cancer cases and controls born in England and Wales as well as in the countries of emigration, showing that no major differences in smoking habits were present between immigrants from the U.K. and the local white population. The authors of these studies concluded that the higher mortality from lung cancer should be ascribed to exposure to air pollutants before emigration. The evidence was strengthened by the observation that the mortality excess was larger among individuals leaving the country after the age of 30 than among those emigrating at a younger age. The studies are consistent in indicating a lung cancer excess of around 40%.

In some respects, the most eligible population for studying the potential carcinogenic effects of air pollution are non-smokers, although recent epidemiological evidence strongly suggests a lung cancer risk from environmental tobacco smoke. The need to adjust also for this potential confounder further complicates the study design of the epidemiological research on the effects of air pollution. No relevant difference in lung cancer rates was found by Doll [19] among non-smokers resident in Greater London, other urban areas and rural districts. Mortality data for England and Wales have been subsequently analysed by Doll [20], who suggested a possible effect on the lung cancer risk in relation to exposure to carcinogens in urban areas. The effect is believed to be small but an interactive effect with smoking and occupational exposure cannot be excluded.

Based on the State of Utah Cancer Registry, Lyon et al. [21] identified male and female lung cancer cases diagnosed from 1967 to 1975 among Mormons (who do not smoke or drink alcohol) and non-Mormons. Lung cancer incidence rate ratios in urban vs rural areas were estimated at 1.8 and 1.2 for men and women among non-Mormons. For Mormons the corresponding rate ratios were 0.9 and 1.0.

Overall descriptive and correlation studies investigating the possible role of air pollution on the aetiology of lung cancer do not provide consistent results and do not permit firm conclusions. Although most of the studies show some association between lung cancer and air pollution, the lack of control for confounding factors, together with the highly imprecise definition of exposure, make it difficult to interpret the data in quantitative terms.

Studies on Populations in Industrial Areas

Populations living in areas close to industries that are suspected of contributing heavily to air pollution have been studied to identify any increased risk of lung cancer which could be related to air pollution. Most of these studies are of ecological nature and often limited by a lack of information on smoking habits and occupational exposures. With few exceptions, these studies did not have access to detailed information on pattern of exposure (particularly historical) nor on level or other characteristics of the exposure. It is therefore difficult to select the most appropriate study population. Too large populations would increase the risk of including many subjects with very low exposures, thus diluting the effect - if any, while small populations will result in a low number of cases and might include a large proportion of residents employed in the industries under investigation.

Several epidemiological investigations have been performed on lung cancer in industrial areas. The studies worthy of mention are the one by Blot and Fraumeni [22], who found a higher lung cancer mortality in areas with chemical, paper and pulp and petroleum industries; the one by Axelsson and Rylander [23], who investigated the possible effects of environmental exposure to chromium due to ferro-chromium alloy industries in Sweden; the one by Shear et al. [24], who analysed one parish in Louisiana which had the highest incidence of lung cancer in the United States and who found an increased risk for residents within 1.2 kilometre from industrial facilities, and the study by Matanoski et al. [25], who found an association with arsenical pesticide production facilities.

Iron and steel foundries and non-ferrous smelting plants are the two types of industries most frequently investigated in relation to the potential lung cancer risk resulting from emissions to the environment. Occupational exposure in iron and steel foundries has been shown to increase the risk of lung cancer [26]. Populations residing near iron and steel foundries have been studied particularly in Scotland. In 3 subsequent studies [27-29], researchers from the University of Dundee have investigated lung cancer mortality in relation to environmental exposure to emissions from iron and steel foundries. The population studied was composed of 3 small communities with old foundries. According to the same methodological approach, the residents in the 3 towns were divided into different subgroups of estimated exposure based on the soil contamination of metals. In all 3 studies, the highest lung cancer mortality was concentrated in the areas estimated to be more exposed to emissions from the foundries and a decreasing pattern of lung cancer risk was observed with decreasing contamination by metals. The lung cancer excess, which ranged from 30% to 100% in some subgroups, was reduced when adjusted for socioeconomic factors, but the decreasing pattern did not change.

The possible effects on lung cancer risk from exposure to emissions from non-ferrous smelters have been studied in various countries. Correlation studies have shown an increased lung cancer mortality in relation to residence near non-ferrous smelters [30-33]. A more than 2-fold increase was reported in some of the studies but the results were inconsistent across sexes and after adjustment for employment at the smelters. Blot and Fraumeni analysed the U.S. mortality data for the period 1950-69 and found an overall increase in lung cancer rates in 31 counties where non-ferrous smelters were located [34]. Using a case-control approach, Lyon et al. [35], Greaves et al. [36] and Rom et al. [37] tested the association between exposure from non-ferrous smelter emissions and lung cancer risk in 3 smelter counties and failed to demonstrate a relationship between residence and exposure. Two further case-control studies were conducted in the U.S. and

Sweden, taking into account potential confounding from employment at the smelter and smoking. Brown et al. [38] found a 2-fold increased risk of lung cancer associated with residence near a zinc-smelter facility with increased exposure to arsenic, cadmium and several other metals. Similar results were found in a case-control study conducted by Pershagen [39] among men living close to a copper smelter with huge arsenic emissions in northern Sweden. The relative risk of lung cancer among residents in the exposed area was 2.3 for non-smokers and 17.5 for smokers. Considering the RR of 8.3 for smokers in the reference area, the results are suggestive of multiplicative interaction between tobacco smoke and ambient air pollution. Further support of an effect from exposure to emissions from smelting facilities on lung cancer risk comes from a study by Frost et al. [40], who reported an association between lung cancer risk in women living near a U.S. smelter and estimated exposure to airborne arsenic levels.

Overall, the studies suggest that emissions from some types of industries may increase the lung cancer risk of the surrounding population. The evidence is strongest for non-ferrous smelters, where arsenic emissions may be of importance. In addition, increased lung cancer risks have generally been observed among persons employed at these industries, who are more heavily exposed to the same agents.

Analytical Studies in Urban Populations

Analytical epidemiological studies generally provide the best opportunity to elucidate causal relationships in human populations. Cohort and case-control studies are the two predominant types of such studies. Both these types use individuals as the unit of observation, in the sense that they contain information on exposure(s) and disease(s) of interest for each study subject. As a rule, the case-control design is more effective when rare diseases are studied. On the other hand, the risks of some types of bias are often greater in case-control than in cohort studies. The available evidence on urban lung cancer risks from *cohort studies* generally comes from studies aimed at investigating the risks of tobacco smoking. This implies that data on smoking are often quite extensive, while the exposure information regarding ambient air pollution is less detailed. Most studies did not include any quantitative information on air pollution levels. Furthermore, information on other potential confounders, such as occupational exposures, is limited.

The first major cohort study with data on lung cancer in relation to urban/rural residence included 187,783 white men from 9 U.S. states who were followed from 1952 to 1955 [41]. A total of 11,870 deaths occurred, including 448 from lung cancer. The age and smoking-standardised death rate for lung cancer was 75 and 59 per 100,000 man years in cities with more than 50,000 inhabitants and rural areas, respectively, corresponding to a relative death rate of about 1.3. The increased risk was seen both in smokers and non-smokers.

Data on smoking habits were obtained in 1957 for 69,868 men from the California Division of the American Legion [42]. In the more polluted Los Angeles and San Diego counties, between 0.3 and 6.7 per cent of the maximum hourly oxidant concentrations exceeded 0.15 ppm (300 µg/m^3) at different locations in 1963. The mortality of the cohort was followed through 1962 and a total of 304 cases of lung cancer were identified. Age and smoking-adjusted mortality rates for lung cancer were 95.4 per 100,000 man years in Los Angeles County and 102 per 100,000 in the San Fransisco Bay area and San Diego counties. In other, less urban, Californian counties the corresponding death rate was 75.5 per 100,000, giving a relative death rate in urban areas of about 1.3. The higher relative death rate in urban areas was present both in non-smokers and smokers and an additive effect of urban living and smoking was suggested.

In 1959, more than one million men and women in 25 U.S. states were interviewed about smoking habits, place of residence, occupational exposures etc. [43]. Over a 6-year follow-up period, 1510 lung cancer deaths among men were observed. Among men with occupational exposure to "dust, fumes, gases or X-rays" there were age and smoking-standardised lung cancer death rates of 1.23, 1.14 and 0.98 in metropolitan areas with more than 1 million people, less than 1 million and non-metropolitan areas, respectively. Corresponding ratios for men without these occupational exposures were 0.98, 0.97 and 0.92, respectively. Data for specific smoking groups were not presented.

In 1963, a sample of 25,444 men and 26,467 women from Sweden responded to a questionnaire on smoking [44]. In a follow-up up to 1972, 116 male and 28 female lung cancer cases were observed. For smokers there was a relative lung cancer death rate of about 1.6 in cities (Stockholm, Gothenburg and Malmö) and 1.2 in towns in comparison with rural areas. Too few cases for a meaningful analysis occurred among women and non-smokers. An extended follow-up of the male part of the cohort through 1979 showed smoking-standardised death rates of 1.4 and 1.1 in cities and towns, respectively (personal communication).

A cohort of 34,440 male British doctors was followed from 1951 to 1971 [45]. Based on residence in 1951, age and smoking-standardised lung cancer death ratios in "conurbations, large towns (50,000-100,000), small towns (<50,000) and rural areas" were calculated at 0.99, 1.07, 0.99 and 0.96, respectively. No information was given on urban/rural rates in different smoking groups.

In a link-up of the Swedish National Census of 1960 and the Cancer Registry 1961-1973, a total of 15,799 male and 4119 female lung cancer cases were identified [46]. Using smoking data available for about 1% of the cohort, Ehrenberg et al. [47] estimated that about 40% and 20% of the lung cancer incidence in males and females, respectively, was "statistically explainable" by urbanisation variables after subtraction of the effects of diagnostic intensity and smoking.

A cohort of 4475 Finnish men was followed from 1964 to 1980 to study effects of migration, marital status and smoking as risk factors for cancer [48]. There was a relative risk for lung or laryngeal cancer of about 1.2 for "urbanised" and 0.7 for "urban" smokers in relation to "rural" smokers among married men. The relative risks for unmarried men and non/past smokers were difficult to interpret because of small numbers.

All *case-control studies* on air pollution and cancer reviewed here contain individual data on smoking and most recent studies also include information on occupational exposures. The exposure information for the cases was often obtained from relatives. Data on ambient air levels for different pollutants were generally rather scanty. Most of the studies were performed in the U.K. and the U.S. and studies from these countries will be discussed together.

The first study from the U.K. included 725 male lung cancer cases and about 12,000 hospital controls without cancer from north Wales and Liverpool who were identified in the period 1952-54 [49]. Six-month average concentrations of smoke were reported at between 200 and 350 $\mu g/m^3$ in the urban study areas and about 50 $\mu g/m^3$ in the rural areas. For benzo(a)pyrene the corresponding levels were between 20 and 80 and about 10 ng/m^3, respectively. There were relative risks of 1.1 to 3.4 in different groups of smokers when urban and rural areas were compared. An additive effect from urban residence and smoking was suggested.

A series of papers on air pollution and lung cancer in north-east England and Northern Ireland was published by Dean and coworkers [50,51]. Monthly average smoke and sulphur dioxide levels reported from one of the areas in 1972 exceeded 100 $\mu g/m^3$. The investigations were of similar design and included from 780 to 2873 men and from 138 to 199 women who had died of lung cancer. Controls were sampled from the living population of the study areas or among those who died from "non-respiratory illness". The case/control ratio ranged from 1/1 to 1/15. In general, increased lung cancer risks were observed in both men and women in urban areas or areas with "high" levels of air pollution. The age and smoking-standardised relative risks mostly ranged between 1.5 and 5. Some findings indicated that the combined effects of urban residence and smoking exceeded additivity.

The first two case-control studies from the U.S. providing data on urban/rural residence and lung cancer were based on a 10% sample of all white male and female lung cancer deaths in 1958 and 1959 [52,53]. Controls were sampled from the general population. A total of 2381 male and 749 female cases were included as well as 31,516 male and 34,339 female controls. Overall age and smoking-standardised mortality ratios of 1.43

and 1.27 were observed comparing urban and rural residence in men and women, respectively. Positive trends in risk with duration of residence were seen for both sexes. In men, the joint effect of smoking and urban residence exceeded additivity, while in women the interaction appeared to be additive.

In Los Angeles County, California, Pike et al. [54] obtained smoking, occupational and residential histories of 1425 male and 576 female lung cancer cases diagnosed in 1972-1975 as well as 445 male and 186 female population controls. There was an increased lung cancer incidence in "high" air pollution areas in males, which appeared to be fully explained by occupational factors. No association was found between duration of residence in the area and lung cancer risk. Benzo(a)pyrene levels of 3 ng/m^3 were reported at the time of the study, but it was estimated that earlier they were 10 to 20-fold higher.

Information on smoking, residence history and occupation was provided by 417 white male lung cancer cases and 752 hospital controls with non-respiratory, non-neoplastic disease admitted to a large hospital in Eire County, New York, between 1957 and 1965 [55]. Two-year average concentrations of total suspended particulates in the early 1960s exceeded 200 µg/m^3 in the most heavily polluted areas of the county. Relative risks of about 1.1 and 1.4 for non-smokers and smokers, respectively, were associated with 50 or more years of residence in areas with "high or medium" levels of air pollution. The combined effect of air pollution and smoking appeared to exceed the sum of the two exposures.

A population-based study in New Mexico included 283 male and 139 female lung cancer cases as well as 475 population controls identified in the period 1980-1982 [56]. Multiple logistic regression models including smoking, occupation and ethnic group revealed no consistent association of residence history variables with lung cancer risk.

Five further case-control studies on air pollution and lung cancer were performed in Japan, Poland, China, Greece and Germany. The study from Japan included 180 male and 79 female lung cancer cases as well as 2241 male and 2475 female population controls identified in 1960-1966 in 2 cities near Osaka [57]. Concentrations of suspended matter in 1965 were reported at 190, 220 and 390 µg/m^3 in "low, intermediate and high" air pollution areas. Corresponding "maximum" benzo(a)pyrene levels were 26, 31 and 79 ng/m^3, respectively. The age and smoking-adjusted relative risks in areas with "high" levels of air pollution were 1.8 and 1.2 in men and women, respectively, compared with low air pollution areas. The increased risks were primarily seen in smokers.

A study including 901 male and 198 female lung cancer cases as well as 875 and 198 female controls with non-respiratory diseases identified from death registers in the period 1980-1985 was performed in the heavily polluted Cracow area in Poland [58]. A combined index of air pollution was used based on total suspended particulates (TSP) and SO_2: Low: TSP < 150 µg/m^3 and SO_2 < 104 µg/m^3; medium: TSP > 150 µg/m^3 or SO_2 > 104 µg/m^3; high: both TSP and SO_2 above these levels. There was a relative risk of 1.46 for men in high air pollution areas compared with subjects in low air pollution areas. A multiplicative interaction was suggested between air pollution, smoking and occupational exposure.

In a population-based study interviews were taken from 729 male and 520 female lung cancer cases diagnosed in 1985-1987 as well as from 788 male and 557 female population controls in Shenyang, China [59]. Ambient air pollution resulted mainly from combustion of coal for home heating and cooking, and from industrial emissions. Monthly average benzo(a)pyrene concentrations of 60 ng/m^3 in the winter were reported. Relative risks adjusted for age, education and smoking of 2.3 and 2.5 in men and women, respectively, were found in areas with a "smoky" outdoor environment, compared with "non-smoky" areas. Corresponding relative risks were 1.5 and 1.4 in "somewhat/slightly smoky" areas.

One hundred and one women with lung cancer and 89 controls with fractures or other orthopaedic conditions were included in a study performed in Athens, Greece [60]. Exposure to air pollution was assessed based on information regarding lifelong residential and employment addresses. Current (1983-1985) air pollution measurements showed daily smoke values frequently exceeding 400 µg/m^3 in the most polluted areas. There seemed to be a positive interaction between air pollution exposure and duration of smoking in a multiple logistic regression model (p=0.1) and contrasting the extreme quartiles of air pollution exposure gave relative risks of 0.81, 1.35 and 2.23 among non-smokers, smokers of 15 years' duration and smokers of 30 years' duration, respectively.

A hospital-based case-control study from 5 German cities included 194 lung cancer cases (146 males and 48 females), 194 hospital controls and 194 population controls [61]. Air pollution exposure was assessed based on the residential history and each county was classified into one of 8 pollution categories for 10-year intervals from 1895 to 1984. A relative risk of 1.16 was observed comparing high and low exposure to ambient air pollution in men (no data were given for women), adjusting for smoking and occupation. Allowing for a latency period of 20 years, the same type of analysis gave a relative risk of 1.82.

In conclusion, it is difficult to interpret the epidemiological evidence on ambient air pollution and lung cancer. Most studies were not originally designed to study this relation which has implications for the detail and quality of the exposure information. Data from measurements of air pollutants were generally limited, making it difficult to compare the findings in different studies and to assess dose-response relationships.

It is clear that the environments under study show great differences in the types of exposures. Emissions resulting from the use of coal and other fossil fuels for residential heating were dominant sources of pollution in some areas, while in others, motor vehicles or industries were more important. It is not possible from the data available to separate effects of residential heating-generated pollutants from those resulting from motor vehicle emissions.

The crude exposure measures used in the epidemiological studies are a major problem. If the imprecision in the exposure assessment is unrelated to the health effects under study, this would lead to underestimation (dilution) of any associations. For example, most of the exposure information provided refers to recent measurements while the pertinent exposures may have occurred decades ago.

Confounding factors are of great concern in evaluating relative risks of the magnitude encountered in the studies of air pollution and cancer, i.e., in the order of 1.5 or lower. Data on smoking habits were available in most of the analytical studies, but there may still be residual confounding from smoking when urban and rural areas are compared [45]. Occupational exposures may also be important confounders and this was often not controlled in the earlier studies. Other potential confounders in urban/rural comparisons of lung cancer risks include diagnostic intensity [47], dietary habits [62] and domestic radon exposure [63]. It is likely that influences of different confounders vary between the populations under study.

A particular problem affecting the case-control studies is the high mortality of lung cancer. This often resulted in the use of proxy respondents for the cases. However, for the controls exposure information was obtained directly from the study subjects in many of the investigations. It is not clear if this difference in the source of data has resulted in biased estimates of relative risks associated with the exposures.

Other Cancers

Many of the ecological studies discussed earlier in this chapter also included cancers other than lung cancer. Some additional investigations on cancer in urban areas focused on all sites taken together or on sites other than the respiratory tract [64-67]. Increased total cancer rates in urban areas were often observed, but the relative risks were generally lower than for lung cancer. For specific sites, the results were less consistent. A few studies have reported increased rates of cancer of other sites than the lung in populations living near industries with emissions of air pollution, such as mesothelioma near asbestos factories [68,69] and angiosarcoma of the liver near vinyl chloride fabrication and polymerisation plants [70].

A few of the analytical epidemiological studies reviewed in the section on lung cancer presented data on urban/rural rates for other sites, controlling for smoking. In the Swedish cohort described by Cederlöf et al. [44], there were positive trends in the incidence of bladder cancer in men and cancer of the uterine cervix in women with increasing urbanisation, both among non-smokers and smokers. The relative risks were of similar magnitude as those observed for lung cancer.

In the study based on the Utah Cancer Registry described above, increased mortality ratios in urban areas were found for cancer of the oral cavity and pharynx, oesophagus, bladder, colon and prostate among non-Mormon males [21]. The relative risks were often of the same magnitude as for lung cancer, and generally highest for tobacco-related sites. For Mormons, the only increase in urban areas was seen for cancer of the colon. Among women, there was an overall increased cancer risk in urban areas for Mormons, with the most pronounced excess for bladder cancer. In non-Mormons there was a higher risk for cancer of the uterine cervix in urban areas, while the opposite was true for Mormons.

In the Swedish census cohort described by Ehrenberg et al. [47], there was a stronger correlation between degree of urbanisation and total cancer risk in women than in men. Overall, about 25% of the total cancer incidence in both men and women was reported to be "explainable" by factors related to urbanisation other than smoking and diagnostic intensity.

For cancer of all sites, there was a positive trend with increasing residence time in urban areas among married men who were non/past smokers in the Finnish cohort described above [48]. No similar trend was seen among married smokers.

It may be concluded that urban/rural differences in cancer rates are often seen for sites other than the respiratory tract. Even though smoking habits were controlled in some of the studies, there may be residual confounding from smoking. Other factors such as diagnostic intensity, occupational exposures and diet may also have contributed. It is not possible to assess in detail the role of ambient air pollution. In some industrial areas, environmental exposures have resulted in increased rates of mesothelioma and angiosarcoma of the liver.

Magnitude of the Effects

The strongest evidence of an effect of air pollution on cancer is seen for lung cancer. Smoking-standardised relative risks comparing urban and rural areas were often in the order of 1.5 or lower in the published studies, and generally higher in men than in women. A relative risk of 1.5 would imply that one third of the cases among the exposed are "attributable" to the exposure. Corresponding attributable risks for relative risks of 1.1 and 1.3 are 9.1% and 23.1%, respectively. The attributable risk for the whole population is lower and depends on the proportion exposed in the population.

Two of the analytical studies on air pollution and lung cancer provided data on attributable risks (or similar measures). In the national Swedish cohort, Ehrenberg et al. [47] reported that some 40% and 20% of the lung cancer incidence in men and women, respectively, was "statistically explainable" by urbanisation variables other than smoking and diagnostic intensity. Smoking explained 85% and 20-40% of the lung cancer incidence in men and women. In the case-control study from the Cracow region, it was estimated that 4.3% of the lung cancers in men and 10.5% in women were attributable to air pollution [58]. Corresponding estimates for smoking and occupational exposure were 74.7% and 20.6% in men, and 47.6% and 8.3% in women.

Cancer risks associated with some of the components of air pollution in urban and industrialised areas have been studied in experimental animals and among occupationally exposed populations. In general, the exposures have been of orders of magnitude higher than those encountered in the general environment. Thus, a number of extrapolation models have been proposed, including the generally used non-threshold "average relative risk model" [71].

The WHO recently evaluated cancer risks in humans exposed to various carcinogens in ambient air [1]. Based on extrapolations from epidemiological data on occupational exposures, the lifetime (70-year) lung cancer risk resulting from exposure to 1 µg/m^3 was estimated at 9×10^{-2} and 4×10^{-3} for benzo(a)pyrene and arsenic, respectively. Assuming a background lifetime risk of lung cancer of 3%, this implies that lifetime exposures of about 170 ng/m^3 of BaP and 4 µg/m^3 of arsenic are necessary to produce relative risks of the order of 1.5. Levels in this range have earlier been recorded for BaP in cities and for arsenic near copper smelters [1], but are somewhat higher than those reported in the epidemiological studies discussed above. It should be kept in mind, however, that exposure information was only provided in a few of the studies and for a very limited number of agents. Furthermore, the exposure data was often based on recent measurements and earlier levels may have been substantially higher.

After reviewing available experimental and epidemiological evidence in 1977, a Task Group estimated that "combustion products of fossil fuels in ambient air, probably acting together with cigarette smoke, have been responsible for cases of lung cancer in large urban areas, the numbers produced being of the order of 5-10 cases per 100,000 males per year" [72]. This would correspond to about 10% of the male lung cancer incidence in such cities, and an even lower proportion of the incidence in the smoking part of the population.

Most of the evidence presented in this review indicates that the lung cancer risk attributable to urban residence is higher than the number estimated by the Task Group in 1977. It is not clear, however, how much of this effect can be attributed to air pollution. Recent data suggest that air pollution-related effects in very heavily polluted areas may be at least as great as those indicated by the Task Group. With increasing urbanisation in many countries it is also expected that the population attributable risks related to urban air pollution will grow.

For effects other than lung cancer the epidemiological evidence in relation to air pollution is less consistent. An overall increase in cancer risk was observed in many studies, and there is room for an effect by air pollution although other explanations seem more plausible. It is clear from chapter 3 that some systemic distribution of carcinogenic and genotoxic air pollutants and their metabolites takes place among those exposed, which raises the possibility of cancer risks in other organs than the respiratory tract.

One way of extrapolating cancer risks is to assume that the relation between total cancer risk and lung cancer risk is the same as in smokers. This implies that the total number of cancers will be 2-3 times as great as the number of lung cancers. Obviously, this estimate is considerably more uncertain than the one for lung cancer.

Interactions

In several studies on lung cancer aetiology a multiplicative interaction between smoking and occupational exposures has been observed. Some examples include asbestos [73], arsenic [74] and radon daughters [75]. Multistage models for carcinogenesis with agents operating at different stages in the cancer induction process may generate this type of interaction. In other studies, the interaction has been less pronounced, more consistent with an additive effect [76,77]. In most studies it was not possible to conclusively reject either an additive or a multiplicative model, mainly because of a small number of non-smoking lung cancer cases resulting in a low statistical power of the tests.

The epidemiological studies on urban air pollution and lung cancer gave somewhat inconsistent results as to the type of interaction with tobacco smoking. Some studies provided evidence of a combined effect exceeding an additive effect, and often compatible with a multiplicative interaction [50,52,55,58,60]. Other studies were more consistent with an additive effect [42,49,53]. In most of the studies urban/rural differences in lung cancer rates were more pronounced or only seen among smokers. For example, the study in Utah revealed increased urban rates for non-Mormons only [21]. A positive interaction between urban air pollution and smoking may contribute to these results.

For industrial air pollution and lung cancer, individual data on smoking were obtained only in 2 studies near non-ferrous smelters

[38,39]. Interaction was evaluated only in the study by Pershagen and suggested a multiplication of the effects of residence in the smelter area and smoking. This was similar to the interaction between arsenic and smoking observed among workers at the same smelter [74].

The available evidence on ambient air pollution and lung cancer suggests there may be an interaction with smoking in excess of an additive effect, although the findings are not entirely consistent. The results have to be interpreted with caution, and there may be bias due to both crude exposure measures and uncontrolled confounding. However, the findings are consistent with data on occupational exposures to high doses of some of the agents present in ambient air pollution. In addition, it may be expected that there are interactions between various components of the pollutant mixture in urban and industrial areas, both of synergistic and antagonistic nature. It is not possible to assess the effects of such interactions in detail, but they may help to explain some of the apparently discrepant findings in the epidemiological studies.

REFERENCES

1. World Health Organization Regional Office for Europe: Air quality guidelines for Europe. WHO Regional Publications, European Series, Vol 23, Copenhagen 1987
2. Tobacco Research Council: Statistics of smoking in the United Kingdom, Todd GF (ed). Tobacco Research Council, London 1972
3. Stocks P: Studies on medical and population subjects. Regional and local differences in cancer death rates. No 1, HMSO, London 1947
4. Curwen MP, Kennaway EL and Kennaway NM: The incidence of cancer of the lung and larynx in urban and rural districts. Br J Cancer 1954 (8):181-198
5. Hoffman EF and Gilliam AG: Lung cancer mortality. Geographical distribution in the United States for 1948-1949. Publ Hlth Rep 1954 (69):1033-1042
6. Haenszel W, Marcus SC and Zimmerer EG: Cancer morbidity in urban and rural Iowa. Publ Hlth Monograph No 37, US Government Printing Office 1956
7. IARC: Cancer Incidence in Five Continents, Vol III. In: Waterhouse J et al (eds). International Agency for Research on Cancer, Lyon 1976
8. Stocks P: Report on cancer in North Wales and Liverpool region. In: British Empire Cancer Campaign 35th Annual Report 1957. Supplement to Part II. British Empire Cancer Campaign, London 1958
9. Mancuso TF, MacFarlane EM and Porterfield JD: Distribution of cancer mortality in Ohio. Am J Public Health 1955 (45): 58-70
10. Levin ML, Haenszel W, Carroll BE: Cancer incidence in urban and rural areas of New York State. JNCI 1960 (24):1243-1257
11. Goldsmith JR: The "urban factor" in cancer: Smoking, industrial exposures, and air pollution as possible explanations. J Env Pathol Toxicol 1980 (3):205-217
12. Trichopoulos D, Hatzakis A, Wynder E, Katsouyanni K and Kalandidi A: Time trends of tobacco smoking, air pollution, and lung cancer in Athens. Environ Res 1987 (44): 169-178
13. IARC: Cancer Incidence in Five Continents, Vol V. In: Muir C et al (eds). Publ No 88. International Agency of Research on Cancer, Lyon 1987
14. Royal College of Physicians: Air Pollution and Health. Pitman Medical and Scientific Publishing Co, London 1970
15. Lawther PJ and Waller RE: Trends in urban air pollution in the United Kingdom in relation to lung cancer mortality. Environ Health Perspect 1985 (22): 71-73
16. Eastcott DF: The epidemiology of lung cancer in New Zealand. Lancet 1956 (i):37-39
17. Dean G: Lung cancer among white South Africans. Br Med J 1961 (ii):1599-1605
18. Dean G: Lung Cancer in Australia. Med J Aust 1962 (i):1003-1011
19. Doll R: Mortality from lung cancer among non-smokers. Br J Cancer 1953 (7): 303-312
20. Doll R: Atmospheric pollution and lung cancer. Environ Health Perspect 1978 (22):23-31
21. Lyon JL, Gardner JW and West DW: Cancer risk and life style; Cancer among mormons from 1967-1975. In: Cairns J, Lyon JL and Skonick M (eds) Cancer Incidence in Defined Populations. Banbury report 4. Cold Spring Harbor Laboratory, New York 1980 pp 3-30
22. Blot WJ and Fraumeni JF: Geographic patterns of lung cancer: Industrial correlation. Am J Epidemiol 1976 (103):539-550
23. Axelsson G and Rylander R: Environmental chromium dust and lung cancer mortality. Environ Res 1980 (23):469-476
24. Shear CL, Seale DB and Gottlieb MS: Evidence for space-time clustering of lung cancer deaths. Environ Health 1980 (35):335-343
25. Matanoski G, Fishbein L, Redmond C, Rosenkranz H and Wallace L: Contribution of organic particulates to respiratory cancer. Environ Health Perspect 1986 (70):37-49
26. IARC: Monographs on the Evaluation of Carcinogenic Risk of Chemicals to Humans, Vol 34. International Agency for Research on Cancer, Lyon 1984 pp 133-190
27. Lloyd OL: Respiratory cancer clustering associated with localized industrial air pollution. Lancet 1978 (i): 318-320
28. Lloyd OL, Smith G, Lloyd MM, Holland Y and Gailey F: Raised mortality from lung cancer and high sex ratios of births associated with industrial pollution. Br J Ind Med 1985 (42):475-480
29. Smith GH, Williams FLR and Lloyd OL: Respiratory cancer and air pollution from iron foundries in a Scottish town: An epidemiological and environmental study. Br J Ind Med 1987 (44): 795-802
30. Newman JA, Saccomanno G, Auerbach O, Archer V, Kuschner M, Grondahl R and Wilson J: Histologic types of bronchogenic carcinoma among members of copper-mining and smelting communities. Ann NY Acad Sci 1975 (271):250-268
31. Pershagen G, Elinder CG and Bolander AM: Mortality in a region surrounding an arsenic emitting plant. Environ Health Perspect 1977 (19):133-137
32. Cordier S, Theriault G and Iturra H: Mortality patterns in a population living near a copper smelter. Environ Res 1983 (31):311-322
33. Xiao HP and Xu ZY: Air pollution and lung cancer in Liaoning Province, People's Republic of China. NCI Monogr 1985 (69):53-58
34. Blot WJ and Fraumeni JF: Arsenical air pollution and lung cancer. Lancet 1975 (22):142-144
35. Lyon J, Filmore JL and Klauber MR: Arsenical air pollution and lung cancer. Lancet 1977 (22):869
36. Greaves WW, Rom WN, Lyon JL, Varley G, Wright DD and Chiu G: Relationship between lung cancer and distance of residences from nonferrous smelter stack effluent. Am J Ind Med 1981 (2):15-23
37. Rom WN, Varley G, Lyon JL and Shopkow S: Lung cancer mortality among residents living near the El Paso smelter. Br J Ind Med 1982 (39):269-272
38. Brown LM, Pottern LM and Blot WJ: Lung cancer in relation to environmental pollutants emitted from industrial sources. Environ Res 1984 (34): 250-261

39 Pershagen, G: Lung cancer mortality among men living near an arsenic-emitting smelter. Am J Epidemiol 1985 (122): 684-694
40 Frost F, Hfarter L, Milham S, Royce R, Smith A, Hartley J and Enterline P: Lung cancer among women residing close to an arsenic emitting copper smelter. Arch Environ Health 1987 (42): 471-475
41 Hammond EC and Horn D: Smoking and death rates - report on forty-four months of follow-up of 187783 men. JAMA 1958 (166):1294-1308
42 Buell P, Dunn JE and Breslow L: Cancer of the lung and Los Angeles type air pollution. Cancer 1967 (20): 2139-2147
43 Hammond EC: Smoking habits and air pollution in relation to lung cancer. In: Lee DHK (ed) Environmental Factors in Respiratory Disease. Academic Press, New York 1972 pp 177-198
44 Cederlöf R, Friberg L, Hrubec Z and Lorich U: The relationship of smoking and some social covariables to mortality and cancer morbidity. Department of Environmental Hygiene, Karolinska Institutet, Stockholm 1975
45 Doll R and Peto R: The causes of cancer: Quantitative estimates of avoidable risks of cancer in the United States today. JNCI 1981 (66):1191-1308
46 The Swedish Cancer-Environment Registry 1961-1973. National Board of Health and Welfare, Stockholm 1980
47 Ehrenberg L, von Bahr B and Ekman G: Register analysis of measures of urbanization and cancer incidence in Sweden. Environ Internatl 1985 (11): 393-399
48 Tenkanen L and Teppo L: Migration, marital status and smoking as risk determinants of cancer. Scand J Soc Med 1987 (15):67-72
49 Stocks P and Campbell J: Lung cancer death rates among nonsmokers and pipe and cigarette smokers. Br Med J 1955 (2):923-929
50 Dean G: Lung cancer and bronchitis in Northern Ireland. Br Med J 1966 (1):1506-1514
51 Dean G, Lee PN, Todd GF and Wicken AJ: Report on a second retrospective mortality study in North-East England. Part 1 & 2. Tobacco Research Council, London 1977 & 1978
52 Haenszel W, Loveland DB and Sirken MG: Lung-cancer mortality as related to residence and smoking histories: White males. JNCI 1962 (28):947-1001
53 Haenszel W and Taeuber KE: Lung-cancer mortality as related to residence and smoking histories: White females. JNCI 1964 (32):803-838
54 Pike MC, Jing JS, Rosario IP, Henderson BE and Menck HR: Occupation: Explanation of an apparent air pollution related localized excess of lung cancer in Los Angeles County. In: Breslow L and Whittemore A (eds) Energy and Health. SIAM-SIMS Conference Series, Philadelphia 1979 pp 3-16
55 Vena JE: Air pollution as a risk factor in lung cancer. Am J Epidemiol 1982 (116):42-56
56 Samet JM, Humble CG, Skipper BE and Pathak DR: History of residence and lung cancer risk in New Mexico. Am J Epidemiol 1987 (125):800-811
57 Hitosugi M: Epidemiological study of lung cancer with special reference to the effect of air pollution and smoking habit. Bull Inst Publ Health 1968 (17):236-255
58 Jedrychowski W, Becher H, Wahrendorf J and Basa-Cierpialek Z: Case-control study of lung cancer with special reference to the effect of air pollution in Poland. J Epidemiol Commun Health 1990 (44):114-120
59 Xu ZY, Blot WJ, Xiao HP, Wu A, Feng YP, Stone BJ, Sun J, Ershow AG, Henderson BE and Fraumeni JF: Smoking, air pollution and the high rates of lung cancer in Shenyang, China. JNCI 1989 (81): 1800-1806
60 Katsouyanni K, Trichopoulos D, Kalandidi A, Tomos P and Riboli E: A case-control study of air pollution and tobacco smoking in lung cancer among women in Athens. Prev Med 1991 (20):271-278
61 Jöckel KH, Ahrens W, Wichmann HE, Becker H, Bolm-Andorff V, Jahn I, Molik B, Greiser E and Timm J: Occupational and environmental hazards associated with lung cancer. Int J Epidemiol 1992 (21):202-213
62 Jedrychowski W, Wahrendorf J, Popiela T and Rachtan J: A case-control study of dietary factors and stomach cancer risk in Poland. Int J Cancer 1986 (37): 837-842
63 Svensson C, Pershagen G and Klominek J: Lung cancer in women and type of dwelling in relation to radon exposure. Cancer Res 1989 (49): 1861-1865
64 Winkelstein W and Kantor S: Stomach cancer: Positive association with suspended particulate air pollution. Arch Environ Health 1969 (18):544-547
65 Demopoulos HB and Gutman EG: Cancer in New Jersey and other complex urban/industrial areas. J Environ Path Toxicol 1980 (3):219-235
66 Robertson LS: Environmental correlates of intercity variation in age-adjusted cancer mortality rates. Environ Health Perspect 1980 (36):197-203
67 Blondell JM: Urban-rural factors affecting cancer mortality in Kentucky, 1950-1969. Cancer Det Prev 1988 (11):209-223
68 Newhouse M and Thompson H: Mesothelioma of pleura and periotoneum following exposure to asbestos in the London area. Br J Ind Med 1966 (22):261-269
69 Magnani C, Borgo G, Betta GP, Botta M, Ivaldi C, Mollo F, Scelzi M and Terracini B: Mesothelioma and non-occupational environmental exposure to asbestos. Lancet 1991 (338):50
70 Brady J, Liberatore F, Harper P, Greenwald P, Burnett N, Davis J, Bishop M, Polan A and Vianna N: Angiosarcoma of the liver: An epidemiologic survey. JNCI 1977 (59): 1383-1385
71 Environmental Protection Agency: Health Assessment Document for Acrylonitrile. US Environmental Protection Agency, Washington, DC 1983
72 Cederlöf, R, Doll R, Fowler B, Friberg L, Nelson N and Vouk V: Air pollution and cancer: Risk assessment methodology and epidemiologic evidence. Report of a Task Group. Environ Health Perspect 1978 (22):2-10
73 Hammond EC, Selikoff IJ and Seidman H: Asbestos exposure, cigarette smoking and death rates. Ann NY Acad Sci 1979 (330):473-496

74 Pershagen G, Wall S, Taube A and Linnman L: On the interaction between occupational arsenic exposure and smoking and its relationship to lung cancer. Scand J Work Environ Health 1981 (7):302-309
75 Archer VE, Wagoner JK and Lundin FE: Uranium mining and cigarette smoking effects on man. J Occup Med 1973 (15): 204-211
76 Pinto SS, Henderson V and Enterline PE: Mortality experience of arsenic exposed workers. Arch Environ Health 1978 (33):325-331
77 Radford EP and St Clair-Renard KG: Lung cancer in Swedish iron miners exposed to low doses of radon daughters. N Engl J Med 1984 (310):1485-1494

The Economics of Controlling Outdoor and Indoor Air Pollution

John D. Graham

Center for Risk Analysis, Harvard School of Public Health, 718 Huntington Avenue, Boston, M.A. 02115, U.S.A.

Economics is concerned with the allocation of scarce resources, both labour and materials, in the pursuit of improving the welfare of citizens. While money is the currency used by economists to express the costs of pollution prevention activities, it is important to recognise money costs as the "opportunity costs" of expending scarce labour and materials on one purpose rather than another. For example, if a factory expends resources to prevent outdoor air pollution, those same resources typically cannot be used to produce products that meet other societal needs. This chapter illustrates how the tools of economics can assist decision makers in their efforts to prevent human cancer by controlling levels of outdoor and indoor air pollution.

The first section of the chapter uses risk assessment to compare the carcinogenic effects of indoor and outdoor air pollution. Quantitative estimates of risk are critical because they permit decision makers to focus scarce prevention resources on the most important sources of carcinogenic air pollution. The second section describes various technical strategies that are available to reduce levels of indoor and outdoor air pollution. The third section presents selected estimates of the cost-effectiveness of cancer prevention strategies, thereby providing a sense of perspective about which cancer prevention strategies are the most promising from the perspective of economic analysis. The chapter concludes with some suggestions about how economic analysis can help decision makers in efforts to reduce human cancer.

Risk Estimation

Risk estimation (sometimes called risk assessment) is the use of scientific information to estimate how much the risk of disease or injury will increase due to exposure to toxic chemicals, radiation, or other harmful agents. In the United States, risk assessment is used to quantify how much excess cancer risk is attributable to air pollution. In theory, numerical estimates of risk can provide an objective basis for determining which sources of pollution are the most serious and which are relatively trivial. Since decision makers have limited resources to invest in cancer prevention, information about the magnitudes of various cancer risks can be quite helpful.

Unfortunately, the challenge of making accurate cancer risk estimates for air pollutants is formidable due to gaps in scientific knowledge. Scientists do not know precisely how much human cancer is caused by indoor and outdoor air pollution [1,2]. Despite the scientific uncertainties, efforts have been made to estimate the carcinogenic risks of air pollution. This section reviews recent estimates made in the United States for selected outdoor and indoor air pollutants.

Risks of Outdoor Air Pollution

The U.S. Environmental Protection Agency has developed a standard procedure for making cancer risk estimates that is now in widespread use [3]. The procedure has the advantage of making use of the growing body of scientific data that is available for specific pollutants. Such data may address emission rates, patterns of atmospheric dispersion and transformation, levels of human exposure, toxicity and epidemiology. Although EPA's procedure still rests on a somewhat weak scientific foundation, it is likely to improve in the years ahead as more knowledge is acquired about the pharmacokinetics of carcinogenic air pollutants and their mechanisms of action in carcinogenesis.

Before describing EPA's approach, it is important to recognise that any procedure for estimating the cancer risks of air pollution must employ assumptions or models in at least two critical stages. Firstly, the procedure must permit extrapolation of biological effects in animals to carcinogenic responses in humans. For most air pollutants, insufficient human data exist to estimate directly how the incidence of human cancer is influenced by changes in exposure to air pollution. Secondly, the procedure must permit extrapolation of biological responses observed at high doses to the much lower doses often experienced in human populations. Since both types of extrapolation (between species and from high to low dose) cannot currently be performed with scientific precision, the U.S. EPA has devised a procedure that is designed to produce a plausible upper bound on the true yet unknown risk attributable to air pollution.

EPA recently examined how much cancer incidence in the United States may be attributable to 90 "toxic" air pollutants emitted from 60 industrial source categories [4]. The list of pollutants does not include the more ubiquitous pollutants (ozone, lead, sulphur dioxide, carbon monoxide, nitrogen dioxide, and particulates) that are regulated in the United States on the basis of non-cancer health effects. Nor does the list include hundreds of other airborne chemicals that have not yet been adequately studied for toxicity and human exposure. The recent EPA report was intended as a scoping study to determine what level of regulatory priority the United States should assign to carcinogenic air pollutants.

Before describing the overall findings of the EPA report, the risk estimates for two pollutants, benzene and formaldehyde, are scrutinised in some detail. Benzene illustrates how data from occupational epidemiology are used in risk estimation while formaldehyde illustrates how data from long-term laboratory animal bioassays are used in risk estimation. Since other chapters in this monograph have discussed exposure and toxicity assessment, the focus here is on EPA's development and use of cancer potency factors (sometimes called "unit risk" factors).

Benzene

EPA's national risk estimate for benzene (181 excess cases of cancer per year in the USA) is based on measured concentrations of 8 micrograms per cubic meter for urban populations and 0.6 micrograms per cubic meter for rural populations. Using relative-risk estimates obtained from occupational epidemiology, EPA predicts that 70 years of exposure to 1 microgram per cubic meter of benzene will increase a person's risk of cancer by as much as 8.3 in a million - or 1 year of exposure will (theoretically) increase risk by as much as 0.119 in a million. Hence, the 185 million urban Americans are estimated to experience as many as 176 benzene-induced cancers each year while the 70 million rural Americans are estimated to experience as many as 5 benzene-induced cancers each year.

The key number in this calculation, the cancer potency factor of 8.3 in a million, is an extrapolation of the excess incidence of leukaemia documented among workers exposed to relatively high and intermittent concentrations of benzene. Although several epidemiological studies of workers have demonstrated that benzene exposure is associated with an excess risk of leukaemia [5-7], EPA's potency factor is based primarily on a particular study of pure benzene exposures sponsored by the National Institute of Occupational Safety and Health (NIOSH) [8].

The NIOSH study reported on a cohort of 1,165 white male workers exposed to benzene after World War II in 2 rubber hydrochloride (Pliofilm) manufacturing plants, one in Akron, Ohio and the other in St Mary's, Ohio. They found a total of 9 leukaemia deaths compared to 2.7 expected (based on the mortality experience of the general U.S.

white male population), or a crude relative risk (RR) of 3.3. Retrospective exposure assessment of these plants suggests a dose-response relationship for benzene-induced leukaemia. The RRs were 1.09 for workers with less than 40 ppm-years of cumulative exposure, 3.22 for workers with between 40 and 200 ppm-years of exposure, 11.86 with between 200 and 400 ppm-years of exposure, and 66.37 with 400 or more ppm-years of exposure. By way of comparison, the average urban dweller in America is exposed to 0.02642 ppm benzene in outdoor air, or 1.8 ppm years of benzene exposure during a 70-year lifetime. The validity of EPA's risk estimate for benzene has been questioned on several grounds.

Firstly, some observers have cautioned against using epidemiological data in risk estimation when a small number of cases determine the relative risk estimates and when exposure information is sketchy [9,39]. Note that the RRs in the NIOSH study are based on 9 cases of leukaemia. Moreover, the exposure assessment for the NIOSH cohort involves a considerable amount of guesswork. Recent efforts to refine the exposure assessments and extend the follow-up period for this cohort have suggested a non-linear dose-response relationship for benzene-induced leukaemia [10]. While this inference requires further validation, the EPA's cancer potency estimate for benzene may be too large.

Secondly, cumulative exposure to benzene may not be the biologically correct measure of exposure. In particular, recent laboratory evidence indicates that intermittent exposure to benzene is more toxic than continuous exposure, holding constant the amount of cumulative exposure [11,12]. The temporal pattern of exposure appears to be at least as important in generating toxic and carcinogenic responses as the absolute amount of benzene administered. Since the workers in the NIOSH cohort were exposed to benzene intermittently, their responses may not be relevant to people who breathe low levels of benzene continuously throughout a lifetime.

Finally, even if cumulative exposure to benzene is a biologically relevant measure of exposure, it does not necessarily follow that cancer risk is proportional to cumulative exposure at low exposure levels. Statisticians have arrived at conflicting conclusions about which dose-response models are appropriate in the case of benzene [13]. Although the hypothesis of a no-effect level cannot be proven or refuted with available data, some scientists believe that bone marrow toxicity is a necessary precursor to benzene-induced leukaemia [14].

Formaldehyde

EPA's national risk estimate for formaldehyde (128 cases of cancer per year in the USA) is based on average outdoor urban concentrations of 3.16 micrograms per cubic meter and average rural concentrations of 1.50 micrograms per cubic meter. These figures are based on recent ambient measurements that are somewhat larger than the earlier EPA figures that had been based on modelling exercises.

EPA predicts that 70 years of exposure to 1 microgram per cubic meter of formaldehyde will increase a person's risk of cancer by 1.3 in 100,000. This unit risk factor is based on the malignant tumour data from the Chemical Industry Institute of Toxicology's long-term rodent bioassay of formaldehyde. (Note that this unit risk factor is about 36% larger than the unit risk factor for benzene.) Given the urban-rural distribution of the U.S. population, EPA predicts that outdoor formaldehyde concentrations are responsible for as many as 109 cases of cancer per year among urban residents and 19 cases of cancer per year among rural residents.

EPA's unit risk factor for formaldehyde is derived from CIIT's longterm inhalation bioassay, which administered formaldehyde to Fischer 344 rats and B6C3F1 mice of both sexes at concentrations of 0, 2, 6 and 15 ppm for 24 months. The incidence of squamous cell carcinomas of the nasal cavity in rats was 0% among controls (0/208), 0% at 2 ppm (0/210), 1% at 6 ppm (2/210), and 50% (103/206) at 15 ppm [15]. Note that the 2.5-fold increase in administered concentration (from 6 to 15 ppm) was associated with a 50-fold increase in the incidence of malignant tumours (1% to 50%). The results in the mice were less dramatic, since the only positive response occurred in the highest exposure group (0%, 0%, 0%, 3.3%, respectively in the 4 exposure groups). EPA used the rat data for purposes of risk estimation.

The unit risk factor is obtained by fitting the rat data to a linearised version of the multistage model. This model, which is now widely accessible through computer software, is a restricted version of the multistage model that compels a linear dose-response relationship at sufficiently low doses. The slope of the dose-response line at low doses is the largest value that does not flunk a statistical test of compatibility with the experimental responses. Thus, while CIIT's cancer incidence data for rats are highly non-linear within the experimental range, the linearised multistage model is still used by EPA to extrapolate carcinogenic risk to exposure levels below the experimental range.

For an intuitive feel of how this procedure works, note first that EPA's unit risk factor of 1.3 in 100,000 for 70 years of exposure to 1 microgram per cubic meter formaldehyde can be expressed as 1.2 in 100,000 for 70 years of exposure to 1 part per billion formaldehyde. Next, recall that a lifetime of exposure to 6 parts per million formaldehyde caused a cancer incidence of roughly 1% among the rats in the CIIT study. Employing a linear extrapolation to 1 part per billion from the incidence observed at 6 ppm, we divide 0.01 by 6000 and obtain a risk of 1.7 in a million for a lifetime exposure to 1 part per billion formaldehyde.

In this case, the linear extrapolation places us within an order of magnitude of the estimate produced by the linearised multistage model. More precisely, EPA's unit risk estimate is about a factor of 7 larger than would result from a simple linear extrapolation of the cancer incidence observed in rats at 6 ppm. Our linear extrapolation would have performed even better as an approximation of EPA's procedure if, instead of using the observed incidence of 1% at 6 ppm, we had used the upper confidence limit on the incidence of cancer observed at 6 ppm. This adjustment would account for the fact that the 1% incidence figure is based on a sample of only 210 rats. Due to sampling error, it is possible that the observed incidence in an infinite sample of rats would be as high as 3 to 4%. Using the 4% figure as an upper bound on the "true" incidence of cancer at 6 ppm, we can make a simple linear extrapolation that comes within a factor of two of the unit risk factor used by EPA for a lifetime exposure to 1 part per billion. More rigorous discussions of the linearised multistage model are available elsewhere [16].

As we saw in the case of benzene, serious criticisms are leveled against such attempts at quantitative risk estimation. The major criticisms of EPA's formaldehyde risk estimate are summarised below. In light of some of these criticisms and new data, EPA is now reexamining its assessment of formaldehyde. Firstly, some scientists believe that it is premature to quantify human cancer risk at low exposure levels on the basis of carcinogenic responses observed in rodents at relatively high exposure levels. This reservation applies not just to formaldehyde but to several hundred chemicals that have tested positive in long-term rodent bioassays. These scientists argue that our scientific understanding of chemical carcinogenesis is too primitive to permit reliable quantitative risk estimation. Our ability to accurately extrapolate responses across species is particularly limited [17].

Secondly, new biological data on formaldehyde seem to indicate that the amount of formaldehyde delivered to target cells in rats and monkeys vanishes as the concentrations of formaldehyde administered to animals decline. This non-linear relationship between delivered and administered doses suggests that EPA's unit risk estimate of formaldehyde overstates risk by several orders of magnitude at exposure levels in the part per billion range [18,19]

Thirdly, some scientists believe that EPA should depart from the standard linearised multistage model in the case of formaldehyde due to the non-linear shape of the experimental data and the known role that cell proliferation plays in the chemical's toxicity. An alternative approach, which is to rely on the maximum likelihood estimate of the multistage model, would retain the non-threshold assumption but predict a non-linear relationship between exposure and cancer incidence at low exposure levels [18,20].

Fourthly, some scientists have criticised EPA for not including benign tumours (polypoid adenomas) and various precursor lesions in the quantitative risk estimate of formaldehyde. Although the CIIT investigators found no evidence that these tumours progress into squamous cell carcinomas, it is possible that

a fraction of them progress into adenocarcinomas. If a fraction of the benign tumours were added to the carcinomas to obtain an overall tumour incidence rate, then EPA's unit risk factor would be larger than it is currently estimated to be [21].
Finally, scientists have reached divergent conclusions about how to interpret the growing body of epidemiological data on formaldehyde. Some interpret the results as providing limited evidence of carcinogenicity in humans, others see the results as negative, and others believe that the human data are uninterpretable. In any event, none of the epidemiological studies have the requisite statistical power to refute or confirm EPA's unit risk estimate for exposure levels in the part per billion range.

Overall EPA Findings

EPA added the risk estimates for 90 pollutants at 60 source categories to obtain a national estimate of cancer incidence due to outdoor air pollution. Their overall estimate is 1,700 to 2,700 excess cases of cancer per year in the USA, or an equivalent of roughly 7 to 11 annual cases of cancer per million population. The authors of the report emphasise that their estimates are not necessarily appropriate as absolute predictions and are intended to be used for comparison purposes.
The largest single source of excess cancer incidence was motor vehicles, which accounted for 58% of total estimated incidence. Large industrial facilities ("point sources") accounted for another 20% of the estimated national incidence while small diffuse facilities such as wood stoves and dry cleaners accounted for the remaining incidence (22%). The 7 pollutants estimated to be responsible for more than 100 annual cases of cancer were benzene, 1,3-butadiene, chloroform, chromium (hexavalent), dioxin, formaldehyde and products of incomplete combustion.

Risks of Indoor Air Pollution

Since indoor air pollution is typically in the control of the household, risk estimates in this section are reported at the individual level. At current mortality rates, a baby born today in the United States has roughly 1 chance in 4 (0.25) of dying from cancer [9]. This is the average American's baseline risk of dying from all causes of cancer (genetic, dietary, occupational and environmental). The baseline risks for most Europeans are probably within a factor of 2 of this value for Americans. Now let us suppose that the average individual is subjected to additional cancer risks from various indoor sources that have been quantified using the standard methods of risk assessment employed by scientists in the United States.
The average indoor radon concentration in the United States, about 50 becquerels per cubic meter (one becquerel is equal to one radioactive decay per second), is associated with an incremental lifetime risk of fatal cancer of about 0.4% or 0.004. This estimate is somewhat uncertain, since it entails extrapolating the elevated lung cancer risks of uranium miners to the residential populations exposed to radon and its decay products [22]. Taken at face value, this rough estimate suggests that indoor radon increases the baseline risk of cancer from about 0.250 to about 0.254. On the other hand, people who live for 20 years in houses that have 1,000 becquerels of radon per cubic meter face an incremental risk of 2 to 3%, or an increase from 0.25 to 0.27 or 0.28. Some analysts have argued that only the small fraction of homes with strikingly elevated radon concentrations should be the targets of prevention activity [23].
While the carcinogenic risks of indoor radon in homes may appear modest, they are remarkably large compared to the predicted risks of outdoor air pollution that typically generate regulatory attention in the United States. For example, major industrial emitters of chemical carcinogens in the United States are increasingly regulated until the incremental lifetime cancer risks of emissions fall below the range from 1 in 10,000 to 1 in 1,000,000 or less, even for a hypothetical person who lives downwind at the factory fenceline breathing outdoor air 24 hours a day for 70 hours [24]. This means that an industrial polluter is not permitted to increase anyone's cancer risk from a baseline value of 0.2500 to 0.2501 or more. Some highly protective regulators will not permit an increase

from 0.250000 to 0.250001, even for the maximally exposed resident. While these tiny increases in cancer risk are not detectable with epidemiological methods, they are assumed to be estimable using mathematical models of risk assessment.

The incremental lifetime cancer risk from the average level of radon in U.S. water supplies is predicted to be about one chance in 100,000, or a slight increase from 0.25000 to 0.25001. Note that this risk is much smaller than the risk estimated from background levels of radon in the basements of U.S. homes [22].

Concern has been raised about the risks of lung cancer faced by non-smokers who live with smokers. One risk assessment based on epidemiological data estimates that an adult non-smoker who lives continuously with a heavy smoker suffers an incremental lifetime cancer risk of 0.005, which means an increase from the baseline risk of 0.250 to 0.255.

Formaldehyde is often a significant indoor air pollutant due to its presence in building materials and its use in urea formaldehyde foam insulation. One risk assessment estimates that a mobile home resident who breathes 0.10 ppm of formaldehyde for 10 years incurs an incremental lifetime risk of cancer of 0.0002 [9] or an increase in the baseline risk from 0.2500 to 0.2502.

Risks in Perspective

In discussing the risks of indoor and outdoor air pollution, it is useful to have a sense of perspective about the magnitude of other mortality risks in daily life. Table 1 displays a spectrum of mortality dangers reported in recent risk assessments. The risks of indoor air pollution, while smaller than the risks of traffic accidents and homicide, are larger than the risks of breathing benzene and formaldehyde in outdoor air. In the United States, a growing number of scientists are suggesting that indoor air pollution is a larger public health problem than outdoor air pollution [25].

Table 1. Comparing selected risks in daily life, USA

Risk description	Probability of outcome
Lifetime risk of fatal cancer, all causes	0.25
Lifetime risk of smoking-related death 2 packs/day, 40 years	0.10
Lifetime risk of homicide, black adult males	0.05
Lifetime risk of fatal car accident	0.02
Lifetime risk of homicide	0.005
Lifetime risk of cancer, non-smoker who lives with heavy smoker	0.005
Lifetime risk of lung cancer in home with average radon levels of 55 Bq/m^3	0.003
Lifetime risk of cancer from inhaling 0.10 ppm HCHO in mobile home, 10 years	<0.0002
Lifetime risk of cancer from inhaling 3 ppb HCHO in urban air	<0.00008
Lifetime risk of radon in U.S. public water supplies	<0.00001
Lifetime risk of being struck and killed by an airplane	0.000005

Source: Center for Risk Analysis, Harvard School of Public Health, 677 Huntington Av., Boston, MA 021151

Strategies to Control Air Pollution

Although cancer is only one of many potential adverse consequences of outdoor air pollution, the risk of cancer may spur decision makers to explore strategies for reducing air pollution. Selection of appropriate strategies will generally depend on what emission control measures are technically and economically feasible for particular sources. In this section, we discuss various pollution control strategies that decision makers may want to consider. Insofar as air pollution is a significant cause of human cancer, public health professionals would regard these strategies as primary disease prevention policies.

Reducing Outdoor Air Pollution

The addition of emission control equipment to stationary and mobile sources of air pollution can result in sharp reductions in the rate of air emissions compared to uncontrolled emission conditions. For example, such equipment has been quite effective in reducing emissions from motor vehicles and electric utilities. Once such equipment is installed, monitoring and maintenance of emission control performance is usually critical to achieving sustained pollution control. While add-on equipment is well-suited for end-of-stack or tailpipe emissions, it is not necessarily effective at reducing various fugitive emissions from the numerous doors, cracks, and leaks present at many production facilities. Such add-on equipment can rarely eliminate the emission problem and may create some new problems of waste disposal. In the long run, economic growth and the increase in the number of pollution sources can outstrip the reductions in emissions that are achieved by add-on equipment.

Innovation in the design of industrial and combustion processes promises more effective emission control than can be achieved by add-on equipment. For example, it is unlikely that fugitive emissions at coke plants throughout the world can be reduced to acceptable levels solely through the addition of add-on emission control equipment. Research and development into new steel making processes that do not require coke production is environmentally attractive. However, such a radical reform of steel making is not yet technically and economically feasible and may take decades to become reality [26]. One of the benefits of applying stringent control requirements to industrial processes is that they can spur research and development into the design of cleaner industrial processes.

Since combustion of fossil fuels (coal and oil particularly) is a major source of air pollution, the development of clean, alternative energy sources must be considered an attractive pollution control strategy. The most feasible alternative today is nuclear power, although its public acceptance varies throughout the world. Solar energy and wind power offer some promise as sources of electricity but are not yet economically competitive in many regions of the world. Natural gas is perhaps the cleanest source of energy and its use is rapidly increasing.

Energy conservation is another promising approach to air pollution control that is not utilised adequately in the residential, industrial, and transportation sectors of the world economy. In the United States, for example, many highly polluted urban areas have weak mass transit systems and little encouragement for car pooling arrangements during commuting hours. While the high and unstable oil prices of the 1970s spurred some efforts at energy conservation, the return to relatively cheap oil in the 1980s has undercut the economic incentive for energy conservation. Several countries in Europe encourage conservation through taxes and fees on gasoline consumption.

In order to stimulate the prevention or reduction of air pollution, decision makers need to recognise air pollution as a public health problem and utilise policy instruments that encourage pollution control. In the United States, command-and-control regulation in the form of detailed emission limits or technology requirements for each source has been the most widely used policy instrument for the last 20 years. The results have been mixed, and many environmentalists are turning to economic incentives or penalties as an alternative approach to curbing air pollution. Taxes or fees on emissions need to be used more widely to discourage emissions and encourage research and development into innovative pollution control methods.

Reducing Indoor Air Pollution

Engineering strategies can be employed to reduce indoor air pollution [28]. Three types of strategies are employed:
- source control, which entails reducing the pollutant emissions from specific indoor sources such as combustion appliances, tobacco smoking, building materials and consumer products;
- enhanced ventilation, which dilutes indoor air with outdoor air to reduce concentrations of indoor air pollutants;
- air cleaning, which actively removes pollutants from indoor air through chemical and physical methods.

Growing concern about indoor air quality has also led to new thinking about appropriate design and maintenance practices for buildings and homes [29]. Careful design of interior space, mechanical systems, and the building envelope can optimise air quality, assuming that proper maintenance practices are followed to meet or exceed design goals for indoor air quality.

Where the emission rate is the primary determinant of indoor concentrations, source controls may be crucial. For example, emissions of formaldehyde and other volatile organic substances can be lessened by changing the way particle board, adhesives and other products are manufactured. While source control strategies may seem the most direct method for preventing indoor air pollution, their potential effectiveness is limited by important practical barriers. It is not always easy to identify the quantitatively important sources of indoor air pollution. Even when sources are identified, it may not be easy for home owners or building managers to control source emissions. For example, the use of particular building materials which cause indoor air pollution may not be easily controlled after the building is constructed. Some source control strategies, such as source substitution and modification of building materials, must be performed by designers, builders, or product manufacturers.

Ventilation strategies are often very promising because they can reduce or eliminate virtually all airborne contaminants, regardless of the source. The ultimate effectiveness of ventilation may be limited by the precise design of ventilation systems and the presence of sources that generate pollutants too rapidly to be addressed by dilution. The opportunities for ventilation may also be constrained by concerns for energy conservation. When outside air requires conditioning for thermal comfort, ventilation can also prove costly.

Air cleaning is often recommended to supplement ventilation control of particulate and reactive gas pollution when dilution is unfeasible or insufficient. Commercial air cleaners have widely varying degrees of effectiveness and need to be properly operated and maintained in order to achieve optimal effectiveness.

The case of indoor radon

Radon, a chemically inert gas, occurs in nature as a decay product of radium-226, the fifth daughter of uranium-238. The uranium decay series is formed in virtually all soil and rock. As radon forms, some atoms leave the soil or rock and enter the surrounding air or water. Since radon has a half-life of about 4 days in which to reach nearby air or water, it is ubiquitous indoors and outdoors. Indoor concentrations of radon are determined by the ease with which air can pass from the soil into a dwelling and by how well the dwelling is ventilated.

Entry of radon from the ground can be reduced substantially by a system of pipes and fans that draw air from (or blow air on) the soil or gravel immediately under the substructure of the house. This ventilation strategy requires an initial capital investment and increased electricity costs to operate the fans continuously. The optimal control strategy for a specific house will depend on the type of structure, the details of the substructure and underlying ground, and the reduction factor desired [22]. Hence, the precise cost of controlling radon will vary from home to home depending upon the severity of the problem, the ease with which the system of pipes is installed, and the home owner's desire to conceal the system of pipes and fans.

Air cleaning devices do not necessarily solve the radon problem. Filter systems and electrostatic precipitators remove particles suspended in air by imparting an electric charge to them, but increase the fraction of the radon decay products that are not attached to airborne particulates. The free decay products appear to cause the greater radiation dosage to the lung [30].

The Costs of Pollution Control

The control of air pollution can be quite costly. Economists have estimated that the total costs of existing outdoor air pollution control programmes in the United States are about $35 billion per year - $15 billion for mobile sources and $20 billion for stationary sources [31]. These cost estimates account for depreciated capital expenditures, operating and maintenance expenditures and a variety of indirect costs such as reduced productivity and innovation. These annual costs could increase by 50% or more by the mid-1990s due to the 1990 Clean Air Act Amendments [32].

Although comparable cost estimates for pollution control are not available on a global basis, it is possible to obtain global information on one significant component of this cost: annual expenditures for new air pollution control equipment. The firm Temple, Barker and Sloane, Inc. has estimated that global expenditures for new air pollution control equipment will approach $5.3 billion in 1989 [33]. These expenditures are divided among Europe (45%), the United States (25%), Japan (15%) and all other nations (15%). As a percentage of Gross National Product, pollution control expenditures in Canada and the United States are smaller than they are in West Germany and Japan.

In light of the substantial costs of pollution control programmes, it is important that such programmes be subjected to cost-effectiveness analysis (CEA). The purpose of CEA is to determine whether programmes are achieving air quality goals at minimum cost or, alternatively, whether fixed investments in pollution control are being allocated in a manner that maximises air quality improvement [34]. To measure programme effectiveness, analysts use either estimates of how much pollution will be removed (e.g., in tons) or estimates of how many cases of cancer will be prevented (which requires quantitative risk estimates). For illustrative purposes, we shall describe several such analyses below.

Controlling Emissions from Motor Vehicles

In most regions of the world, motor vehicles are a significant source of air pollution. Since stationary and mobile sources emit many of the same pollutants, a critical question becomes which sources can be controlled in the most cost-effective fashion. The answer to this question will vary among nations and over time due to differences in technology and incremental estimates of cost and emission control effectiveness.

In the United States, economists have estimated the incremental cost of controlling hydrocarbons, carbon monoxide and nitrogen dioxide from stationary and mobile sources. They have determined that the marginal cost of removing an extra ton of pollution from motor vehicles through design change has been greater than the marginal cost of reducing the same amount of pollution from various stationary sources. For example, the estimated marginal cost per ton of emissions reduced for America's 1981 new car emission standards was about $400 - or more than twice as large as the cost per ton of removing the same pollutants from stationary sources ($160 per ton) [34]. Interestingly, these cost-effectiveness comparisons have not deterred American policy makers from requiring progressively stricter tailpipe emission standards for new cars. The U.S. Congress has adopted new vehicle emission standards for the mid-1990s that may transcend the current technological capabilities of vehicle and engine manufacturers.

Unless the use of motor vehicles can be curtailed significantly, emissions must be reduced by curtailing the amount of pollution emitted from the tailpipe. Economists have also compared the cost-effectiveness of 2 different strategies for achieving this goal: tightening new vehicle emission standards or requiring states to implement motor vehicle inspection and maintenance programmes. The latter policy can in principle address all vehicles on the road while the former policy must operate gradually as cleaner new vehicles replace dirty old vehicles.

In the United States, the basic finding has been that the cost per ton of emission reduction is lower for stringent inspection and maintenance than for tighter new vehicle emission standards [35]. The difficulty with this comparison is that one of the unmeasured costs of inspection/maintenance, the inconvenience to vehicle owners, has a high degree of salience among America's elected politicians. Thus, America continues to require ever more stringent new vehicle emission standards, even though emission control performance deteriorates as vehicles age since motorists do not maintain the equipment. This problem explains in part the motivation behind proposals to convert motor vehicles from gasoline to alternative fuels such as methanol.

In addition to tailpipe pollution, motor vehicles also emit pollution during the process of refueling gasoline tanks. Refueling emissions, which are volatile organic compounds, are a contributor to the smog problem and may increase the incidence of cancer among people who inhale the vapours. The control options include: 1) require gasoline stations to "control at the pump" through installation of stage II vapour recovery systems; and 2) require vehicle manufacturers to redesign fuel tanks with "on-board canisters" that capture gasoline vapours and reuse them.

The cost-effectiveness analyses of this question have not reached a definitive conclusion but they have shed light on the key decision factors [36]. Taking into account both estimated emission control effectiveness and the costs of new equipment and maintenance, it appears that control at the pump is more cost effective (i.e., lower cost per unit of emission control) than the on-board canisters. Moreover, controls at the pump can be applied selectively in geographical areas where the smog problem is particularly serious.

In the final analysis, the potential cancer risks from inhaling gasoline vapours become an important decision factor. A serious cancer threat would tilt the analysis in favour of the more expensive on-board canister since it is more effective. If, however, smog control is the only anticipated health benefit, then the analysis tends to favour controls at the pump in those regions with severe smog problems.

Unfortunately, the existing scientific evidence on the potential carcinogenic risks of inhaling unleaded gasoline vapours is not adequate to make reliable estimates of the human risk [37]. In light of the scientific uncertainties, the decision has become politicised in the United States and the ultimate resolution is not yet apparent.

The example of refueling emissions illustrates that while cost-effectiveness analysis can offer insight into the choice of prevention strategies, the analytic tool cannot substitute for a lack of scientific understanding of the relationship between air pollution and human cancer. In this respect, the measures of effectiveness used by economists are often dependent on the scientific underpinnings of cancer risk estimates.

Controlling Emissions from Stationary Sources

In controlling emissions from major industrial facilities, cost-effectiveness analysis has played an important role in identifying which emissions within industry can be prevented most cheaply. For example, reducing emissions from smokestacks through process changes and add-on equipment has generally been less expensive than reducing fugitive emissions from leaks, valves and doors [38]. Nor are the costs of emission control uniform across plants within the same firm or across firms within the same industry. Factors such as the age of a plant, its original design and upkeep, and operating practices can influence the marginal costs of emission control.

In light of the above considerations, economists have shown that it is not necessarily cost effective for regulators to try to specify a uniform level of pollution control for firms within an industry or even for all plants within a single firm. Since the marginal costs of emission control may vary among plants and firms, it is less expensive to achieve any specified emission control objective by allowing some firms/plants to emit more pollution than others. Although such an approach might seem inequitable, it can offer enormous reductions in the overall cost of pollution control.

Rather than require each emission source at a plant to be controlled through specified methods, EPA has begun to use plantwide standards ("bubbles") that allow plant managers to identify and implement the most cost-effective methods of emission control. In the iron and steel and petrochemical industries, the use of plantwide standards has resulted in a 20% reduction in the cost of emission control compared to source-specific standards. Even larger savings have been identified in the chemical industry if corporate managers are permitted to trade emissions among plants [32]. Such "trading" schemes allow companies to continue emissions at plants with large marginal costs of control if less costly emission reductions can be accomplished at plants that have already satisfied source-specific standards.

The same concepts of cost-effectiveness can be implemented on an industry-wide basis by permitting firms to buy and sell the permission to pollute. Rather than achieve an industry-wide emission goal through plant-specific standards, the government might sell the rights to pollute to firms and allow these rights to be bought and sold in a competitive market. Under such a pollution-rights scheme, firms with relatively large marginal costs of emission control would buy pollution rights from firms that find it relatively cheaper to curtail their emissions. The government can control the total amount of emissions from the industry by restricting the number of permits that are available for sale. In the final analysis, each firm compares the cost of buying an emission permit to the cost of emission control.

One of the difficulties with both "bubble" and "trading" policies occurs when companies would prefer to control pollutant A rather than pollutant B. Unless both pollutants are of equal carcinogenic potency, it does not necessarily make sense to allow such flexibility in the emission control process. Moreover, the same pollutant may be easier to control at plant A than at plant B but the population densities around the 2 plants may not be equivalent. Hence, cost-effectiveness considerations must be pursued with an understanding of the ultimate implications for public health. Once again, these implications can be known only as the scientific basis of risk estimation improves in the future.

Cost-Effectiveness Comparisons

In order to gauge the relative cost-effectiveness of air pollution control as a cancer prevention strategy, it is useful to have a common metric that can be used to assess diverse strategies. One metric typically used by economists is the ratio of the costs of a strategy to the expected increase in longevity (due to reduced cancer incidence). Since the costs and enhanced longevity may occur at different points in time, the ratio is often expressed as the present value of economic costs per year of expected life saved. The present-value adjustment is made by either discounting future longevity benefits at a rate of, say, 5% per year, or annualising up-front costs using a 5% interest rate.

In Table 2, cost-effectiveness estimates are presented for selected cancer prevention and treatment strategies. The estimates in Table 2 indicate the cost per year of life saved for each cancer prevention strategy. Readers should recognise that these estimates are no more reliable than the estimates of programme effectiveness and cost that serve as the inputs to the cost-effectiveness ratios. Since the estimates are based on published studies of varying quality, the estimates reported here should be considered accurate within, at best, one order of magnitude.

Indoor air pollution control is neither the most cost-effective not the least cost-effective strategy for achieving cancer prevention. It ranks behind several underutilised medical screening and management strategies but ranks well ahead of various programmes to reduce human exposure to occupational and environmental carcinogens produced by industry. These estimates suggest that controlling indoor radon levels, at least in high-risk homes, is more cost-effective than controlling indoor formaldehyde levels through a ban on installation of urea-formaldehyde foam insulation. This comparison should be made with caution since indoor formaldehyde levels can also cause discomfort and irritation among some residents at fairly low levels of exposure (e.g., around 0.25 ppm).

Table 2. Cost/life year saved estimates for various strategies to prevent and treat cancer

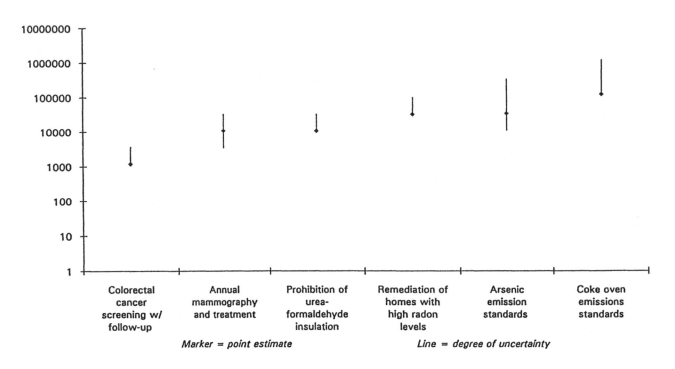

Marker = point estimate *Line = degree of uncertainty*

Source: Harvard Center for Risk Analysis, Cost-Effectiveness Database, 1992

LIVESAVING STRATEGIES AND TARGET POPULATIONS FOR TABLE 2

Lifesaving strategy	Target population
One haemoccult screening for colorectal cancer with follow-up tests if screen is positive	55 years and older, asymptomatic for colorectal cancer
Annual screening programme for breast cancer (clinical mammography) and biopsy and surgery for treatment of cases	Asymptomatic women, aged 40-64
Prohibition of manufacturing or sale of urea-formaldehyde foam insulation in the U.S.	Persons living in uninsulated residences
Remediate all homes with radon levels in excess of 150 Bq/m^3 (8.11 pCi/L)	4 million homes with radon levels about 150 Bq/m^3
National emission standards for inorganic arsenic emitted by primary copper smelters	Individuals living/working within 20 km of primary copper smelting, high arsenic emitting plants
Coke oven emission standards	Population within 20 km of plants

Conclusion

In order to optimise the allocation of scarce human and material resources, economic analysis should be applied to the control of indoor and outdoor air pollution. Some sources and types of air pollution deserve more priority because they are predicted to cause significant excess cancer risks. While numerous technical strategies can be implemented to reduce air pollution, some strategies are far more cost-effective than others. In judging which investments in cancer prevention are worthwhile, it is instructive to compare the estimated cost per life year saved from pollution control to comparable estimates of the cost effectiveness of cancer screening and treatment.

REFERENCES

1. Pershagen G and Simonato L: Epidemiological evidence on air pollution and cancer. In: Tomatis L (ed) Air Pollution and Human Cancer. European School of Oncology Monograph Series. Springer Verlag, Berlin 1990 pp 63-74
2. Gough M: Estimating cancer mortality. Environ Sci Technol 1989 (23):925-930
3. Anderson EL, and the Carcinogen Assessment Group: Quantitative approaches in use to assess cancer risk. Risk Analysis 1983 (3):277-295
4. US Environmental Protection Agency: Cancer Risk from Outdoor Exposure to Air Toxics. External Review Draft. Research Triangle Park, North Carolina 1989; updated in 1990
5. Aksoy M: Benzene Carcinogenicity. CRC Press, Boca Raton, FL 1988
6. Vigliani EC, Saita G: Benzene and leukemia. N Engl J Med 1964 (271):872-876
7. Ott GM et al: Mortality among individuals occupationally exposed to benzene. Arch Environ Hlth 1978 (33):3-10
8. Rinsky RA et al: Benzene and leukemia: An epidemiological risk assessment. N Engl J Med 1978 (23 April):1044-1049
9. Graham JD, Green LC, Roberts MJ: In Search of Safety: Chemicals and Cancer Risk. Harvard University Press, Cambridge, MA 1988 p 163
10. Paustenbach DJ et al: Reevaluation of benzene exposure for the Pliofilm (rubberworker) cohort (1936-1976). J Toxicol Environ Hlth 1992 (36):177-231
11. Cronkite E: Chemical leukogenesis: benzene as a model. Sem Hematol 1987 (24):2-11
12. Irons RD (ed) Toxicology of the Blood and Bone Marrow. Raven Press, New York 1985
13. Thorslund TW et al: Quantitative Re-evaluation of the Human Leukemia Risk Associated with Inhalation Exposure to Benzene. Final Report, Clement Associates, Inc, Fairfax VA, 1988
14. Goldstein GD: Clinical hematotoxicity of benzene. In: Mehlman MA (ed) Benzene: Occupational and Environmental Hazards - Scientific Update. Princeton Scientific Publishing Co, Princeton NJ 1989
15. Kerns WD et al: Carcinogenicity of formaldehyde in rats and mice after long-term inhalation exposure. Cancer Res 1983 (43):4382-4392
16. Sielken RL: The capabilities, sensitivity, pitfalls, and future of quantitative risk assessment. In: McColl RS (ed) Environmental Health Risks: Assessment and Management. University of Waterloo Press, Ontario, Canada 1987
17. Crouch E, Wilson R: Interspecies comparison of carcinogenic potency. J Toxicol Environ Hlth 1978 (5):1095-1118
18. Starr TB, Buck RD: The importance of delivered dose in estimating low-dose cancer risk from inhalation. Fundament Appl Toxicol 1984 (4):740-753
19. Hawkins N, Graham JD: Expert scientific judgement and cancer risk assessment: a case study of pharmacokinetic data. Risk Analysis 1988 (8):615-625
20. US Dept of Labor: Occupation Exposure to Formaldehyde. Federal Register 1985 (50):50458+
21. Wolff SK et al: Choice of experimental data for use in quantitative risk assessment: an expert-judgment approach. J Toxicol Ind Hlth (in press)
22. Nero AV: Elements of a strategy for control of indoor radon. In: Nazaroff WM and Nero AV (eds) Radon and its Decay Products in Indoor Air. John Wiley and Sons, New York 1988 pp 459-485
23. Mossman KL, Sollitto MA: Regulatory control of indoor radon. Hlth Physics 1984 (60):169-176
24. Rosenthal A, Gray GM, Graham JD: Legislating acceptable cancer risk from exposure to toxic chemicals. Ecology Law Quarterly 1992 (19):269-362
25. McCarthy JF, Bearg DW, Springler JD: Assessment of indoor air quality. In: Samet JM and Spengler JD (eds) Indoor Air Pollution: A Health Perspective. The Johns Hopkins University Press, London 1991 p 91
26. Graham JD, Holtgrave DR: Coke oven emissions: a case study of technology-based regulation. Risk: Issues in Health and Safety 1990 (1):243-272
27. Rosenthal A, Sawey MJ, Graham JD: Incinerating Municipal Solid Waste: A Health Benefit Analysis of Controlling Emissions. Report to the US Congressional Research Service, Washington, DC, 1989
28. US Environmental Protection Agency: Report to Congress on Indoor Air Quality, Volume II, Assessment and Control of Indoor Air Pollution. EPA/400/1-89/001C, 1989
29. Sexton K: Indoor air quality: an overview of policy and regulatory issues. Science, Technology and Human Values 1986 (11):53-67
30. Samet JM, Nero AV: Indoor radon and lung cancer. New Engl J Med 1989 (320):591-594
31. U.S. Environmental Protection Agency: Environmental Investments: The Cost of a Clean Environment. Washington DC 1990 pp 2-3

32 American Council for Capital Formation: U.S. Environmental Policy and Economic Growth: How Do We Fare? Center for Policy Research, Washington DC 1992
33 Copeland G, Associate, Temple, Barkin and Sloane, Inc: Letter to John D. Graham, 5 October 1989. See also: OECD: Pollution Control and Abatement Expenditures in OECD Countries: A Statistical Compendium. OECD Environment Monograph No 38, November 1990
34 White LJ: The Regulation of Air Pollutant Emissions from Motor Vehicles. AEI, Washington DC 1982 p 85
35 Thompson MS: Benefit-Cost Analysis for Program Evaluation. Sage, New York 1980 pp 221-249
36 US EPA: Evaluation of Air Pollution Regulatory Strategies for the Gasoline Marketing Industry. Washington DC, July 1984
37 Health Effects Institute: Gasoline Vapor and Human Cancer. Cambridge, MA 1985; supplement, 1988
38 Graham JD, Holtgrave D: Coke Oven Emissions: A Case Study of Technology-Forcing Regulation. Report to the US Congressional Research Service, Washington DC, 1989
39 International Agency for Research on Cancer: Overall Evaluation of Carcinogenic Risks, Suppl 7. An Updating of IARC Monographs Vols 1-42. IARC Monographs on the Evaluation of Carcinogenic Risks to Humans. Lyon, 1987